Oncologic Emergencies

CLINICAL ONCOLOGY MONOGRAPHS

Series Editors

John W. Yarbro, M.D., Ph.D.
Richard S. Bornstein, M.D.
Michael J. Mastrangelo, M.D.

HUMAN MALIGNANT MELANOMA
  edited by Wallace H. Clark, Jr., M.D., Leonard I. Goldman, M.D.,
  and Michael J. Mastrangelo, M.D.

ONCOLOGIC EMERGENCIES
  edited by John W. Yarbro, M.D., Ph.D., and Richard S. Bornstein, M.D.

Oncologic Emergencies

Edited by John W. Yarbro, M.D., Ph.D.

Professor of Medicine
University of Missouri School of Medicine
Columbia, Missouri

Richard S. Bornstein, M.D.

Chief, Division of Oncology
Mt. Sinai Hospital
Cleveland, Ohio

GRUNE & STRATTON
A Subsidiary of Harcourt Brace Jovanovich, Publishers
New York   London   Toronto   Sydney   San Francisco

Library of Congress Cataloging in Publication Data

Main entry under title:

Oncologic emergencies.

(Clinical oncology monographs)
Includes bibliographical references and index.
1. Cancer—Complications and sequelae.
2. Medical emergencies. I. Yarbro, John W.
II. Bornstein, Richard S. III. Series. [DNLM:
1. Neoplasms—Complications. 2. Neoplasms—
Therapy. 3. Emergencies. QZ 266 O575]
RC262.O52   616.99'4025   80-26259
ISBN 0-8089-1317-4

Grune & Stratton, Inc.
111 Fifth Avenue
New York, New York 10003

Distributed in the United Kingdom by
Academic Press, Inc. (London) Ltd.
24/28 Oval Road, London NW1

Library of Congress Catalog Number 80-26259
International Standard Book Number 0-8089-1317-4
Printed in the United States of America

Contents

Contents

Preface

Our capacity to treat the cancer patient effectively has increased markedly in the past two decades. Cure rates for many tumors and long-term control rates for other tumors have improved. But these advances have necessitated an increase in the complexity and toxicity of cancer management. Thus, we have added the complication of multimodal cancer management to the already numerous complications of the cancer itself.

Similarly, our capacity to deal with the intensive care needs of cancer patients has also expanded. We now have the therapeutic potential to reverse temporarily many life-threatening events that in the past were usually terminal.

This improved therapeutic potential has focused renewed attention on the life-threatening complications associated with cancer. It is the purpose of this volume to address those special problems that fall into the general category of oncologic emergencies.

Emergencies may arise in three distinct clinical settings, each of which requires a somewhat different viewpoint and approach. First, a patient not known to have cancer may present with a severe life-threatening complication—for example, superior vena cava syndrome in lung cancer or lymphoma. Here one must combine the initial diagnosis and staging with appropriate emergency treatment, and do so in such a manner as to preserve any curative therapeutic options. Second, an emergency may arise during the course of treatment of a known cancer patient, and in this situation it is important to avoid, if possible, any compromise in the already selected therapeutic regimen. Third, an emergency may arise in a clearly terminal patient, in which case the approach to treatment is likely to be quite different. The decision to intervene with the full force of modern technology must be based not merely on a careful diagnostic assessment but on a careful *prognostic* assessment as well.

The first responsibility of the physician faced with an oncologic emergency is a careful evaluation of what the prognosis will be after the emergency has been dealt with. This must be accomplished *before* emergency management has been decided upon, because decisions in the first minutes to hours have a way of setting the tone of patient management for days and weeks to come. The psychological mind-set of family, nurses, house staff, and other physicians is often determined by decisions made at the very outset of an emergency, and if such decisions are inappropriate they may be regretted over weeks or even months of painful and expensive artificial prolongation of life. The aggressiveness of management of the emergency should be directly proportional to the probability of cure or long-range remission of the cancer, and this decision can best be made by an experienced oncologist thoroughly familiar with the course of illness of the particular patient under treatment. Certain questions must be addressed simultaneously with the considerations related to the presenting emergency:

1. What is the tumor cell type, stage, and present extent?
2. What surgery, radiation, and/or chemotherapy has the patient already had?
3. Does there remain an effective therapy likely to produce a good remission?
4. What will be the treatment plan for this patient *after* the emergency is over?
5. What is the realistic probability of cure or long-term control?

Careful attention to these questions will place the presenting crisis in its proper perspective. For example, Stage IV Hodgkin's disease has a 50 percent probability of cure at the time of first treatment; a hemorrhagic or infectious complication, therefore, should be approached with an aggressive and optimistic view. Even when the first attempt at cure of Hodgkin's disease has failed, subsequent attempts may be successful. On the other hand, with pancreatic cancer or advanced head and neck malignancy when the usual modalities have failed to prevent tumor progression, the ultimate prognosis is quite poor even though the emergency may be "treatable." This question is, of course, inextricably linked with the question of medical ethics, but the point for emphasis is the importance of an *early* and accurate prognostic assessment.

A second point deserves emphasis and follows logically from the early development of a postemergency treatment plan. Some of the complications of cancer can be reversed only when the cancer itself is controlled. In other cases, management of the emergency may delay or interfere with definitive therapy of the cancer. For these reasons, attention must be given to the initiation at the earliest possible time of definitive antitumor therapy. The decision to delay "toxic" cancer treatment until the complication has been managed and the patient "stabilizes" may on occasion be wise and prudent; more often, however, the most effective approach is early definitive therapy.

In addition to the potentially curable cancer patient who may be successfully managed in an emergency situation, there are numerous patients for whom the quality of life can be substantially improved even though they are not curable. For example, successful management of compression of the spinal cord or of intercranial metastases can alter the quality of the remaining life in many patients, even though it may not alter the ultimate survival. Appropriate management of pathological fractures can, in a similar manner, mean the difference between an ambulatory patient who is reasonably active and a bedfast invalid.

Finally, one must be constantly alert to the fact that not all emergencies in the cancer patient relate to the cancer or its treatment. Cancer patients are vulnerable to the usual medical problems, and one must guard against the tendency to blame any new acute symptom complex on the recurrence of a previously diagnosed cancer.

John W. Yarbro, M.D., Ph.D.
Richard S. Bornstein, M.D.

Contributors

JANET M. BLANCHARD, M.D., *Chief Resident, Department of Plastic Surgery, Cleveland Clinic Foundation, Cleveland, Ohio*

CLARA D. BLOOMFIELD, M.D., *Professor of Medicine and Director, Masonic Leukemia Treatment Center, University of Minnesota Hospitals, Minneapolis, Minnesota*

FRANCES E. BULL, M.D., *Professor of Medical Oncology, Department of Internal Medicine, University of Michigan Medical Center, Ann Arbor, Michigan*

J. GREGORY CAIRNCROSS, M.D., *Fellow in Neuro-Oncology, Memorial Sloan-Kettering Cancer Center, New York, New York*

GEORGE P. CANELLOS, M.D., *Chief of Medical Oncology, Sidney Farber Cancer Institute, Boston, Massachusetts; Associate Professor of Medicine, Harvard Medical School, Boston, Massachusetts*

STEPHEN K. CARTER, M.D., *Director, Northern California Cancer Program, Palo Alto, California*

ROBERT B. CATALANO, PHARM. D., *Coordinator of Clinical Research, Department of Medical Oncology, American Oncologic Hospital, Fox Chase Cancer Center, Philadelphia, Pennsylvania; Clinical Assistant Professor of Pharmacy, Philadelphia College of Pharmacy and Science, Philadelphia, Pennsylvania*

GARY COHEN, M.D., *Clinical Associate in Medicine, Sidney Farber Cancer Institute, Boston, Massachusetts; Clinical Fellow in Medicine, Harvard Medical School, Boston, Massachusetts*

ROBERT W. CRICHLOW, M.D., *Department of Surgery, Dartmouth Medical School, Hanover, New Hampshire*

MICHAEL A. FRIEDMAN, M.D., *Associate Professor of Medicine, Cancer Research Institute, University of California, San Francisco, California*

MARC B. GARNICK, M.D., *Assistant Professor of Medicine, Harvard Medical School, Boston, Massachusetts; Assistant Physician, Sidney Farber Cancer Institute, Boston, Massachusetts; Junior Associate in Medicine, Brigham and Women's Hospital, Boston, Massachusetts*

xi

DUANE K. HASEGAWA, M.D., *Instructor, Department of Laboratory Medicine and Pathology and Department of Pediatrics, University of Minnesota Hospitals, Minneapolis, Minnesota*

EDWARD S. HENDERSON, M.D., *Chief, Department of Medical Oncology, Roswell Park Memorial Institute, Buffalo, New York*

DONALD J. HIGBY, M.D., *Associate Chief, Department of Medical Oncology, Roswell Park Memorial Institute, Buffalo, New York*

DAVID D. HURD, M.D., *Assistant Professor of Medicine, Section of Medical Oncology, Department of Medicine, Masonic Cancer Center, University of Minnesota, Minneapolis, Minnesota*

B. J. KENNEDY, M.D., *Professor and Director, Section of Medical Oncology, Department of Medicine, Masonic Cancer Center, University of Minnesota, Minneapolis, Minnesota*

STEVEN J. KETCHEL, M.D., *Clinical Oncologist, Tuczon, Arizona*

ALAN S. KLIGER, M.D., *Associate Professor of Medicine, Yale University School of Medicine, New Haven, Connecticut*

MELVIN J. KRANT, M.D., *Professor of Medicine, University of Massachusetts Medical Center, Worcester, Massachusetts*

DAVID H. LOVETT, M.D., *Fellow in Nephrology, Yale University School of Medicine, New Haven, Connecticut*

ROBERT J. MAYER, M.D., *Assistant Professor of Medicine, Harvard Medical School, Boston, Massachusetts; Assistant Physician, Sidney Farber Cancer Institute, Boston, Massachusetts; Associate in Medicine, Brigham and Women's Hospital, Boston, Massachusetts*

CARLOS A. PEREZ, M.D., *Director, Division of Radiation Oncology, Mallinckrodt Institute of Radiology, Washington University, St. Louis, Missouri*

JEROME B. POSNER, M.D., *Chairman, Department of Neurology, Memorial Sloan-Kettering Cancer Center, New York, New York*

MARSHALL POSNER, M.D., *Fellow in Medical Oncology, Sidney Farber Cancer Institute, Boston, Massachusetts; Clinical Fellow in Medicine, Harvard Medical School, Boston, Massachusetts*

CARY A. PRESANT, M.D., F.A.C.P., *Director, Department of Medical Oncology, City of Hope National Medical Center, Duarte, California*

VICTORIO RODRIGUEZ, M.D., *Clinical Oncologist, Soutwest Oncology Associates, San Antonio, Texas*

PHILIP F. ROY, A.C.S.W., *Social Worker, Palliative Care Service, University of Massachusetts Medical Center, Worcester, Massachusetts*

JOSEPH R. SIMPSON, M.D., *Associate Radiation Oncologist, Division of Radiation Oncology, Mallinckrodt Institute of Radiology, Washington University, St. Louis, Missouri*

JAMES G. SISE, M.D., *Department of Surgery, Dartmouth Medical School, Hanover, New Hampshire*

EZRA STEIGER, M.D., F.A.C.S., *Staff Surgeon, Department of General Surgery, Cleveland Clinic Foundation, Cleveland, Ohio*

ATHANASIOS THEOLOGIDES, M.D., PH.D., *Professor of Medicine, University of Minnesota, School of Medicine, Minneapolis, Minnesota*

ROBY C. THOMPSON, JR., M.D., *Professor and Head, Department of Orthopedic Surgery, University of Minnesota, School of Medicine, Minneapolis, Minnesota*

ALBERT L. VAN AMBERG, M.D., *Instructor in Medicine, Washington University School of Medicine, St. Louis, Missouri*

Oncologic Emergencies

1

NEOPLASTIC CARDIAC TAMPONADE

Athanasios Theologides

Cardiac tamponade in a patient with malignant neoplastic disease is a serious oncologic emergency, requiring prompt recognition and management. It may cause death in a patient who has a potentially controllable tumor with a rather good life expectancy.[1] Death occurs when the pumping action of the heart is so much restricted that there is a marked drop in the cardiac output, followed rapidly by circulatory collapse. In many patients with cancer this medical emergency is not recognized. Even when suspected, a fatalistic approach dominates the clinical management.

Neoplasm is the most frequent cause of cardiac tamponade. In a series reported in 1979, it was the primary cause of 57.7 percent of patients with tamponade.[2] In most cases it follows gradual and surreptitious progression of a neoplastic pericardial effusion, but occasionally it may represent the first manifestation of a malignant solid tumor or even a leukemia.[2-11] Accumulation of malignant fluid in the pericardium is the most common cause of neoplastic cardiac tamponade, but occasionally it is secondary to a combination of pressure and constriction from a tumor mass and fluid. Rarely, it may result from a tumor that encases the entire heart in a thick, constrictive, neoplastic hull.[8] Postirradiation pericarditis with fibrosis, effusion, or a combination of both may also cause cardiac tamponade.[12] Although in these instances the tumor is indirectly responsible for the tamponade's genesis, a discussion of the resulting postradiotherapy tamponade will be included in this chapter. Unfortunately, in the prospective studies published there is an inadequate number of patients to show the incidence of overt cardiac tamponade in patients with neoplastic and postirradiation pericarditis.

Definition

The term *cardiac tamponade* describes a state of compression of the heart. In clinical medicine the term is used when a significant rise in the intrapericardial pressure interferes with the function of the heart as a pump, leading to overt impairment of the systemic circulation.[13,14] When etiologically related to cancer, it may be called *neoplastic cardiac tamponade.*

The severity of cardiac tamponade depends upon the rate of pericardial fluid accumulation, the distensibility of the pericardium, the fluid volume, and the tempo of compression of the heart.[1] The pericardium stretches gradually when the rate of fluid accumulation is slow, and the heart can tolerate a higher degree of compression if the compression develops at a slow pace.[15,16] For these two reasons, several liters of fluid may be present in chronic tuberculous pericarditis without significant hemodynamic decompensation.[17] However, with a rising intrapericardial pressure, a critical point of cardiac compression is reached. This, in turn, precipitates a breakdown in the cardiocirculatory compensatory mechanisms.[17,18] The critical point may be reached earlier in neoplastic pericarditis because of thickening of the pericardium with tumor and impaired distensibility. It may also occur earlier, even with a small intrapericardial volume of slowly accumulating fluid, if there is constriction of the intravascular volume due to a variety of reasons.

Etiology

Benign tumors of the pericardium or mediastinum, most commonly teratomas, fibromas, and angiomas, may occasionally cause cardiac tamponade.[19] Primary malignant tumors of the pericardium, most commonly mesotheliomas and sarcomas, frequently have a clinical course characterized by rapid accumulation of massive amounts of bloody pericardial fluid, leading to tamponade.[20-28] Secondary involvement of the pericardium with tumor may result from either direct invasion by a primary tumor in adjacent structures or metastases from a distant primary tumor through lymphatic or hematogenous spread. The pericardium is subject to metastases from almost any primary malignant tumor. The metastases are usually multiple and very rarely have solitary metastatic lesions been observed.[29-49] Neoplastic growths that most commonly involve the pericardium include those of the lung and breast, leukemia, Hodgkin's and non-

Hodgkin's lymphomas, melanomas, gastrointestinal primaries, and sarcomas.

The incidence of combined metastases to the pericardium and the heart has ranged from 0.1 to 21 percent of cancer autopsies.[1] In some studies, metastases to both the pericardium and the heart have been analyzed separately and have been found to roughly equal the proportion of patients who had metastases to the heart only or to the pericardium only.[31,35] The types of pericardial involvement observed have been direct extension, diffuse nodular metastatic lesions, localized or diffuse infiltration with thickening of the pericardium, bloody or cloudy effusion, and obliterative or constricting pericarditis.[32-36] In roughly one third of the patients, pericardial involvement was the primary cause of death.[38] A significant proportion of the remaining patients had pericardial involvement as a contributing cause of death.

The symptoms and signs of neoplastic pericarditis are similar to those of pericardidis with other etiologies. Despite the clinical seriousness of the metastases, however, the neoplastic involvement of the pericardium may be totally asymptomatic and the lesions may be discovered as incidental findings at autopsy.[32] Less than 30 percent have cardiac symptoms and many systemic symptoms may be attributed to the general manifestations of a widespread neoplastic disease. This was found in one study in which the diagnosis of secondary malignancy in the pericardium was made antemortem in less than 10 percent of the patients.[38]

Radiation-induced heart disease is a well-known complication of megavoltage radiotherapy, especially if 4,000 or more rads are given to a considerable area of the heart.[50] The injury to the pericardium may manifest itself as an acute pericarditis either during the course of the treatment or a few weeks to months after its completion. Pericarditis in a chronic form becomes overt clinically a few months to 20 years after the treatment.[50-63] In one series 92 percent of the pericardial effusions occurred in the first 12 months after the end of radiation therapy.[61] The incidence of radiation pericarditis has varied from 3.4 to 29.6 percent in reported series, depending on the diagnostic criteria and frequency and duration of observation of the irradiated patients.[50,61]

Acute forms are of the inflammatory or effusive type; chronic forms are of the effusive and/or constrictive types. The acute inflammatory effusive forms are frequently self-limited, subsiding without residual constriction. The chronic effusive or constrictive types may gradually lead to cardiac tamponade and death.[53] In one series, effusion remained stable or regressed in 4 patients, while in 8 others it progressed to constriction and tamponade.[50] Features of effusive or constrictive pericarditis might be present in a chronic form. Because of the insidious onset of the effusion or the fibrous thickening of the pericardium, the condition might not be suspected until the full-blown picture of cardiac tamponade develops.

The differential diagnosis between radiation-induced pericarditis and progressive malignant disease with pericardial involvement is difficult. In a patient with pericarditis the presence of pneumonitis in a chest roentgenogram in areas of the lungs included in the radiation field suggests the diagnosis of postirradiation pericarditis if the heart is also included in the field. The pericardial fluid findings may not be helpful in the differential diagnosis between benign and malignant effusion. The fluid is often bloody and may have a high protein content in postirradiation pericarditis, and the cytology may be negative in the presence of primary or secondary cancer of the pericardium.

When a thickened pericardium hampers the diastolic filling of the ventricles, it is said that a mechanical state of constrictive pericarditis exists.[64] Constrictive pericarditis may develop as a direct effect of cancer studding the pericardium with metastatic lesions or as an indirect result from complications of radiotherapy that produce a fibrous thickening of the pericardium.[56–58,65–70] Again, the diagnosis might be missed until some obvious features of cardiac tamponade appear. On the other hand, findings suggestive of cardiac tamponade may follow the displacement and compression of the heart by an extracardiac tumor in the absence of pericardial effusions.[71]

Pathophysiology

The progressive elevation of intrapericardial pressure interferes with the ventricular expansion and hampers the filling of the heart in diastole, resulting in a drop in the stroke volume.[13,14] The rapid rise in ventricular diastolic pressure results in early reduction of the AV gradient, in a premature closure of the atrioventricular valves, and in a shorter than normal myocardial fiber length at systole that further diminishes stroke volume. In addition to the pressure in both ventricles, the mean left atrial, pulmonary venous, pulmonary arterial, right atrial, and vena cava pressures also increase.

In an effort to maintain a normal cardiac output, various compensatory mechanisms come into play: the heart empties more completely with each contraction; the heart rate increases as a result of the Bainbridge reflex; an arteriolar vasoconstriction in the vascular bed of the skeletal muscles appears in order to maintain arterial pressure and venous return, and finally, there is an increase in blood volume as a result of the decreased renal flow that consequently increases sodium and water retention. This increase in volume is largely distributed to the systemic venous portion of the circulation.[14]

With an increasing intrapericardial pressure, a critical stage is reached when the tachycardia and peripheral vasoconstriction can no longer counterbalance a falling stroke volume. There is a continued fall in cardiac output and arterial pressure, and a decrease in venous return; the ventricular filling pressure gradient becomes even smaller. A vicious cycle is set into motion that may rapidly lead to total circulatory collapse and death. However, when the rate of fluid accumulation is slow and the pericardium has time to stretch, the total accumulated volume remains relatively stable because of efficient reabsorption. Thus, the intrapericardial pressure does not rise to very high levels, the compensatory mechanisms may remain effective in maintaining cardiac output, and the vicious cycle leading to circulatory collapse may not be established. The latter situation can be designated clinically as chronic tamponade. It is a precarious state and can progress as any moment to overt circulatory failure.

Clinical Manifestations

The following symptoms have been observed in patients with tamponade of various etiologies: extreme anxiety and apprehension; a precordial oppressive feeling or actual retrosternal chest pain with dyspnea of various degrees; and true orthopnea and paroxysmal nocturnal dyspnea that are uncommon, with the patient possibly assuming a variety of positions to get some relief from the chest pain and the dyspnea. A common position is to lean forward to adopt a knee–elbow posture. Often prominent are cough, hoarseness of voice, hiccups, and occasionally gastrointestinal manifestations such as dysphagia, nausea, vomiting, and epigastric or right hypochondriac abdominal pain that is probably the result of visceral congestion.[13-18,72-74]

The patient's face may appear ashen and pale, especially in the patient with cancer who may be anemic. The patient may perspire profusely, have a cold skin, and have an impaired consciousness presenting as mild confusion all the way to a deep coma. There may be intermittent grand mal-type seizures; breathing may be rapid, shallow, and occasionally laborious; and there may be peripheral cyanosis due to venous spasm and low cardiac output. Moreover, neck veins are usually engorged and the distended jugular veins permit bedside estimation of the central venous pressure, which is always elevated in cardiac tamponade. The Kussmaul's sign (a rise in venous pressure with inspiration) is rarely seen in tamponade. There may occasionally be striking facial plethora and a full neck due to edema (Stoke's collar). The carotid pulses may be small, the radial pulse is very soft and compressible, the systolic blood pressure is usually low, and the pulse pressure is decreased. However, even normal values of systolic, diastolic, and pulse pressures are consistent with tamponade of moderate degree.

An extremely useful finding for the diagnosis and also for the follow-up evaluation of tamponade is the presence of pulsus paradoxus, but it should be kept in mind that this finding may be observed in other conditions as well. Although a greater than 10 mm Hg drop with inspiration is considered significant, it appears that the absolute decrease is related to the height of the systolic pressure. For this reason pulsus paradoxus has been defined recently as a more than 10-percent decrease in systolic arterial pressure with inspiration rather than any absolute value.[75] However, pulsus paradoxus may be absent in tamponade with hypovolemia and in the presence of atrial septal defect, of significant aortic insufficiency, and when the left ventricular diastolic pressure is intrinsically elevated and exceeds the right ventricular diastolic pressure throughout the respiratory cycle.[76,77] (Needless to say, paradoxical pulse is difficult to assess when there is cardiac arrhythmia and severe hypotension). Pulsus alternans, which is often associated with myocardial impairment, rarely occurs in tamponade, but an alternation of heart sounds, murmurs, and friction rub may be observed in the presence of electrical alternans. We have observed a very pronounced alternation in the intensity of the first heart sound in one patient who had electrical alternans.

Examination of the chest might reveal bilateral pleural effusion; inspection and palpation of the precordium may reveal weakness or absence of the cardiac impulse. On percussion of the heart there might be a marked increase of precordial dullness (flatness) to the right and the left of the sternum and a decrease in relative cardiac dullness, while significant tachycardia and arrhythmias may be present on auscultation. In general, heart sounds are weak and distant with pericardial effusion. With a malignant neoplastic effusion the heart sounds might remain clear and loud, probably due to good sound transmission through neoplastic bridges connecting the visceral and parietal layers of the pericardium. The early diastolic sound that is so characteristic of constrictive pericarditis is generally absent in pericardial effusion with tamponade. Rarely, however, a third sound may be present. A pericardial friction rub (usually exopericardial) may persist, and the Ewart sign may be detected. Examination of the abdomen may reveal ascites, as well as hepatomegaly with a positive hepato-jugular reflux. Moreover, presacral or ankle edema may also be found. As the heart compression progresses, the peripheral vascular findings of shock may appear in the presence of neck vein distention and increased venous pulsation.

Electrocardiographic Findings

The electrocardiogram may demonstrate the usual nonspecific changes of pericardial effusion such as low voltage, sinus tachycardia, arrhythmia, elevation of the ST segment, and various T-wave changes. A finding, considered almost pathognomonic of cardiac tamponade, is that of the total or simultaneous electrical alternans involving both atrial and ventricular complexes. It should originate in the same pacemaker, and it should be independent of periodic extracardiac phenomena.[13,78-83] This alternation in the configuration of the P wave, as well as the QRS-T complex, is seen more often in pericardial effusion with a stiff pericardium. Approximately two thirds of the reported cases of total alternans were in patients with tamponade caused by massive pericardial effusion in neoplastic pericarditis. For this reason, an electrical alternans in the patient with cancer is considered virtually pathognomonic for neoplastic cardiac tamponade. Ventricular alternation (only QRS) is more common but less specific; it is seen in patients with myocardial failure of different etiologies. Again, in the patient with a primary or a metastic intrathoracic cancer and a marked and persistent ventricular alternans this finding may be considered as strong evidence of cardiac tamponade. In addition to the well-known 1:1 or exact alternans, a 1:1 and 3:1 alternans, which may be only ventricular or total, have been observed in neoplastic cardiac tamponade.[82]

The alternation usually disappears soon after the removal of a small volume (about 50 ml or a little more, physiologically a critical increment) of the pericardial fluid, even in cases when there is a large effusion. A disappearance of the electrical alternans may occur spontaneously or be observed even in the presence of fluid increase.[79]

Roentgenological Signs

The chest roentgenogram may be helpful in the diagnosis of pericardial effusion or even pericardial thickening. An enlarged heart shadow, and especially cardiomegaly with a normal pulmonary vascular pattern and clear lung fields, is very suggestive of pericardial effusion. The "water-bottle heart" is also considered a typical finding, and the bulging and globular shapes with shortening and widening of the mediastinal "pedicle" and a loss of the normal arcuate borders are characteristics.[13] Rarely, even without special techniques, epicardial fat lines may be demonstrated and from this the relation of the epicardium to the myocardial border can be established. In the presence of pericardial effusion, fluoroscopy will demonstrate that the cardiac borders hardly pulsate though the aortic pulsations are vigorous.[16] In this respect, cinefluorography, roentgenokymography, and electrokymography are more objective than plain fluoroscopy. However, it should be kept in mind that a normal chest roentgenogram does not exclude the possibility of a life-threatening effusion or pericardial thickening, and this is especially true in neoplastic pericarditis.[18]

Echocardiography

The use of ultrasound for the detection of pericardial effusion has been recognized as the simplest, safest, and most reliable diagnostic study.[84-88] The fluid between the epicardium and the pericardium is demonstrated as an echo-free space that separates the heart wall echo from a pericardial echo.

In addition to the demonstration of fluid, the echocardiographic study may provide diagnostic findings of cardiac tamponade. Such findings are an abnormal cardiac motion, an inspiratory decrease in the E-F slope, an inspiratory augmentation of right ventricular filling, and (probably) the presence of fluid behind the left atrium.[89-93] An echogram may detect a pericardial tumor, which occasionally can mimic a pericardial effusion.[94,95]

Other Diagnostic Studies

The following studies were used frequently in the past for the diagnosis of pericardial effusion or thickening of the pericardium, but the introduction of echocardiography has either decreased their need or replaced them completely.

Angiocardiogrpahy, either positive contrast (radiopaque media) or negative contrast (pneumoatriography with carbon dioxide) could outline one of the heart chambers and visualize an increase in thickness of the shadow of the wall. However, false-positive results may be obtained when the contrast dye is injected into a peripheral vein and not directly into the right atrium through a cathether.[96]

Radioisotope scanning of the heart has been used for the diagnosis of pericardial effusion. A macroaggregated[131] human serum albumin (RISA) is injected intravenously, and a precordial photoscan is obtained. The area outlined in the scan is compared with the cardio-pericardial silhouette of a plain chest roentgenogram, and discrepancies in the transverse diameter of the heart between the roentgenogram and the scan are suggestive of pericardial effusion or significant pericardial thickening.

Cardiac catheterization with angiography has been used in patients with suspected constrictive pericarditis. The catheter is inserted into the right atrium and an ordinary chest film or fluoroscopy will indicate pericardial thickening when the catheter tip, touching the atrial wall, is separated from the heart shadow border by a distance of more than 5 mm.

If a diagnostic pericardiocentesis is performed, the introduction of air into the pericardial space has long been used to examine the pericardial and cardiac surfaces, the thickness of the pericardium, and the presence of free or loculated fluid. Pericardial tumors have been demonstrated with this approach, although there were instances of false-positive results.[97,98] Injection of contrast dye into the pericardial sac can be dangerous, since it may induce a reactive hyperproduction of fluid that would lead to tamponade.[98]

The simplest hemodynamic study is the measurement of the central venous pressure with a catheter positioned in the superior vena cava. Concomitant right-heart and left-heart catheterization and measurement of the intrapericardial pressure give a complete profile of the cardiocirculatory changes, but all these studies rarely are necessary for diagnostic purposes.

Diagnosis

The diagnosis of neoplastic pericarditis with effusion is frequently missed prior to the development of significant hemodynamic impairment or circulatory collapse. Malignancy may not be considered in the etiologic assessment of a new case of pericarditis.[99] Pericardial fluid, removed for diagnostic purposes, should be examined not only biochemically but also cytologically. Malignant cells have been detected in 18–87 percent of patients with neoplastic effusion.[99–101] When bloody fluid is removed during pericardiocentesis, it is difficult to ascertain immediately if it represents hemorrhagic fluid from the pericardial sac or blood from the cardiac chambers. With the electrocardiographic monitoring during the procedure, the appearance of ST segment elevation or ventricular extrasystoles indicates contact of the exploring needle with the myocardium or penetration into a chamber. The injection of Decholin (dihydrocholic acid) has been used to differentiate the site of aspiration. When a bitter taste develops just seconds after the injection, it denotes the intracardiac position of the needle. It should be remembered also that the malignant hemorrhagic fluid rarely clots and always has a lower hematocrit than venous blood. Recently, the simultaneous measurement of pCO_2 and of pO_2 of central venous blood and pericardial fluid has been proposed as a useful and rapid bedside method to confirm the site of aspiration during pericardiocentesis.[102] Furthermore, echocardiographic contrast studies during the pericardiocentesis have been proposed as helpful in making the differentiation.[103]

The diagnosis of cardiac tamponade is not difficult once the condition is considered clinically. In a patient with cancer the diagnosis should be considered when there is dyspnea, clouded sensorium, thready pulse or pulsus paradoxus, elevated systemic venous pressure, and a low systolic blood pressure. An echocardiogram will demonstrate sizable pericardial effusion and the previously described findings diagnostic of tamponade. But since the condition is a medical emergency, the diagnosis frequently has to be made rapidly at the bedside without the benefit of an echocardiogram and other studies, except for an ECG. If the ECG shows total or ventricular electrical alternans in such a patient, this constitutes an absolute indication for immediate pericardiocentesis because of the risk of sudden death.

Unfortunately, the diagnosis of tamponade is very often missed. In one reported series, the diagnosis was missed by the first physician in 11 of the 17 cases of acute tamponade, and in a few instances it was missed by more than one examiner.[15]

A condition that may create some diagnostic difficulties is the subacute effusive-constrictive periocarditis with tamponade observed in patients with neoplastic pericarditis and in patients following irradiation with the heart in the field. The condition can be diagnosed when right heart catheterization is performed in conjunction with pericardiocentesis. The diagnostic hallmark is the persistence of hemodynamic findings of cardiac compression after the removal of pericardial effusion.[104,105]

Management

In cardiac tamponade there is always the possibility of sudden death. When the condition is diagnosed and while preparing for an emergency pericardiocentesis, supportive therapy to sustain life should be instituted immediately. In order to expand the venous blood volume and improve cardiac filling, intravenous fluid should be started right away. The volume expander may be normal saline or whatever is available, such as 5-percent human serum albumin, Dextran, or blood. Frequently a needle puncture of an extremity vein is very difficult because of the severe venous spasm. Oxygen should be administered when there is dyspnea and peripheral cyanosis. Positive pressure breathing is contraindicated, since it raises both the intrapleural and the intrapericardial pressures; thus reducing venous return to the heart.[13] Pharmocologic intervention that will increase the cardiac output is indicated in many instances. During experimental cardiac tamponade the following agents were administered as intravenous infusion and increased the cardiac output: isoproterenol, phenoxybenzamine, nitroprusside combined with blood transfusion, hydralazine, and dopamine.[106] However, more clinical studies are needed in this area for evaluating the timing, dosage combinations, and potential adverse effects of these agents. Clinically, isoproterenol given intravenously has the advantages of stimulating cardiac contraction, dilating the resistant arterioles, and decreasing heart size. In this way it may increase cardiac output and support the circulation in cardiac tamponade.[14] In patients with shock a pressor drug such as norepinephrine or methoxamine, or a combined infusion of isoproterenol and norepinephrine, may be used.[14] Needless to say, more pharmacologic studies on cardiocirculatory support are needed in neoplastic cardiac tamponade.

The only life-saving treatment for tamponade that is effective immediately is removal of the fluid.[107] Pericardiocentesis should be performed as soon as possible when there is impairment of consciousness, cyanosis, dyspnea, shock, or a rising peripheral venous pressure above 130 mm H_2O, a pulsus paradoxus exceeding 50 percent of the pulse pressure, or a falling pulse pressure below 20 mm Hg.[13] There is a certain risk in the procedure involving complications such as cardiac arrhythmias and hemorrhage from an injured coronary vessel. Even sudden death has been observed.[108] The pericardial puncture, of course, should be done under electrocardiographic and blood pressure monitoring

After the aspiration of the first 50–100 ml of fluid, the electrical alternation may disappear and there may be improvement in the pulsus paradoxus and the peripheral venous pressure. Moreover, with additional fluid removal the peripheral cyanosis clears, the breathing improves, the pulse becomes stronger and slower, and the arrhythmias may disappear.[13] It is advisable to remove the maximum possible quantity of fluid even with a relatively rapid rate of aspiration.

The fluid may reaccumulate following the initial pericardiocentesis, and the cardiac tamponade may recur within 24–48 hours. Therefore, additional therapeutic approaches should be planned and initiated. One approach to provide short-term management of a rapidly accumulating pericardial effusion is to insert an indwelling pericardial catheter during the first pericardiocentesis.[109-111] It provides a concurrent way to instill agents into the pericardial sac. For a more prolonged control a pericardial pleural window should be considered. Its record of success has been quite good and the procedure is well tolerated, even by the weakened patient with cancer.[112-115] In one series pericardial tamponade was reported to have been relieved by a window from 3.5 to 13 months.[112] The window is not always effective in preventing reaccumulation of fluid, and the window may rapidly close due to adhesions, thus creating the need for further drainage procedures.[116] Occasionally there are technical problems in establishing a pleuropericardial window, especially when a tumor encases the heart and the pericardium. The choice between the placement of an indwelling pericardial catheter or the creation of a window is controversial, because there are advantages and disadvantages in both.

Because of surgical difficulties, pericardiectomy for the treatment of cardiac tamponade due to cancer is rarely advisable or feasible. Furthermore, when the life expectancy of the patient is limited because of the type and extent of the cancer, such a major intervention may not be justifiable. On the other hand, primary pericardiectomy is the treatment of choice for radiation-induced constrictive pericarditis or pericardial effusion that has failed to respond to corticosteroid therapy or other measures and has led to tamponade.

Another approach to control the recurrence of pericardial effusion is to obliterate the pericardial space with an injection into the space of talcum, various chemotherapeutic agents, or radioactive isotopes. Tetracycline hydrochloride has been effective in some patients.[117] Quinacrine has been instilled, but its effectiveness cannot be evaluated in many reported cases because chemotherapy was given concomitantly or radiotherapy was administered to the heart.[118] The intrapericardial administration of mechlorethamine (nitrogen mustard), triethylenethiophosphoramide (Thiotepa) and other alkylating agents, 5-fluorouracil and amethopterin (methotrexate) have also been reported as effective in controlling pericardial effusions.[40,118-121] However, deaths have also occurred immediately after instillation of nitrogen mustard into the pericardial sac.

Encouraging results have been reported with intrapericardial installation of radioactive phosphorus (^{32}P), yttrium (^{90}Y), and gold (^{198}Au).[39,122,123] Only a small number of patients with a variety of tumors treated with these isotopes have been reported on so that at this point meaningful conclusions about the rate and degree of effectiveness of this therapeutic modality cannot be drawn.

Radiotherapy may also control a malignant pericardial effusion. More than 50 percent of patients with pericardial effusion secondary to malignant invasion from a variety of primaries respond to this treatment.[39,44,109,124] A combination of external beam irradiation plus intrapericardial installation of radioactive phosphorus has also been tried.[125]

Depending on the tumor, systemic therapy (chemotherapy, hormonotherpay, and immunotherapy) should be initiated in addition to the local therapeutic approaches to control all the lesions, including the pericardial ones. In responsive tumors, such as lymphomas and breast cancer, the results may be very satisfactory.

The criteria used to judge response have varied widely, and attempts have been made to standarize such criteria.[117,122] A response may be considered good when there is a decrease or disappearance of pericardial effusion lasting 30 days or more; absence of symptoms of pericardial tamponade for more than 30 days; and no requirement for pericardiocentesis for 30 days after initiation of local and/or systemic treatment.[117,122]

Prognosis

The prognosis of neoplastic cardiac tamponade has been very grave with limited survival in the small number of cases reported. The presence of total electrical alternans is an especially unfavorable prognostic sign, even when the alternans disappears after pericardiocentesis. Most of the patients died a few days after its apppearance, despite an improvement following the removal of fluid.[82] However, unusual long-term survival in patients with neoplastic tamponade has been reported, as well as cases of spontaneous remission of malignant pericardial effusion.[126,127]

The presence of malignant pericardial effusion without overt tamponade has a better prognosis. In one study the mean survival time from initiation of treatment to death or to the last follow-up examination was 12.8 months for 5 patients and 15–16 months for 4 patients who responded to treatment.[118] Other authors concluded that the appearance of pericardial effusion in patients with cancer does not necessarily represent a short, terminal phase of the disease.[128] With an optimistic attitude and aggressive management of the neoplastic pericarditis and pericardial effusion, the incidence of fatal cardiac tamponade will probably decrease.

References

1. Theologides A: Neoplsatic cardiac tamponade. Sem Oncol 5:181–192, 1978
2. Anderes U, Heierli B, Follath F: Herztamponade bei malignen tumoren. Schewiz Med Wschr 109:791–793, 1979
3. Goldman, BS, Pearson FG: Malignant pericardial effusion: Review of hospital experience and report of a case successfully treated by talc poudrage. Canadian J Surg 8:157–161, 165
4. De Backer G, Van Hove W, Pannier R: Tamponnade cardiaque: Première manifestation d'une tumeur maligne. Coeur Med Interne 11:411–418, 1972
5. Delaye A, Amoros JF, Trigano JA: Péricardite liquidienne "chirurgicale" révélatrice d'une néoplasie gastrique. Nouv Press Med 3:2747, 1974
6. Brown SE, Harder HI, Brown AF: Bronchiolo-alvelolar carcinoma presenting as pericardial effusion with tamponade. West J Med 124:500–502, 1976
7. Chia BL, DaCosta JL, Ransomme GA: Cardiac tamponade due to leukaemic pericardial effusion. Thorax 28:657–659, 1973
8. Spodick DH, Kumar S: Subacute constrictive pericarditis with cardiac tamponade. Dis Chest 54:62–66, 1968
9. Westfried M, Mandel D, Alderete, MN, et al: Sipple's syndrome with a malignant pheochromocytoma presenting as a pericardial effusion. Cardiology 63:305–311, 1978
10. Damuth TE, Bush CA, Leier CV: Adenocarcinoma of the lung: Pericardial tamponade as the major presenting feature. Ohio State Med J 75:25–27, 1979
11. Levitt LJ, Ault KA, Pinkus GS, et al: Pericarditis and early cardiac tamponade as a primary manifestation of lymphosarcoma cell leukemia. Am J Med 67:719–723, 1979
12. Hurst DW: Radiation fibrosis of pericardium, with cardiac tamponade. Canad Med Assoc J 81:377–380, 1959
13. Spodick DH: Acute cardiac tamponade: Pathologic physiology, diagnosis and management. Prog Cardiovasc Dis 10:64–96, 1967
14. Hancock EW: Cardiac tamponade. Med Clin North Am 63:223–237, 1979
15. Williams C, Soutter L: Pericardial tamponade: Diagnosis and treatment. Arch Intern Med 94:571–584, 1954
16. Shabetai R: Cardiac tamponade and constrictive pericarditis. Med Ann Dist Columb 41:635–637, 1972

17. Spodick DH: Observations in cardiac tamponade: Physiological considerations. Bull Tufts N Engl Med Center 2:191–197, 1956

18. Pories WJ, Gaudiani VA: Cardiac tamponade. Surg Clin North Am 55:573–589, 1975

19. Marsten JL, Cooper AG, Ankeney JL: Acute cardiac tamponade due to perforation of a benign mediastinal teratoma into the pericardial sac: Review of cardiovascular manifestations of mediastinal teratomas. J Thoracic Cardiovasc Surg 51:700–707, 1966

20. McDonald S Jr: Primary endothelioma of the pericardium. J Path Bacteriol 43:137–141, 1936

21. Dawe CJ, Wood DA, Mitchell S: Diffuse fibrous mesothelioma of the pericardium. Cancer 6:794–808, 1953

22. Thomas J, Phythyon JM: Primary mesothelioma of the pericardium. Circulation 15:385–390, 1957

23. Chaves E: Primary malignant mesothelioma of the pericardium. Report of a case. Dis Chest 47:663–666, 1965

24. Coulie R, Meersseman F, Kremer R, et al; Tumeurs malignes primitives du péricarde. Acta Cardiol 22:128–145, 1967

25. Sytman AL, MacAlpin RN: Primary pericardial mesothelioma: Report of two cases and review of the literature. Am Heart J 81:760–769, 1971

26. Argianas E, Melissinos K, Drivas G, et al: Mesothelioma of the pericardium with cholesterol pericarditis. Angiology 25:297–299, 1974

27. Bevilacqua G, Mariani M: Clinico-pathological correlations in a case of primary angiosarcoma of the pericardium. Europ J Cardiol 2:495–504, 1975

28. Poole-Wilson PA, Farnsworth A, Braimbridge MV, et al: Angiosarcoma of pericardium: Problems in diagnosis and management. Brit Heart J 38:240–243, 1976

29. Yater WM: Tumors of the heart and pericardium: Pathology, symptomatology and report of nine cases. Arch Int Med 48:627–666, 1931

30. Heninger BR: Clinical aspects of pericardial metastasis. Ann Intern Med 7:1359–1369, 1934

31. Scott RW, Garvin CF: Tumors of the heart and pericardium. Am Heart J 17:431–436, 1939

32. Lamberta F, Nareff MJ, Schwab J: Metastatic carcinoma of the pericardium. Dis Chest 19:528–536, 1951

33. Bisel HF, Wróblewski F, LaDue JS: Incidence and clinical maniffestations of cardiac metastases. JAMA 153:172–715, 1953

34. DeLoach JF, Haynes JW: Secondary tumors of heart and pericar-

dium. Review of the subject and report of one hundred thirty-seven cases. Arch Intern Med 91:224–249, 1953

35. Goudie RB: Secondary tumours of the heart and pericardium. Brit Heart J 17:183–188, 1955

36. Gassman HS, Meadows R Jr, Baker LA: Metastatic tumors of the heart. Am J Med 19:357–365, 1955

37. Cohen GU, Peery TM, Evans JM: Neoplastic invasion of the heart and pericardium. Ann Intern Med 42:1238–1245, 1955

38. Thurber DL, Edwards JE, Achor RWP: Secondary malignant tumors of the pericardium. Circulation 26:228–241, 1962

39. Hirsch DM Jr, Nydick I, Farrow JH: Malignant pericardial effusion secondary to metastatic breast carcinoma: A case of long-term remission. Cancer 19:1269–1272, 1966

40. Kornreich F, Block P: Les atteintes péricardiques au cours d'affections neoplasiques. Acta Cardiol 22:426–443, 1967

41. Guerrin J, Cabanne F, Wilkening M, et al: Péricardite néoplasique suraiguë, seule manifestation clinique évolutive d'une tumeur du sein. Bull Cancer 55:293–298, 1968

42. Brian S, Hochman A, Levij IS, et al: Clinical diagnosis of secondary tumors of the heart and pericardium. Dis Chest 55:202–208, 1969

43. Cantrell EG, Templeton AC: Malignant obliteration of the pericardial cavity, secondary to ovarian cancer. East Afr Med J 46:174–178, 1969

44. Terry LN Jr, Kligerman M: Pericardial and myocardial involvement by lymphomas and leukemias. The role of radiotherapy. Cancer 25:1003–1008, 1970

45. McFadden RR, Dawson PJ: Adenocarcinoma arising in a Ghon complex and presenting with massive pericardial effusion. Chest 62:520–523, 1972

46. Wharter J, Storck D, Schuh D: Péricardite hémorragique révélatrice d'une tumeur de Grawitz. Souffle tumoral rénal. Ann Med Interne 123:381–386, 1972

47. Birmann L, Jossot G, Ravault M-Ch, et al: Au sujet des péricardites liquidiennes d'origine maligne. Bull Soc Sci Méd Luxembg 111:201–209, 1974

48. Eissa MH, Khalil AM, Kadry SM: Secondary malignant tumors of heart and pericardium. J Egypt Med Assoc 58:337–349, 1975

49. Petersen CD, Robinson WA, Kurnick JE: Involvement of the heart and pericardium in the malignant lymphomas. Am J Med Sci 272:161–165, 1976

50. Stewart JR, Cohn KE, Fajardo LF, et al: Radiation-induced heart disease. A study of 25 patients, Radiology 89:302–310, 1967

51. Blumenfeld H, Thomas SF: Chronic massive pericardial effusion following roentgen therapy for carcinoma of withdrawal. Ann Intern Med 80:593–599, 1974

61. Martin RG, Ruckdeschel JC, Chang P, et al: Radiation-related pericarditis. Am J Cardiol 35:216–220, 1975

62. Cénac A, Gaudeau S, Vernant P: Épanchements péricardiques et radiothérapie médiastinale: Quatre observations. Nouv Press Méd 4:185–187, 1975

63. Schneider JS, Edwards JE: Irradiation-induced pericarditis. Chest 75:560–564, 1979

64. Wood P: Chronic constrictive pericarditis. Am J Cardiol 7:48–61, 1961

65. Wallace JJ, Logue RB: Metastatic carcinoma as a cause of constrictive pericarditis. Am Heart J 31:223–230, 1946

66. Fischer JW: Neoplastic involvement of pericardium producing the syndrome of constrictive pericarditis. Am Heart J 35:813–819, 1948

67. Slater SR, Kroop IG, Zuckerman S: Constrictive pericarditis caused by solitary metastatic carcinosis of the pericardium and complicated by radiation fibrosis of the mediastinum. Am Heart J 43:401–412, 1952

68. Mohiuddin AB: Constrictive pericarditis. An analysis of seventeen cases. Dis Chest 51:298–303, 1967

69. DeParis M, Manigand G, Sors C, et al: Les péricardites constrictives d'origine néoplsaique. A propos d'une observation anatoma-clinique. Presse Méd 75:1008–1012, 1967

70. Hancock EW: Constrictive pericarditis: Clinical clues to diagnosis. JAMA 232:176–177, 1975

71. Wynne J, Markis JE, Grossman W: Extrinsic compression of the heart by tumor masquerading as cardiac tamponade. Cath Cardiov Diag 4:81–85, 1978

72. Beck CS: Acute and chronic compression of the heart. Am Heart J 14:515–525, 1937

73. Singh A, Krishan I: Cardiac tamponade following secondary pericardial carcinosis in malignant melanoma. Ind Heart J 19:394–396, 1967

74. Stein L, Shubin H, Weil MH: Recognition and management of pericardial tamponade. JAMA 225:503–506, 1973

75. Reddy PS, Curtiss EI, O'Toole JD, et al: Cardiac tamponade: hemodynamic observations in man. Circulation 58:265–272, 1978

76. Winer HE, Kronzon I: Absence of paradoxical pulse in patients with cardiac tamponade and atrial septal defects. Am J Cardiol 44:378–380, 1979

77. Antman EM, Cargill V, Grossman W: Low-pressure cardiac tamponade. Ann Intern Med 91:403–406, 1979
78. Spodick DH: Electric alternation of the heart: Its relation to the kinetics and physiology of the heart during cardiac tamponade. Am J Cardiol 10:155–165, 1962
79. Lawrence LT, Cronin JF: Electrical alternans and pericardial tamponade. Arch Inter Med 112:169–172, 1963
80. Bashour FA, Cochran PW: The association of electrical alternans with pericardial effusion. Dis Chest 44:146–153, 1963
81. Raftopoulos J, Costeas F: L'alternance électrique dans les péricardites malignes. Arch Mal Coeur 59:1413–1420, 1966
82. Niarchos AP: Electrical alternans in cardiac tamponade. Thorax 30:228–233, 1975
83. Sbarbaro JA, Brooks HL: Pericardial effusion and electrical alternans: echocardiographic assessment. Postgrad Med 63:105–112, 1978
84. Feigenbaum H, Waldhausen JA, Hyde LP: Ultrasound diagnosis of pericardial effusion. JAMA 191:711–714, 1965
85. Klein JJ, Segal BL: Pericardial effusion diagnosed by reflected ultrasound. Am J Cardiol 22:57–64, 1968
86. Gramiak R, Nanda NC, Gross CM: Echocardiography in acquired cardiac and pericardial disease. Sem Roentgenol 10:291–297, 1975
87. Riba AL, Morganroth J: Unsuspected substantial pericardial effusions detected by echocardiography. JAMA 236:2623–2625, 1976
88. Markiewicz W, Glatstein E, London EJ, et al: Echocardiographic detection of pericardial effusion and pericardial thickening of malignant lymphoma. Radiology 123:161–164, 1977
89. D'Cruz IA, Cohen, HC, Prabhu R, et al: Diagnosis of cardiac tamponade by echocardiography. Changes in mitral valve motion and ventricular dimensions, with special reference to paradoxical pulse. Circulation 52:460–465, 1975
90. Vignola PA, Pohost GM, Curfman GD, et al: Correlation of echocardiographic and clinical findings in patients with pericardial effusion. Am J Cardiol 37:701–705, 1976
91. Settle HP, Adolph RJ, Fowler NO, et al: Echocardiographic study of cardiac tamponade. Circulation 56:951–959, 1977
92. Ravindra Nathan MP, Lipat G, Sanders M: Unusual echocardiographic findings in pericardial tamponade. Am Heart J 98:225–227, 1979
93. Hagel KJ: Echocardiographic findings in cardiac tamponade. Acta Medica Scandia (Supp) 627:217–223, 1979

94. Millman A, Meller J, Motro M, et al: Pericardial tumor or fibrosis mimicking pericardial effusion by echocardiography. Ann Inter Med 86:434–436, 1977

95. Lin TK, Stech JM, Eckert WG, et al: Pericardial angiosarcoma simulating pericardial effusion by echocardiography. Chest 73:881–883, 1978

96. Kirkwood JR, Abbott JA: Complete angiography vs right atriography. Diagnosis of pericardial effusion. JAMA 219:1201–1202, 1972

97. Chen JTT, Peter RH, Orgain EJ, et al: The pitfalls in interpreting artificial pneumopericardium. Am J Roentgenol Radium Ther Nucl Med 116:91–96, 1972

98. Bartecchi CE, Fogel TJ, McIlroy RH: Pericardial tumors. A useful technique for diagnosis. Ricky Mtn Med J 70:47–50, 1973

99. Agner RC, Gallis HA: Pericarditis. Differential diagnostic considerations. Arch Intern Med 139:407–412, 1979

100. Johnson WD: The cytological diagnosis of cancer in serous effusions. Acta Cytologica 10:161–172, 1966

101. Zipf RE Jr, Johnston WW: The role of cytology in the evaluation of pericardial effusions. Chest 62:593–596, 1972

102. Balakrishnan S, Hartman CW, Grinnan GLB, et al: Pericardial fluid gas analysis in hemorrhagic pericardial tamponade. Ann Thoracic Surg 27:55–58, 1979

103. Chandraratna PAN, First J, Langevin E, et al: Echocardiographic contrast studies during pericardiocentesis. Ann Inter Med 87:199–200, 1977

104. Hancock EW: Subacute effusive constrictive pericarditis. Circulation 43:183–192, 1971

105. Mann T, Brodie BR, Grossman E, et al: Effusive-constrictive hemodynamic pattern due to neoplastic involvement of the pericardium. Am J Cardiol 41:781–786, 1978

106. Fowler NO: Physiology of cardiac tamponade and pulsus paradoxus. II: Physiological, circulatory and pharmacological responses in cardiac tamponade. Mod Conc Cardiovasc Dis 47:115–118, 1978

107. Kilpatrick ZM, Chapman CB: On pericardiocentesis Am J Cardiol 16:722–728, 1965

108. Cassell P, Cullum P: The management of cardiac tamponade. Brit J Surg 54:620–626, 1967

109. Lokich JJ: The management of malignant pericardial effusions. JAMA 224:1401–1404, 1973

110. Flannery EP, Gregoratos G, Corder MP: Pericardial effusions in patients with malignant diseases. Arch Intern Med 135:976–977, 1975

111. Wei JY, Taylor GJ, Achuff SC: Recurrent cardiac tamponade and large pericardial effusions: Management with an indwelling pericardial catheter. Am J Cardiol 42:281–282, 1978

112. Hill II GH, Cohen BI: Pleural pericardial window for palliation of cardiac tamponade due to cancer. Cancer 26:81–93, 1970

113. Fredriksen RT, Cohen LS, Mullins CB: Pericardial windows or pericardiocentesis for pericardial effusions. Am Heart J 82:158–162, 1971

114. Henri A, Welsch W, Klastersky J: Traitement chirurgical d'un tamponnement cardiaque causé par une péricardite néoplasique. Acta Cardiol 28:95–98, 1973

115. Lajos IZ, Black HE, Cooper RG, et al: Pericardial decompression. Ann thoracic Surg 19:47–53, 1975

116. Chandraratna PAN, Aronow WS: Limitations of surgical methods of pericardial drainage. Echocardiographic observations. JAMA 242:1062–1063, 1979

117. Davis S, Sharma SM, Blumberg ED, et al: Intrapericardial tetracycline for the management of cardiac tamponade secondary to malignant pericardial effusion. New Engl J Med 299:1113–1114, 1978

118. Smith FE, Lane M, Hudgins PT: Conservative management of malignant pericardial effusion. Cancer 33:47–57, 1974

119. Weisberger AS, Levine B, Storaasli JP: Use of nitrogen mustard in treatment of serous effusions of neoplastic origin, JAMA 159:1704–1707, 1955

120. Suhrland LG, Weisberger AS: Intracavitary 5-fluorouracil in malignant effusions. Arch Intern Med 116:431–433, 1965

121. Terpenning M, Orringer M, Wheeler R, et al: Intrapericardial nitrogen mustard with catheter drainage for the treatment of malignant effusions. Proc Am Assoc Cancer Res 20:286, 1979

122. O'Bryan RM, Talley RW, Brennan MJ, et al: Critical analysis of the control of malignant effusions with radioisotopes. Henry Ford Hosp Med J 16:3–14, 1968

123. Clarke TH: Radioactive colloidal gold Au[198] in the treatment of neoplastic effusions. Northwest Univ Med School Quar Bull 26:98–104, 1952

124. Cham WC, Freiman AH, Carstens HB, et al: Radiation therapy of cardiac and pericardial metastases. Radiology 114:701–704, 1975

125. Martini N, Freiman AH, Watson RC, et al: Malignant pericardial effusion. NY St J Med pp. 719–721, 1976

126. Duflo B Durigon M, Guerre J, et al: Péricardite hémorragique récidivante révélatrice d'un adénocarcinome probablement ovarien.

Survie de quatre ans après péricardectomie. Sem Hôp Paris 49:3459–3462, 1973
127. Kusnoor VS, D'Souza RS, Bhandarkar SD, et al; Malignant pericardial effusion. J Assoc Phys India 21:101–104, 1973
128. Biran S, Brufman G, Klein E, et al: The management of pericardial effusion in cancer patients. Chest 71:182–186, 1977

2

MANAGEMENT OF PATHOLOGIC FRACTURES

David D. Hurd
Roby C. Thompson
B. J. Kennedy

Pathologic fractures and impending pathologic fractures are an increasingly common problem in the management of patients with cancer. Though improved treatments have prolonged survival, the development of metastatic bone disease has not been prevented.[3,17,28] Since uncontrolled metastatic cancer is an ultimately fatal process, palliation of symptoms becomes a primary goal when treating the patient with a pathologic fracture. Evaluation and management of the patient must be carried out by standards that are different from those usually applied to the treatment of fractures of traumatic origin.[32] Yet the appropriate treatment of these patients can be rewarding in relieving pain and restoring the patient to a more functional lifestyle.

Since the overwhelming majority of pathologic fractures are due to metastatic tumors rather than to primary bone tumors, we will concentrate on the various aspects of the evaluation and management of pathologic fractures and the prevention of potential fractures due to metastatic disease.

Supported in part by National Institutes of Health Grant No. CA 19527, the Masonic Hospital Fund, Inc., and the Minnesota Medical Foundation.

The authors wish to thank Carole Thomas and Dagmar Kamprud for their assistance in the manuscript preparation.

Metastatic Bone Disease

The true incidence of metastatic cancer to bones has been estimated in the literature to be from 27 percent[27] to 85 percent.[21] In two extensive autopsy series, Abrams[1] reported an overall incidence of 27.2 percent and Johnston[23] reported an overall incidence of 32.5 percent of bone metastases in patients dying with cancer. Certain tumors have a high incidence of bone involvement: breast 49 percent[40] to 73 percent[1]; prostate 47 percent[40] to 70 percent[27]; lung 23 percent[40] to 44 percent[23]; kidney 23 percent[1] to 32 percent[40]; and thyroid 25 percent.[20] Others with a lower incidence include ovary 9.4 percent, colo-rectal 10.7 percent, pancreas 12.5 percent, and stomach 10.9 percent.[1] Based on the frequency of the primary tumors, over 75 percent of all metastases found in bone in the adult are accounted for by cancers of the breast, lung, prostate, GI tract, and kidney. In the pediatric age group, neuroblastoma, retinoblastoma, rhabdomyosarcoma, Wilms' tumor, and leiomyosarcoma are the tumors found most frequently metastasizing to bone.[41]

The distribution of bone metastases within the skeleton and hence the areas at risk for pathologic fracture correspond to the areas of bone marrow production and the areas of highest blood flow in bone. In the adult, the bones most frequently affected by metastases are the vertebrae, pelvis, ribs, proximal long bones, skull, and sternum. It is rare to find metastatic disease below the knees or elbows, and lung primaries account for about one half of all cases when it does occur in those locations.[29] A small minority of patients present with a single bone metastasis,[23] and this finding will have significance in the overall diagnostic workup and treatment strategy.

Metastases most commonly gain access to bone via the vascular system, although direct extension from an adjacent primary may occur. The venous system appears to be more important in the transport of malignant cells than the arterial system. Arteries are relatively resistant to invasion by tumor,[10] and if a large artery is penetrated, the outcome is usually extensive bleeding rather than the establishment of tumor emboli. Tumor cells can enter the arterial system via venous return or the lymphatic drainage of the thoracic duct. After traversing the cardiopulmonary circulation, tumor cells can then enter the systemic circulation. However, the environmental factors of rapid blood flow and high pressures found in the arterial system have unfavorable influences on the survival of detached tumor cells.[10]

Of greater significance in the establishment of bone metastases is the network of valveless veins known as Batson's plexus[4] that interconnect the vertebral venous system with the thoracic, abdominal, and pelvic veins. This system of slow-moving blood preserves the viability of the free-floating neoplastic cells and further explains the distribution of bone metastases. With increased intra-abdominal, intrapelvic, or intrathoracic pressures (such as in coughing, sneezing, or straining) tumor cells can be forced to travel in a retrograde manner via Batson's plexus to establish metastatic foci in the vertebrae, pelvic bones, ribs, skull, etc.

Diagnosis

For the patient with a malignancy at high risk for bone metastases, baseline and periodic evaluation of the skeletal system is an important part of the management for the early detection of metastatic disease. A bone scan is more sensitive than plain x-ray films for the detection of early disease. Up to 30 percent of the bone matrix may be replaced with tumor before routine x-ray films will disclose the lesion. However, in malignancies such as multiple myeloma, where pure lytic lesions are found, a skeletal survey may be more useful than a bone scan in determining the extent of bone involvement. In the high-risk patient, if a bone scan is done every 6 months for the first 2 years and yearly thereafter, early detection of metastatic bone lesions may be accomplished. Any suspicious areas on scan should be further evaluated by plain x-ray films of those areas, and if no lesion is evident, tomograms may be needed to demonstrate the lesion.

Clinical laboratory tests which are useful in the monitoring of patients for bone metastases include serum alkaline phosphatase, calcium and phosphorus determinations, and (in patients with prostatic carcinoma) acid phosphatase fractionation.

A careful history and physical examination done on a periodic basis in the cancer patient will often lead to the diagnosis of metastatic disease in bone. Back, neck, or extremity pain in the patient with a history of a preexisting malignant disease should be considered a metastatic process until proven otherwise. Pain can often precede x-ray changes by several weeks. The pain is usually insidious in onset, and when present at night or not relieved with bedrest, it is highly suspicious of a metastatic deposit. When the lesion is near a joint or in a weight-bearing bone, activity usually makes the pain worse. Patients with cancer should be educated in the signs and symptoms of bone metastases to avoid delays in seeking medical evaluation of their complaints. When symptoms are ignored, lesions can progress to the point that minor trauma can cause a pathologic fracture and further complicate the management of the patient. In 10–13 percent[3,11,42] of all pathologic fractures, the fracture will be the presenting symptom of a previously undiagnosed malignancy. In those cases, a thorough history, a physical examination, and simple laboratory studies will usually lead to the accurate diagnosis of the underlying primary lesion.

The therapeutic implications of finding metastatic disease in the bone are numerous and will greatly influence the overall management decisions for the patient. If present at the time of diagnosis, metastases will often alter the approach to the primary tumor; if diagnosed while on systemic therapy, metastases may indicate a need to alter therapy; and if diagnosed at a time remote from the treatment of a primary tumor, the bone lesions will require a more definitive diagnosis before therapeutic decisions can be made. Irrespective of the decisions on systemic treatment, each lesion must be evaluated regarding the potential need for localized therapy to either prevent or treat complications from a bone metastasis.

Bone Biopsy in Metastatic Disease

The need for a bone biopsy in the patient with metastatic bone disease must be considered in two separate categories, i.e., the patient with a previously diagnosed malignant disease and no known metastasis, and the patient with no known primary disease but evidence of metastatic bone disease on x-ray or bone scan. In the first instance the initial presence of a destructive bone lesion suggesting metastasis may indicate the need of a biopsy for diagnostic confirmation in order to allow selection of appropriate therapy. Most radiotherapists will not proceed with radiation treatments unless a positive diagnosis is established, and the selection of chemotherapy or hormonal therapy can better be determined by establishing an accurate diagnosis. Biopsy is especially important when the lesion appears at a time remote from the treatment of the initial primary. Since the incidence of second primaries is quite common, it cannot be assumed that the bone lesion is metastatic from the previous primary, and histologic confirmation reinforces the nature of the new lesion.

In the management of patients with breast cancer, the estrogen receptor status of the tumor tissue is helpful for directing the choice of therapy. Biopsy of a metastatic breast lesion would be indicated not only if the estrogen receptor status of the primary were unknown, but also to determine the estrogen receptor status of the metastasis, since it will not necessarily correspond to that of the primary.

Diagnosis is paramount to selection of appropriate treatment in the patient with radiographic evidence of metastatic bone disease and no known primary site. When a readily accessible lesion is present this should be the site of initial biopsy, whether it be skin or bone. The biopsy is very useful in expediting the diagnostic workup when the primary tumor is not readily determined by the initial evaluation. The use of percutaneous needle biopsy may be employed for lesions in the long bones and pelvis, with little morbidity. Similar techniques are useful in the spine but may be more complicated.

In addition to the above criteria, special situations may dictate the need for a diagnostic biopsy in order to determine appropriate therapy. For example, in the immunosuppressed patient with a gynecologic or urologic malignancy who develops a spine lesion associated with a chronic urinary tract infection, it may be difficult to differentiate a septic focus from a metastatic focus based on the usual parameters of fever, elevation of the sedimentation rate, and the x-ray characteristics of the lesion. A bone biopsy in this situation would be essential in defining the problem and directing therapy. For patients with Paget's disease, a bone biopsy is indicated when there is clinical suspicion of sarcomatous degeneration.

Pathologic Fractures

One third of all patients with cancer will develop bone metastases, but only 25 percent of these patients will actually develop pathologic fractures (or about 8 percent of all patients with cancer will develop pathologic fractures). Because of the distribution of metastatic deposits in bone, the majority of fractures will occur in the vertebrae, ribs, and pelvis, and only 20 percent of the pathologic fractures will involve the long bones.[34] From a functional and therapeutic viewpoint, long-bone fractures are much more important than the majority of fractures occurring in other locations. However, a discussion of the incidence and management of fractures in other areas is pertinent before further discussing the treatment of long-bone pathologic fractures.

Spine

The spine is the most frequent site of bone involvement by metastatic disease[6] when the vertebral system is considered in its entirety. It is also the most frequent site for pathologic fractures. Solid-tumor metastases easily gain access to the vertebral venous system via Batson's plexus. Additionally, the vertebral bodies, being a major source of bone marrow production in the adult, have a higher risk for involvement by a metastatic process. In Fornasier's[15] series, breast cancer, lymphoma, lung cancer, and multiple myeloma were the tumors most commonly found in the vertebral system, and breast cancer, prostate cancer, multiple myeloma, and lymphoma had the highest incidence of multiple vertebral involvement. Overall, the lumbar vertebrae are the most frequently involved vertebrae by metastatic tumor, and the thoracic and cervical vertebrae follow in descending order.[6] Fornasier reported that breast cancer more frequently metastasized to L2 than other vertebrae, with T9 being the next most common. Craig[9] found that breast cancer most commonly involved L3, L2, and L4, in that order. Lung cancer most frequently involved T12 in Fornasier's series. Multiple myeloma, by the nature of the disease, has no vertebral preference. Tumorous involvement of the C1 and C2 vertebrae is extremely rare and in two thirds of the cases is due to metastatic deposits from lung, breast, prostate, or thyroid primaries or involvement by multiple myeloma or lymphoma.[13] The most significant sign of involvement of the atlantoaxial articulation is loss of rotation of the neck, though several other symptoms suggesting upper cervical involvement include cervical pain, torticollis, positive Lhermitte's sign, paraesthesias, weakness, spasticity, ataxia, vertebral artery insufficiency, and respiratory symptoms.[13]

Most patients with cervical involvement are best treated with external immobilization using a cervical collar when spinal stability is not threatened, or a halo cast or vest when stability is at risk, while systemic therapy and/or radiotherapy for the underlying tumor is instituted. In a minority of cases where complete anterior and posterior bone destruction is present, operative stabilization is necessary. Dunn[12] reported a series of 24 patients in which methylmethacrylate and wires were used to stabilize the cervical spine. The only indication for methylmethacrylate usage in that series was in patients with metastatic or primary tumors who had limited life spans, yet could be expected to withstand surgery and were troubled by severe neck pain and/or progressive deformity or instability which was likely to, or already had, produced a neurologic deficit. Seventeen of 24 patients improved following surgery, and seven remained stable. Of significant advantage in this group using methylmethacrylate was the early mobilization (20/24) of the patients.

Most of the painful compression fractures in the vertebral system can be treated conservatively with analgesics and braces until the pain from the acute process subsides. It is unusual for compression fractures per se to cause a neurologic deficit, but loss of stability of the spine due to a destructive metastatic focus, or extra dural extension of the tumor, will lead to signs of nerve root or cord compression. The thoracic spine is the major area of cord compression, whereas the cervical and lumbar areas are less frequently involved. Signs or symptoms of paraesthesia, hypoesthesia, weakness, sphincter incompetence, and muscle atrophy require a diagnostic myelogram and definitive therapy. Symptoms heralding a poor prognosis from neurologic recovery are rapid progression of symptoms, sphincter involvement, compromise of the vascular supply, and thoracic involvement. Good prognostic signs include a lesion in the cauda equina and a short duration of symptoms prior to diagnosis. Treatment will depend upon the location and type of primary. For radiosensitive tumors (breast, lung, lymphoma, myeloma, thyroid), patients usually respond well to radiation alone. However, neurologic symptoms may temporarily become worse due to edema. This may be controlled for a short time by the use of adrenocorticosteroids.

When decompression laminectomy is indicated for acute neurologic sequelae, consideration should be given to concomitant stabilization with Harrington rods and methylmethacrylate. This will allow earlier mobilization of the patient without danger of further loss of spinal stability secondary to tumor destruction of the bone combined with laminectomy.

In the treatment of painful compression fractures and painful metastatic deposits, localized irradiation to the spine is beneficial in relieving pain. Eisen[14] has suggested that total spinal radiation should be given instead of localized therapy, since in his series of metastatic breast cancer to the spine 41 percent of patients receiving treatment to localized areas required subsequent irradiation to other lesions. The theoretical advantage of treating the whole spine would be to reduce or eliminate microscopic foci and hence reduce the risk of development of subsequent compression fractures, cord lesions, or painful progressive disease. This form of therapy, however, is not advocated by the majority of radiotherapists. Furthermore, consideration must be made to the myelosuppression of total spinal radiation and its impact on future chemotherapy.

Sternum

Very little has been written about the incidence of sternal metastases and pathologic fractures of the sternum. Urovitz et al.[38] reviewed 412 autopsy cases of malignant disease and found 63 cases of sternal involvement. Of these, breast cancer, lymphoma, and lung cancer were the most common, with the body of the sternum more frequently involved than the manubrium. This is in distinction to Kinsella's[24] review which found thyroid, kidney, and breast cancers to be the most common malignancies involving the sternum, with the manubrium more often affected than the body. There were 19 pathologic fractures in Urovitz's series in which breast cancer was the most common cause (10 cases). Lymphoma (2), multiple myeloma (2), colon (1), kidney (1), cervix (1), and tonsil (1) accounted for the remainder of the fractures of the body of the sternum, and the only pathologic fracture of the manubrium was due to an Ewing's sarcoma. Characteristic of pathologic fractures of the sternum is the greater deformity and the slower healing as compared to fractures of traumatic origin. Treatment is usually palliative irradiation for pain control while systematic therapy for the underlying primary is administered.

Ribs

The incidence of rib fractures is quite high, being the third most common area of bone involvement by metastatic disease. Both direct extension, most commonly from a lung or breast primary, and hematogenous spread lead to metastatic foci in ribs. Pain is the most common symptom of rib involvement by a metastatic process. The pain is usually constant and dull and can be aggravated by respiration. Rib fractures can result from minor trauma to the chest wall or from the stresses of coughing or sneezing. Rarely will a pathologic rib fracture lead to underlying pleural or pulmonary damage, though the tumor deposit could continue to grow and erode onto the pleural surface, thus leading to a malignant effusion. The treatment for painful rib fractures is the proper use of analgesics and palliative radiation therapy as well as systemic therapy for the primary. Splinting the rib cage is generally of little value, and may hasten the demise of the patient.

Clavicle

Pathologic fractures of the clavicle are best treated by immobilization and external beam irradiation. If pain persists due to improper healing, consideration can be given to either operative fixation to prevent the movement of the fracture segments, or surgical removal of the clavicular segment involved.

Small Bones of the Hands and Feet

Pathologic fractures due to metastatic cancers of the small bones of the hands and feet are extremely uncommon. Treatment is immobilization, with a brace or cast depending upon the location of the fracture. Adjunctive treatment with irradiation or systemic therapy should be employed, and if no response then excision, internal fixation, or curettage and packing with bone cement may be necessary to obtain relief of pain and to restore a more functional limb for the patient.

Long-Bone Fractures

The management of a patient with a pathologic long-bone fracture requires the coordinated efforts of the oncologist, the orthopedic surgeon, and the radiotherapist.[31] Treatment of long-bone fractures can be by either operative or nonoperative means. The immediate goal is the stabilization of the fracture segments to reduce pain and to enable fracture healing to occur. Nonoperative intervention may include the use of a brace, splint, cast, sling, or crutches in conjunction with radiation and/or chemotherapy.

In the treatment of bone metastases prior to fracture, radiation therapy is a useful modality for pain control. In some cases, reossification of the lesion will occur. However, because radiation retards the healing process by interrupting chondrogenesis and callus formation,[7] radiation is of value in pathologic fractures only when prolonged stabilization is insured so that the slower process of osteogenesis can lead to bone healing. The selection of operative and nonoperative intervention for the stabilization of the fracture segments will depend on the fracture site and the nature of the fracture. If an operative intervention is selected, pre- or postoperative radiation is usually given, though some feel that radiotherapy is of little benefit unless the tumor is radiosensitive.[11] Metallic prosthetic devices and methylmethacrylate will not decrease the effectiveness of radiation by acting as a shield, nor will the presence of a metallic orthopedic appliance enhance the radiation effect by reflection of the irradiated beam. Likewise, ionizing radiation has no deleterious effect on the stability of the methylmethacrylate.

Operative intervention usually means open reduction and fixation of the fracture segments by either external or internal metallic fixation with or without the use of methylmethacrylate. The selection of the operative approach and the merits and specific application of the many different prosthetic orthopedic devices are beyond the scope of this chapter and are best left to the judgment of the orthopedic surgeon involved in each case. Methylmethacrylate bone cement, which has only had recent clinical application, has greatly influenced the approach to the problem. Fractures which previously were not considered amenable to operative fixation due to extensive destruction of bone by metastatic deposits can now be treated with curettage of the tumor and packing with bone cement to allow stabilization for the metallic prosthetic device. For more specific discussion of fixation approaches and the use of methylmethacrylate, several reviews are available.[2,8,17,18,37,39]

Operative intervention can also mean amputation of the affected limb. Specific indications for amputation include pain not controllable by any other means; fungation of the tumor with the resultant problems of infection and difficulties with nursing care; arterial occlusion of the limb by the tumor that is not treatable by more conservative measures; and in some cases when a solitary metastasis to bone from a renal primary is found and no other disease can be defined.[16] Additional surgical therapy may involve oophorectomy, adrenalectomy, or hypophysectomy in the patient with breast cancer.

A compilation of several series on long-bone fractures[11,22,25,34,36,37] indicates that the lower extremity is the site of involvement in slightly more than two thirds and the upper extremity in less than one third of pathologic long-bone fractures. The sites of fracture are almost exclusively the femur and humerus, with the tibia and fibula accounting for 2–8 percent of long-bone fractures and the radius and ulna 1–2 percent. As with other pathologic fractures, breast cancer is responsible for nearly 50 percent of all long-bone fractures, with kidney, lung, lymphoreticular malignancies, prostate, and multiple myeloma accounting for 70 percent of the remaining fractures.[18,22,25,32,34]

Rarely is an operative intervention necessary in the treatment of forearm or lower-leg fractures, Rather, proper immobilization and protection with bulky dressings, casts, splints, slings, or crutches are adequate, while nonsurgical modalities are directed toward the control of the lesion.

In the humerus, the most common site of fracture is between the proximal and middle two thirds. Humeral lesions can be treated by either an operative or nonoperative approach, depending upon the nature and extent of the lesion. The majority of humeral fractures are initially treated conservatively with nonoperative immobilizaiton while therapy with radiation and/or chemotherapy is given. Though some patients will benefit with relief of pain and restoration of function, others will need operative intervention to relieve symptoms. Some will benefit from neither approach and will need narcotic analgesics for palliation of pain.

In the femur, as in the humerus, the most common sites of fracture occur in the proximal portion with the femoral head and neck accounting for about one third, the trochanteric region less than one half, and the femoral shaft about one fifth of the pathologic fractures.

It has been demonstrated by several authors[17,18,22,32,34,36,37] that operative fixation of a femoral fracture is preferable if the patient is a candidate for surgical intervention. The goals in operative intervention are to relieve pain, shorten hospitalization, restore ambulation, make nursing care easier, facilitate other modes of treatment, and to improve the overall morale of the patient. Early mobilization prevents or reduces the risk of developing decubitus ulcers or thrombophlebitis, as well as hypercalcemia. The goal is not necessarily the prolongation of life by an operative intervention, since that depends more upon the underlying tumor and its response to other treatment modalities. Rather, the goal of the operation is to improve the quality of remaining life for the patient.[11] In selecting a patient for operative intervention, the orthopedic surgeon must be convinced that it will be more beneficial than any nonsurgical treatment; the bone proximal and distal to the fracture site must be adequate to support metallic fixation with or without the use of methylmethacrylate in order to insure stability of the extremity; and the procedure must facilitate the general care of the patient.[30] Life expectancy of the patient should not be a consideration unless the patient is expected to die within a few days.[42] Absolute contraindications to surgery include altered levels of consciousness that negate the need for pain control and a systemic illness that precludes the use of general anesthesia.[42] Such things as hypercalcemia, the nature of the primary tumor, the degree of metastatic spread, pleural effusions, or ascites are not contraindications per se to an operative intervention.

Preoperative Evaluation

The preoperative evaluation of the patient with a neoplastic fracture is different than that for the patient with a traumatic fracture. Though one uses good medical management as far as evaluating the pulmonary, cardiac, and renal status, it is essential to pay specific attention to the hepatic function, the coagulation profile, the calcium level, the bone marrow status, the general skeletal system, and the potential problems that may arise because of the chemotherapy or radiotherapy with which the patient may have been treated. There is usually no urgency for immediate operative fixation, and the patient can be kept comfortable by traction immobilization and analgesics while this evaluation is undertaken.

A complete coagulation profile including prothrombin time, partial thromboplastin time, and thrombin time in conjunction with evaluation of the platelet count and review of the peripheral smear should be done. Since release of tissue thromboplastins from a tumor or in association with a pathologic fracture may activate the clotting cascade via the Alternative Pathway, signs and symptoms suggesting a disseminated intravascular coagulopathy must be specifically sought. Additionally, coagulation factor deficiencies may be present due to liver dysfunction from metastatic disease and will need to be corrected prior to any operative procedure.

Bone marrow reserve and function must be evaluated. A complete blood count and a careful history of the patient's chemotherapy program, as well as details of previous irradiation to major hematopoietic areas, will be important. Neoplastic fractures can be vascular, and extra blood loss can be anticipated. Pre- and postoperative support with platelets and red blood cells may be needed. Neutropenia, often induced by prior chemotherapy or radiotherapy, may lead to an increased risk for a postoperative infection. Wound healing can be retarded as a result of a recent course of chemotherapy.

Though hepatic metastases are not an absolute contraindication to an operation, the overall liver function and reserve will be important from the standpoint of selection of the anesthetic agents and anesthetic approach. The adrenal and pituitary status must be kept in mind in patients with breast cancer who may have had prior operative hormonal manipulations.

Hypercalcemia is often a complication of widespread bone disease, and immobilization caused by a femoral fracture will make it worse. By improving ambulation through operative fixation of a pathologic fracture, the risks for hypercalcemia are often reduced. For existing hypercalcemia, management with mithramycin will rapidly reduce the hypercalcemia and improve the patient's status for immediate surgery.

Finally, the evaluation of bones other than the one involved in the actual fracture is necessary. For example, if a fractured tibia is to be managed with a cast or brace with crutches for ambulation, the upper extremities must be evaluated to avoid a pathologic fracture with crutch weight-bearing, and the contralateral lower limb must be evaluated since it will be carrying an increased load. Additionally, high-risk lesions for fracture may be found during the preoperative evaluation, and these should be treated prophylactically at the same operative setting rather than exposing the patient to repeated anesthetic exposure.

Prophylactic Management

Some assessment as to risk for fracture must be made when a metastatic lesion is discovered in a long bone, since the time course between the discovery of a metastatic lesion in bone to the time of actual fracture can be quite variable, or may not occur at all. Lesions at low risk for fracture usually require no intervention, whereas prophylactic treatment of a high-risk lesion should be carried out whenever the lesion is discovered.

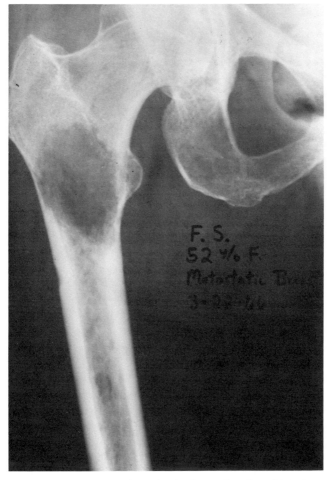

Fig. 1a. *A metastatic focus in the femoral neck and intertrochanteric area has eroded the medial cortex which resists compression stress of the adductor muscles.*

Prophylactic fixation is usually less traumatic for the patient, allows ambulation sooner, and decreases the time in the hospital as compared to patients treated after the fracture actually occurs.

High-risk areas for fracture include diphyseal lesions in major long bones when at least one cortex is destroyed on two views, and when unicortical destruction in long bones is noted if the involved cortex is on the compression side of the bone (Fig. 1a,b). Since long bones are strongest

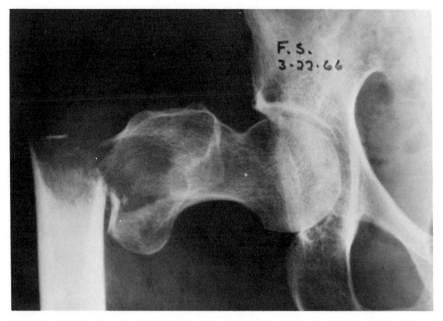

Fig. 1b. *In the process of abducting and externally rotating the hip for a lateral x-ray, a pathologic fracture occurred.*

under compression, these lesions will tend to greatly weaken the load-bearing property of the bone. Additionally, subchondral bone erosion in major weight-bearing joints (e.g., acetabular or tibial plateau) will produce pathologic fractures unless the joint is unloaded or structurally protected by external or internal devices.

In a retrospective study of metastatic breast cancer, Beals[5] found that fractures in the femur occurred in over 50 percent of the cases when a well-defined lytic lesion of 2.5 cm in diameter involved the femoral cortex, or when a lesion of that size was painful regardless of its bony location. Others have also found that pain is a useful indicator of an impending fracture. [42] Risk of fracture is also dependent upon the nature of the primary tumor involving the bone. Rapidly progressing lesions are at a higher risk for fracture than slowly growing lesions. Lytic lesions will more predictably fracture than mixed lytic and blastic lesions, and purely blastic lesions will uncommonly cause pathologic fractures. Zickel[42] also noted that lesions of the femur that developed from a previously undiagnosed primary and lesions secondary to lung cancer were high-risk lesions for fracture.

During radiotherapy or chemotherapy bone pain may be markedly reduced before any reossification occurs.[35] As a result, the patient may become more active, bearing weight or subjecting the involved bone to more stress, and fractures may then occur. This may be avoided by warning the patient that it takes several weeks to months to regenerate new bone, and in the meantime continued caution is needed.

Survival

Survival after prophylactic fixation is longer[42] than survival following fixation of an actual pathologic fracture. However, this might only reflect earlier intervention in the natural progression of the underlying tumor rather than a real increment in survival. Survival following a pathologic fracture is dependent upon the nature of the underlying tumor and its responsiveness to treatment rather than upon the choice of management of the fracture. Operative fixation of a major long-bone fracture is usually preferred since it provides better stabilization, better pain control, and more rapid return of function for the patient. Breast cancer and multiple myeloma patients live longer following a fracture,[18,22] while those with lung cancer[32,42] and undifferentiated tumors[32] have a poorer prognosis. Patients with breast cancer who have had prior adrenalectomy, although survival was longer prior to fracture, had a shorter survival following a pathologic fracture than in those who had not had prior adrenalectomy.[26,36] Schurman and Amstutz[36] also reported shorter average survivals following humeral fractures (6.5 months) than for femoral fractures (10.1 months) in breast cancer, but Douglass[11] could find no difference in survival between upper- and lower-extremity fractures in nonbreast cancer patients.

When a pathologic fracture was the first sign of an underlying tumor, the patients have done poorly, with a median survival of 1–2 months.[32,42] This is predominantly a reflection of the underlying tumor type, with lung cancer being the most common tumor in this group of patients. No difference in survival has been shown if a patient has single or multiple pathologic fractures.[26]

Other Considerations

Operative intervention of a pathologic fracture is not without risks and complications, but the potential benefits from operative fixation outweigh the risks when the patients are selected appropriately and managed carefully. It has been speculated that the intramedullary fixation of a pathologic fracture or impending fracture could lead to spread of tumor locally, as well as the possibility of widespread dissemination of tumor emboli that gained access to the vascular channels during operative manipulation.[33] Although free cancer cells have been recovered from the inferior vena cava during operative fixation of femoral fractures,[19] the clinical significance of this finding has not been demonstrated. In addition to tumor emboli, fat embolization is a risk in pathologic fractures, as it is in fractures of traumatic origin. Signs and symptoms suggesting fat embolization must be sought so that the appropriate treatment can be given.

General anesthesia has been demonstrated to have a temporary adverse effect on the host's immune defense mechanisms, and this theoretically could contribute to the risk of tumor growth and spread. Clinical relevance of this in the management of pathologic fractures is not known.

Tumor fungation through the operative wound is an uncommon complication of surgical fixation of a pathologic fracture. When it occurs, consideration should be given to amputation of the limb if the lesion adversely affects the management of the patient.

Summary

Periodic evaluation of the skeletal system should be done in patients with tumors known to metastasize to bone with a high frequency. When a lesion is found, an assessment of fracture risk is necessary. For those at high risk for fracture, evaluation for prophylactic treatment is indicated. Following long-bone fractures, open fixation is the preferred treatment for the femur if the patient is an operative candidate. Preoperative evaluation of the cancer patient with a pathologic fracture will be more extensive than for the patient with a traumatic fracture. Special attention must be paid to the status of the patient's liver function, coagulation profile, bone marrow reserve, previous chemotherapy or radiation treatment, and the status of the remaining skeletal system in order to anticipate potential problems in the peri- and postoperative periods. The fact that a patient may have a limited life expectancy should not dissuade an operative approach, and the major goal to be achieved is the maintenance of the quality of remaining life for the cancer patient.

References

1. Abrams HL, Spirc R, Goldstein N: Metastases in carcinoma. Cancer 3:74–85, 1950
2. Anderson JT, Erickson JM, Thompson RC, et al: Pathologic femoral

shaft fractures comparing fixation techniques using cement. Clin Orthoped 131:273–278, 1978

3. Anderson JT, Thompson RC, McMahon JE, et al: Total hip replacement in disseminated neoplastic disease. Surg Gynecol Obstet 144:560–562, 1977

4. Batson OV: The role of vertebral veins in metastatic process. Ann Int Med 16:38–45, 1942

5. Beals RK, Lawton GD, Snell WE: Prophylactic internal fixation of the femur in metastatic breast cancer. Cancer 28:1350–1354, 1974

6. Bhalla SK: Metastatic disease of the spine. Clin Orthoped 73:52–60, 1970

7. Bonarigo BC, Rubin P: Nonunion of pathologic fracture after radiation therapy. Radiology 88:889–898, 1967

8. Carlson DH, Adams R: The use of methylmethacrylate in repair of neoplastic lesions in bone. Radiology 112:43–46, 1974

9. Craig FS: Metastatic and primary lesions of bone. Clin Orthoped 73:33–38, 1970

10. del Regato JA: Pathways of metastatic spread of malignant tumors. Semin Oncol 4:33–38, 1977

11. Douglass HO, Shukla SK, Mindell E: Treatment of pathological fractures of long bones excluding those due to breast cancer. J Bone Joint Surg 58-A:1055–1061, 1976

12. Dunn EJ: The role of methylmethacrylate in the stabilization and replacement of tumors of the cervical spine. Spine 2:15–24, 1977

13. Dunn EJ, Anas PP: The management of tumors of the upper cervical spine. Orthoped Clin North Am 9:1065–1080, 1978

14. Eisen HM, Bosworth JL, Ghossein NA: The rationale for whole spine irradiation in metastatic breast cancer. Radiology 108:417–418, 1973

15. Fornasier VL, Horne JG: Metastases to the vertebral column. Cancer 36:590–594, 1975

16. Francis K: The role of amputation in the treatment of metastatic bone cancer. Clin Orthoped 73:61–63, 1970

17. Harrington KD, Johnston MO, Turner RH, et al: The use of methylmethacrylate as an adjunct in the internal fixation of malignant neoplastic fractures. J Bone Joint Surg 54-A:1665–1676, 1972

18. Harrington KD, Sim FH, Enis JE, et al: Methylmethacrylate as an adjunct in internal fixation of pathological fractures. J Bone Joint Surg 58-A:1047–1055, 1976

19. Hoare JR: Pathologic Fractures. Proceedings of the Northwest Metropolitan Orthopaedic Club. J Bone Joint Surg 50-B:232, 1968

20. Holland JF, Frei E: Cancer Medicine. Philadelphia, Lea and Febiger, 1973

21. Jaffe HL: Tumors and Tumorous Conditions of the Bones and Joints. Philadelphia, Lea and Febiger, 1958
22. Jensen TM, Dillon WL, Reckling FW: Changing concepts in the management of pathological and impending pathological fractures. J Trauma 16:496–502, 1976
23. Johnston AD: Pathology of metastatic tumors in bone. Clin Orthoped 73:8–32, 1970
24. Kinsella TJ, White SM, Koucky RW: Two unusual tumors of the sternum. J Thoracic Surg 16:640–667, 1947
25. Krebs H: Management of pathologic fractures of long bones in malignant disease. Arch Orthoped Trauma Surg 92:133–137, 1978
26. Marcove RC, Yang D-J: Survival times after treatment of pathologic fractures. Cancer 20:2154–21558, 1967
27. Mercer W, Duthie RB: Orthopedic Surgery (ed 6). Baltimore, Williams and Wilkins, 1964
28. Mickelson MR, Bonfiglio M: Pathological fractures in the proximal part of the femur treated by Zickel nail fixation. J Bone Joint Surg 58-A:1067–1070, 1976
29. Mulvey RB: Peripheral bone metastases. Am J Roentgen 91:155–160, 1964
30. Murray JA, Parrish FF: Surgical management of secondary neoplastic fractures about the hip. Orthoped Clin North Am 5:887–901, 1974
31. Nussbaum H, Allen B, Kagan AR, et al: Management of bone metastasis—multidisciplinary approach. Semin Oncol 4:93–97, 1977
32. Parrish FF, Murray JA: Surgical treatment for secondary neoplastic fractures, a retrospective study of ninety-six patients. J Bone Joint Surg 52-A:665–686, 1970
33. Peltier LF: Theoretical hazards in the treatment of pathologic fractures by the Kuntscher intramedullary nail. Surgery 29:466–472, 1951
34. Perez C, Bradfield JS, Morgan HC: Management of pathologic fractures. Cancer 29:684–693, 1972
35. Ryan JR, Rowe DE, Salciccioli GG: Prophylactic internal fixation of the femur for neoplastic lesions. J Bone Joint Surg 58-A:1071–1074, 1976
36. Schurman DJ, Amstutz HC: Orthopedic management of patients with metastatic carcinoma of the breast. Surg Gynecol Obstet 137:831–836, 1973
37. Sim FH, Daugherty TW, Ivins JC: The adjunctive use of methylmethacrylate in fixation of pathological fractures. J Bone Joint Surg 56A:40–48, 1974
38. Urovitz EPM, Fornasier VL, Czitrom AA: Sternal metastases and associated pathological fractures. Thorax 32:444–448, 1977

39. Wang G-J, Reger SI, Maffeo C, et al: The strength of metal reinforced methylmethacrylate fixation of pathologic fractures. Clin Orthoped 135:287–290, 1978
40. Warren S, Meissner WA: Neoplasms, in Anderson WAD (ed): Pathology (ed 5). St. Louis, C. V. Mosby, 1966, pp 400–429
41. Wirth CR: Metastatic bone cancer, in Hickey RC (ed): Current Problems in Cancer, Vol 3, No. 11. Chicago, Year Book, 1979, pp 1–36
42. Zickel RE, Mouradian WH: Intramedullary fixation of pathological fractures and lesions of the subtrochanteric region of the femur. J Bone Joint Surg 58-A:1061–1066, 1976

3

SUPERIOR VENA CAVA SYNDROME

Joseph R. Simpson
Carlos A. Perez
Cary A. Presant
Albert L. Van Amburg

Traditionally two emergencies for the radiation oncologist are the occurrence of superior vena cava syndrome and spinal cord compression secondary to malignant disease. The object of this chapter is to help define those situations in which superior vena caval obstruction is truly an emergency, requiring treatment first and histological diagnosis second; to review the etiologies involved and diagnostic steps available; and to outline the most effective therapeutic strategies. The long-term prognosis of patients with malignant superior vena caval obstruction will also be discussed.

Anatomy of the Mediastinum

A review of the anatomy of the mediastinum is quite helpful in understanding the pathophysiology of the superior vena cava (SVC) syndrome. Classically, the mediastinum is divided into four regions: (1) *superior*, lying above the level of the pericardium and containing the thymus in front, the esophagus and aorta behind, and the great vessels related to the heart and pericardium in between; (2) *anterior*, lying in front of the pericardium and behind the sternum, and containing part of the thymus; (3) *middle*, containing the pericardium, heart, adjacent parts of the great ves-

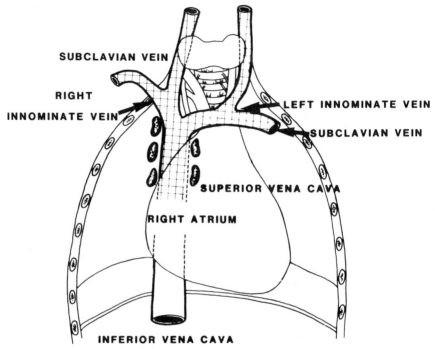

Fig. 1. *Schematic representation of the formation of the SVC.*

sels, and the main bronchi, and (4) *posterior,* lying behind the pericardium and containing the esophagus and thoracic aorta.

Loose connective tissue, often infiltrated with fat, pervades the mediastinum and surrounds and suspends the organs within it. This tissue becomes more fibrous and rigid with age, and therefore the structures tend to be less mobile.[8]

The superior vena cava descends in a right paratracheal location to enter the superior mediastinum. Just above the pericardium, the left innominate vein joins the right to form the superior vena cava, which empties into the right atrium (Fig. 1).

The location of the lymph node groups within the mediastinum plays an important role in the pathophysiology of superior vena cava obstruction. There are three main groups: an anterior, an intermediate (trachealbronchial), and a posterior group.[14] The anterior group is located in the upper half of the thorax along the thoracic portion of the phrenic nerve. These nodes are further divided into right and left groups, distributed on the anterior surface of the great vessels of the thorax including the aortic arch and vessels arising from it, the innominate veins, and the superior vena cava. On the right side, there are nodes situated between the vena cava on the right border of the convexity of the arch of the aorta and the trachea. These nodes lie medial to the right phrenic nerve and communicate with the right paratracheal nodes. Thus, the superior vena cava, with a thin wall and low intravascular pressure, is a collapsible vessel surrounded by solid structures such as the trachea, vertebral bodies, sternum, and lymph nodes which form a compartment which is relatively rigid.

Pathophysiology of Superior Vena Cava Syndrome

There are three mechanisms that usually account for the occurrence of superior vena cava syndrome: (1) occlusion due to extrinsic pressure, (2) invasion of the vein wall by neoplasm, or (3) intraluminal thrombosis. Benign lesions may result in this syndrome due to extrinsic pressure,

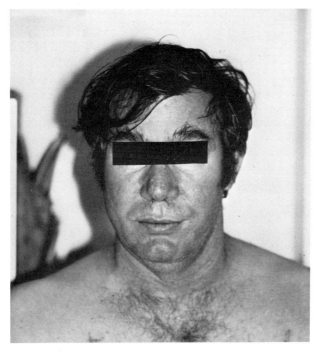

Fig. 2. *Plethoric face of a patient with SVC syndrome.*

whereas malignant disease may occlude the vessel by extrinsic pressure or direct invasion of the vein wall. The clinical picture is due to venous hypertension in areas normally drained by the superior vena cava or its tributaries. Pressure measurements have been taken and values greater than 150 mm saline are reported in most patients.[28] Delayed circulation time, development of venous collaterals, and associated manifestations of the primary process causing the obstruction also form part of the syndrome complex. The severity of symptoms depends upon the rapidity, degree, and location of obstruction, and upon the development and adequacy of collateral circulation. Symptoms, which are quite variable, may include headache, nausea, dizziness, visual changes, hoarseness, stridor, stupor, respiratory distress, and syncope or convulsions. The symptoms are typically increased by bending forward or by assuming a horizontal position and patients may sleep sitting up because of dyspnea on recumbency. The common signs are a plethoric face (Fig. 2), dilated venous channels over the neck, trunk or upper extremities (Figs. 3,4), a change in collar size, and cyanotic or flushed skin. The majority of patients will have had symptoms for less than 1 month with another 20 percent being symptomatic as long as 2 months. There are numerous cases, however, of malignant superior

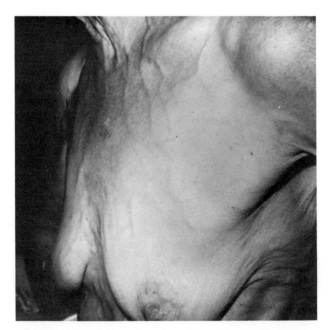

Fig. 3. *Dilated thoracic veins of a patient with SVC syndrome.*

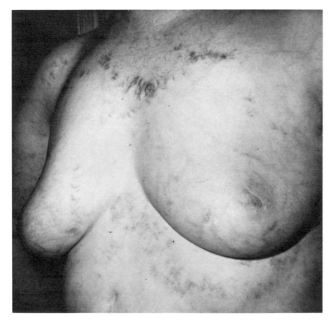

Fig. 4. *Cutaneous telangiectasias in SVC syndrome.*

vena cava syndrome in which the patients are relatively asymptomatic. In general, a slowly developing obstruction, such as is seen with a benign lesion, is well tolerated, whereas a rapidly occurring obstruction, as from a malignancy, produces more acute symptoms. In general, when the collateral channels are given enough time, sufficient blood is shunted around the obstruction to avoid major symptoms under basal conditions.

Epidemiology and Etiology

As mentioned, superior vena cava obstruction has been associated with both benign and malignant conditions. Recent reports in the literature suggest that there has been a definite decrease in the relative frequency of benign causes. In a 1954 report, 48 percent of the causes of SVC syndrome were nonmalignant. Aortic aneurysms accounted for 29 percent of the benign lesions, while the second largest contributor was mediastinitis, including tuberculous, pyogenic, and syphylitic lesions. Thrombosis, including traumatic, spontaneous, or propagating, accounted for 6.5 percent. Pericarditis was listed as the cause in two patients (0.7 per-

Table 1
Superior Vena Cava Syndrome:
Primary Anatomical Diagnosis

	Number of Patients	Percent	Total
Bronchogenic Carcinoma			67
Stage III	63	94	
Recurrent	4	6	
Malignant Lymphoma			14
Stage II	7	50	
Stage III	2	14	
Stage IV	5	35	
Other			
Breast (adenocarcinoma)			1
Heart (Kaposi's sarcoma)			1
Testicle (metastatic seminoma)			1
Total			84

Table 2
Superior Vena Cava Syndrome:
Primary Pathological Diagnosis

	Number of Patients	Total
Bronchogenic Carcinoma		67
Small-cell undifferentiated	31	
Epidermoid carcinoma	17	
Large-cell undifferentiated	10	
Adenocarcinoma	8	
Malignant, NOS	1	
Malignant Lymphoma		14
Lymphocytic	5	
Histiocytic	4	
Mixed	3	
Unclassified	2	
Other		3
Kaposi's sarcoma (heart)	1	
Adenocarcinoma (breast)	1	
Metastatic seminoma (testicle)	1	
Total		84

cent), and mitral stenosis in one.[32] Subsequent reports of benign etiologies have included infectious agents,[6,24] substernal thyroid,[5] and sarcoidosis.[12] In contrast, a review by Adar et al. of 33 SVC cases in Israel from 1955 to 1972 showed that approximately 80 percent were associated with malignant conditions,[1] while Lokich cited a 90-percent association.[18] Current studies show the most prevalent malignancy is bronchogenic carcinoma, with small-cell undifferentiated carcinoma (oat cell) the most common subtype, while malignant lymphomas are second in frequency.[18,19,23] Other frequent malignant causes are esophageal, colon, testicular, and breast cancers.[23,36]

In a series of 84 patients treated at the Mallinckrodt Institute of Radiology (MIR), 67 had bronchogenic carcinoma, 14 had malignant lymphoma, and 3 had other malignant conditions (Table 1). The patients with malignant lymphoma, when subdivided by clinical stages, were fairly evenly divided between localized (Stage II) and disseminated (Stages III and IV) disease.

Table 2 lists the pathological diagnosis for all patients. Approximately 46 percent of the patients with bronchogenic carcinoma had the small-cell undifferentiated histologic subtype and 25 percent had epidermoid carcinoma. There was an equal distribution of histological subtypes within the malignant lymphomas, with five cases classifed as lymphocytic, four as histocytic, three as mixed, and two as unclassified. Three patients in this series had other solid tumors: Kaposi's sarcoma, adenocarcinoma of the breast, and metastatic seminoma.

Clinical Manifestations and Physical Findings

The clinical symptoms most commonly associated with SVC syndrome are dyspnea, cough, orthopnea, facial swelling, headaches, drowsiness, vertigo, and hoarseness. In the MIR series, the presenting symptoms were shortness of breath (43 percent), facial swelling (43 percent), and swelling of the trunk or upper extremities (40 percent). Chest pain, cough, and dysphagia were less frequently reported—approximately 20 percent each. Approximately 20 percent of the patients had symptoms for less than 3 weeks prior to admission, and an additional 35 percent had symptoms between 3 and 4 weeks. In 15 patients (18 percent) the symptoms had been present for 5–8 weeks, and in an additional 15 patients (18 percent) for over 8 weeks.

The physical findings of the 84 patients are listed in Table 3. The most frequent findings were distention of the thoracic veins (67 percent), neck-

Table 3
Superior Vena Cava Syndrome:
Physical Findings

	Number	Percent
Thorax-vein distension	56	67.0
Neck-vein distension	49	59.0
Edema of face	47	56.0
Tachypnea	34	40.0
Plethora of face	16	19.0
Cyanosis	13	15.0
Edema of upper extremities	8	9.5
Paralyzed true vocal cord	3	3.5
Horner's syndrome	2	2.3

vein distention (59 percent), facial edema (56 percent), and tachypnea (40 percent). In other series, too, the most prominent signs have also been edema of the face, neck, and upper extremities, as well as prominence of the superficial venous collaterals of the neck, chest, and abdomen.[25]

Methods of Diagnosis

The diagnosis of SVC obstruction is made from the clinical signs listed above. Tissue diagnosis is desirable, and if clinically feasible should be an early step in evaluating the patient. If there is no previous history of malignancy, one must realize that there is an approximately 80-percent chance that the underlying disease is bronchogenic carcinoma or malignant lymphoma. Furthermore, the most common bronchogenic carcinoma will be the small-cell undifferentiated cell type, which can be widely disseminated. Therefore, a diagnosis can often be made from a peripheral lymph node or bone marrow biopsy (Fig. 5). Lokich and Goodman[18] have recommended that a tissue biopsy be performed when abnormal tissue is readily available for biopsy, or when the clinical manifestations are mild or slowly progressive. If these criteria are not met, however, they favor early therapeutic intervention in this oncologic emergency. One must remember, however, that tissue diagnosis is necessary if further therapy after radiation therapy is to be given. In acute sitautions, there should not be a delay of therapy while attempting a tissue diagnosis. As Lockich and Goodman have cogently stated,[18]

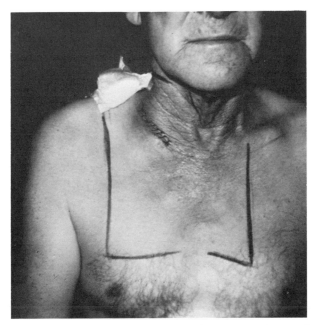

Fig. 5. *Patient with SVC syndrome following scalene node biopsy.*

. . . the pitfalls in the management of SVC syndrome relate to overzealous efforts to establish the site of obstruction and to determine a specific histopathologic diagnosis. (These efforts) may lead to life-threatening complications, such as respiratory obstruction, aspiration, and hemorrhage.

The methods available for tissue diagnosis, in addition to the ones mentioned above, are sputum cytology, bronchoscopy, transbronchial biopsy, percutaneous needle biopsy, cervical mediastinal exploration, and thoracotomy. Table 4 lists the methods of diagnosis used in the MIR series. Bronchoscopy and biopsy were used most frequently, but only yielded a diagnosis in 28 out of 45 patients (62 percent) and, in our experience, had a much lower yield in patients with lymphoma. Thoracotomy and biopsy were performed in 19 patients, with a positive diagnosis being obtained in all. Mediastinoscopy and biopsy were done in 11 patients, and a positive biopsy was obtained in 9 (81 percent). Scalene node biopsies were done in 22 patients with 50 percent positive, while 19 patients had palpable supraclavicular nodes biopsied with 84 percent positive. Sputum cytology was positive in 15 of 24 patients (63 percent) and bron-

Table 4
Superior Vena Cava Syndrome: Methods of Diagnosis

	Number of Patients	Positive Results		Negative Results
		Number	Percent	Number
Thoracotomy & Biopsy	19	19	100	
Mediastinoscopy & Biopsy	11	9	81	2
Bronchoscopy & Biopsy	45	28	62	17
Lymph Node Biopsy				
Scalene	22	11	50	11
Supraclavicular (palpable)	19	16	84	3
Cytology				
Sputum	24	15	63	9
Bronchial washings	12	6	50	6
Pleural effusion	4	4	100	

chial washings in 6 of 12 patients (50 percent). Pleural fluid for cytology was obtained in four patients and was positive in all four.

Radiographic Studies and Findings

In every patient suspected of having superior vena cava syndrome, as in other cardiorespiratory emergencies, PA and lateral radiographs of the chest should be routinely obtained. In the group of 84 patients analyzed at Washington University, 49 (58 percent) were found to have a right superior mediastinum mass on chest x-ray films (Table 5), a finding most often secondary to small-cell undifferentiated carcinoma of the lung or malignant lymphoma.

Hilar adenopathy, either on the right side or bilateral, and evidence of associated mediastinal adenopathy was present in 20 additional patients. Conventional tomograms or computed tomography of the thorax may facilitate the delineation of the mediastinal or hilar masses. In addition, in patients suspected of having a chronic inflammatory process, the presence of calcium in the paratracheal or hilar lymph nodes may be of help in influencing the radiologist to consider this diagnostic possibility.

Phlebography of the superior vena cava is *infrequently* done, although it may be very helpful in localizing the site and degree of obstruction, and venous pressure can be measured in the upper extremities at the time of insertion of the catheter. Phlebography has been used to distinguish between vascular and nonvascular lesions, to define operability, and to as-

Table 5
Superior Vena Cava Syndrome: Chest X-Ray Findings

	Bronchogenic Cancer	Lymphoma	Total	
Superior mediastinal mass (± pleural effusions or pulmonary lesions except right upper lobe)	20	12	32	
Superior mediastinal and hilar mass	11	2	13	49 (67%)
Superior mediastinal and right upper-lobe mass	2		2	
Superior mediastinal, right upper lobe and hilar mass	2		2	
Right hilar (or parahilar) mass				
with atelectasis	6		6	
without atelectasis	13		13	
Bilteral hilar adenopathy	1		1	
Other				
Left upper lobe mass	2		2	
Right middle lobe mass	1		1	
Right pleural effusion	1		1	
Total	59*	14	73	

*Pretreatment chest x-rays were not available for review on 11 patients with bronchogenic carcinoma.

sess the extent of the obstruction, as well as its hemodynamics in case of suspected superior vena cava syndrome. By defining the site and extent of the venous obstruction, it also provides important information for radiotherapy treatment planning as the portals can be more accurately designed. The procedure is performed by simultaneous injection of hypaque or a similar iodine-containing contrast material (30–40 ml, 45-percent concentration) into both subclavian veins through a small polyethylene catheter which is introduced into the basilic vein using the Seldinger technique. If obstruction is severe and there is significant arm edema, it may be difficult to get the Seldinger needle into the basilic vein. Sometimes, this may be overcome by elevation of the arms for a few hours prior to the procedure, or alternatively using a different vein for the initial catheter insertion. Multiple sequential x-ray films are taken in the frontal and lateral positions with a rapid changer at 1-second intervals. This not only provides better anatomical detail, but a clearer hemodynamic picture. The technique as currently employed is no more hazardous or time consuming

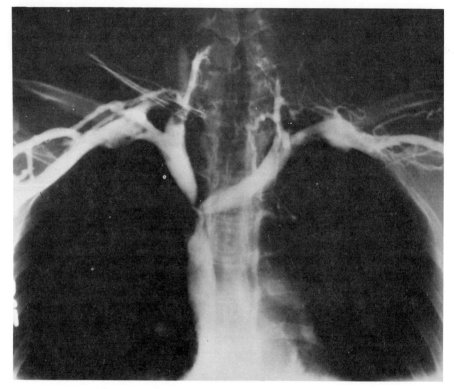

Fig. 6. *Phlebogram demonstrating obstruction of the SVC at its origin.*

than an intravenous pyelogram. In six patients on whom this procedure was performed at Washington University, marked obstruction of the superior vena cava was demonstrated in all cases (Fig. 6).

In addition to elucidating the nature of the obstruction (intravenous thrombosis versus external pressure), the phlebogram is helpful in establishing the presence of collateral circulation and its effectiveness in maintaining appropriate blood flow.

In the first 14 cases reported by Howard when a diagnosis was in doubt, conformation was obtained in 6.[15] Furthermore, in the first 45 phlebograms obtained by that author, it was shown that the obstruction could be proximal to the superior vena cava and involve the subclavian veins. For this reason he suggested that the term superior vena cava obstruction was restrictive and inaccurate and should be discarded in favor of a more suitable term such as "mediastinal obstruction."

Phlebography may also provide prognostic information based upon the degree of collateral information. In Howard's series of 48 patients, 21 had no collateral circulation, and 50 percent were dead within 3 months. In contrast, 80 percent of those in whom there was collateral circulation survived longer than 3 months. Howard furthermore believes that collateral circulation is associated with a better response to radiation therapy, since only one patient with a good collateral circulation failed to respond completely to radiotherapy, while 50 percent of those without good collaterals lacked a complete response.[15]

Short-lived radioisotope tracers, such as technetium-99m pertechnetate, have been used recently instead of phlebography to identify the site of the obstruction. This procedure can be performed without any significant discomfort, morbidity, or mortality. In a series of 20 patients with obstruction of the superior vena cava, Maxfield and Meckstroth[20] reported excellent correlation with the radiographic vascular studies in those patients in whom both procedures were performed. The advantage of the radioisotope method is that it can be used for serial evaluation of the regression of tumor and improvement of blood flow after radiotherapy.[11,31]

Methods of Therapy

Radiation Therapy

Radiation to generous chest portals encompassing the mediastinum, hila, and any adjacent pulmonary parenchymal lesion should be initiated as soon as practicable. All gross tumors with a 2-cm margin should be included. As bronchogenic carcinoma is the most frequent cause of superior vena cava syndrome and supraclavicular nodes are at risk for invasion with upper-lobe lesions or superior mediastinal adenopathy, supraclavicular lymph nodes should routinely be treated even if there are no palpable nodes initially (Fig. 7).

The total dose of irradiation should be in the range of 4000–5000 rad, depending upon the histology of the underlying tumor and the general condition of the patient. In malignant lymphoma, lower doses will be effective, whereas bronchogenic carcinoma should receive the higher dose range. We have found that the dose of radiation therapy showed only minimal correlation with tumor regression and symptomatic improvement (Table 6). However, since this was not a randomized study, it could be related to the initial stage of the disease and the administration of the higher dose of irradiation to patients with a more favorable general condition and initial response to therapy. Fifty percent of the patients receiving less than 2000 rads had a response, whereas those receiving 2000–4000

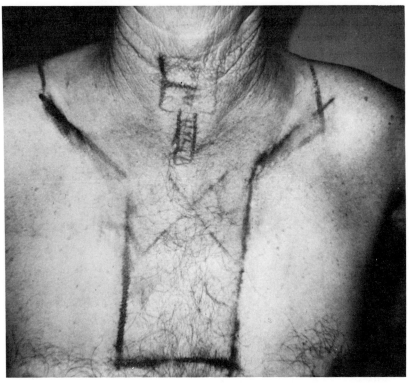

Fig. 7. *Example of irradiation portal for treatment of SVC syndrome.*

rads had response rates in the range of 72–89 percent. Four patients with bronchogenic carcinoma treated with doses of 6000 rads all showed complete tumor regression (100-percent response).[23] Several authors have reported on the use of high initial daily fractions of 400 rad for 3–4 treatments followed by conventional fractionation at 180–200 rad/day to the desired total tumor dose.[2,7,23,27] Others have preferred smaller, more conventional doses of radiation throughout the treatment course.[19] In our patients with bronchogenic carcinoma there was no significant difference in survival between the patients treated with a high dose initially and those receiving conventional irradiation (Fig. 8). Small initial radiation doses with gradual increase to standard fractionation based upon the fear of exacerbation of superior vena cava syndrome because of radiation edema are not indicated because of the unlikely occurrence of such phenomena. The spinal cord should not be irradiated with doses above 4000–4500 rad, since some of these patients survive for long periods of time (Fig. 9).

Table 6
Superior Vena Cava Syndrome: Number of Patients at Levels of Irradiation and Reponse for Bronchogenic Carcinoma

Dose (rads)	XRT and Chemotherapy					XRT Only				
	Number of Pts.	Responses No.	Percent	No. Known Local Relapse (not evaluable)	Duration of Response (months)	Number of Pts.	Responses No.	Percent	No. Known Local Relapse (not evaluable)	Duration of Response (months)
100–1999	4	2	50	0 (1)	14	1	0	—	—	—
2000–3999	4	3	75	1 (3)	5, 3, 3	17	14	82	3 (9)	—
4000–6000	13	9	69	4 (9)	3, 5, 5, 5, 15, 66	27	24	89	5 (22)	—
6000+	0	—	—	—	—	4	4	100	0 (4)	—
Totals	21	14		5 (13)		49	42		8 (38)	

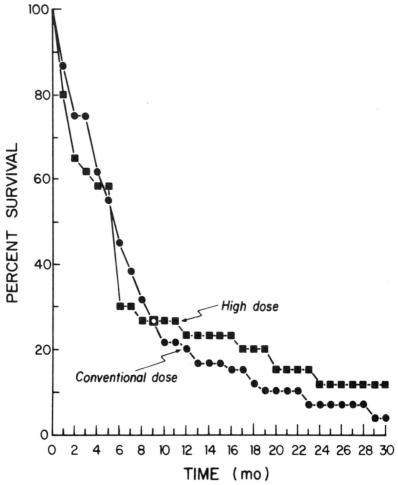

Fig. 8. *Survival of patients with SVC obstruction caused by bronchogenic carcinoma: Initial high-dose vs conventional-dose radiation therapy.*

Chemotherapy and Combined Therapy at Washington University

In 18 of our 67 patients with lung cancer, chemotherapy was administered concurrently with radiation therapy. One patient with adenocarcinoma received cyclophosphamide and methotrexate intravenously, while the remaining 17 patients received one or two intravenous doses of 10–15 mg of nitrogen mustard. Histological subtypes of bronchogenic carcinoma in the 18 patients included small-cell undifferentiated carcinoma (9 pa-

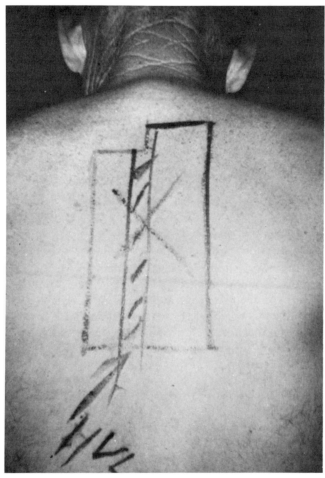

Fig. 9. *Posterior radiation portal with spinal cord block outlined.*

tients), epidermoid carcinoma (2 patients), adenocarcinoma (5 patients), and large-cell undifferentiated carcinoma (2 patients).

None of the 14 patients in our series with malignant lymphoma received chemotherapy concurrently with their radiation.

Supportive Therapy

Patients in this series were frequently treated with diuretics and corticosteroids. Supplemental oxygen was administered for shortness of breath and/or hypoxemia. Anticoagulants and fibrinolytic therapy have also been employed by others.[18,30]

In patients with severe symptoms or signs, elevation of the chest and head was maintained until symptomatic relief was apparent. Additional supportive measures such as tracheostomy, intubation, administration of anticonvulsants, and mannitol infusion may sometimes be required. Although caution was used in watching for tracheal edema, respiratory arrest, convulsions, and coma, these life-threatening syndromes resulting from tracheal, bronchial, or cerebral edema were not observed in our series.

Results of Therapy

Symptomatic Relief and Tumor Regression

Radiation therapy is highly effective in relieving superior vena cava syndrome. The delivery of an adequate radiation dose, at least 4000 rad, appears to be the single most important treatment approach. In our study, over 70 percent of those 31 patients treated with radiation alone had good-to-excellent symptomatic improvement. For those receiving a dose greater than 4000 rad, such responses were noted in 90 percent. Longacre[19] reported relief of superior vena cava syndrome in 74 percent of 31 patients treated after 1961 who received an average tumor dose of 4000 rad. This contrasted with a 46-percent response rate in patients treated before that time, whose dose averaged 2900 rad. Survival and median survival were also considerably longer in the higher-dose group. Levitt[17] reported 28 patients who were randomized between radiotherapy alone and radiotherapy plus nitrogen mustard for treatment of malignant superior vena cava obstruction. Eleven patients completed therapy in each group and complete relief of symptoms was obtained in 9 of the 11 patients (82 percent) treated with radiation alone, as well as in 9 of 11 patients completing treatment plus nitrogen mustard combined with radiation. Davenport[3] has found subjective and objective responses to radiation therapy in 90 percent of a group of 35 patients. Similarly, Slawson and Scott[34] reported subjective relief in 86 percent (36 of 42) of patients with SVC secondary to bronchogenic carcinoma treated with radiation therapy. Objective evidence of tumor regression can be documented on serial chest x-rays (Figs. 10 A through 11 B). We have observed different rates of objective tumor response depending upon tumor histology[23] (Fig. 12).

Survival

In the series of patients treated at Washington University, over 80 percent of those treated with radiation alone had symptomatic improvement with a median survival of 7 months. The over-all survival of the 84

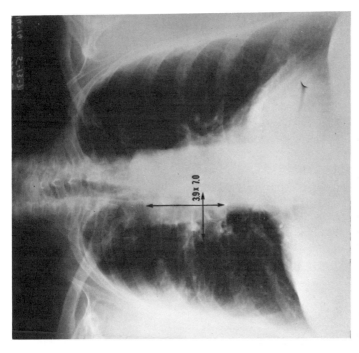

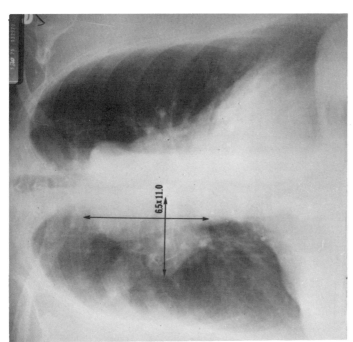

Fig. 10. *Pre- (left) and post- (right) treatment radiographs of patients with SVC secondary to lung cancer.*

61

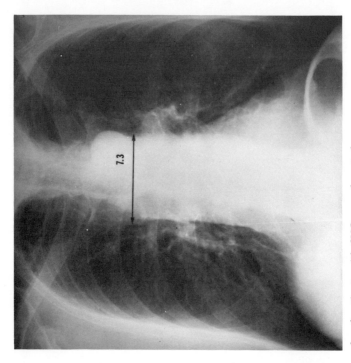

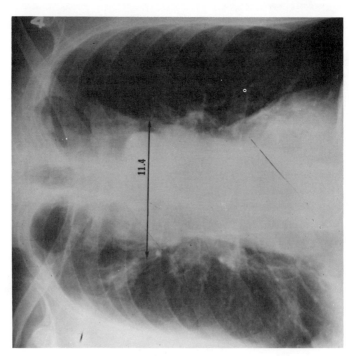

Fig. 11. *Pre- (left) and post- (right) treatment radiographs of patients with SVC secondary to lung cancer.*

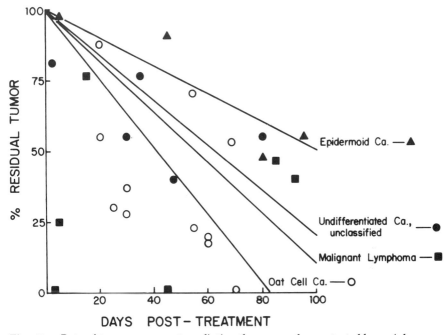

Fig. 12. *Rate of tumor response to radiation therapy as demonstrated by serial x-rays, depending upon histology.*

patients was approximately 25 percent at 1 year and 12 percent at 30 months following initial therapy (Fig. 13). Of interest, 50 percent of the group with malignant lymphoma survived 30 months, in contrast to only 6 percent of the group with bronchogenic carcinoma. Forty-three percent of patients with lymphoma lived 5 years. Nineteen percent of patients with lung cancer survived 1 year, and of 2 of 67 patients (3 percent) survived 5 years (Fig. 14).

Combined Therapy

As we have previously reported,[23] the addition of chemotherapy to radiation therapy in patients with bronchogenic carcinoma was not associated with improved results. Excellent or good responses were observed in 37 of 52 patients treated with radiation therapy alone (71 percent), while 11 of 18 patients (61 percent) receiving chemotherapy plus radiation therapy had an excellent or good response. In patients who received greater than 4000 rad, responses were observed in 9 of 13 patients with combination therapy (69 percent) versus 28 of 31 (90 percent) treated with radiation therapy alone. Furthermore, recurrence of superior vena cava syndrome

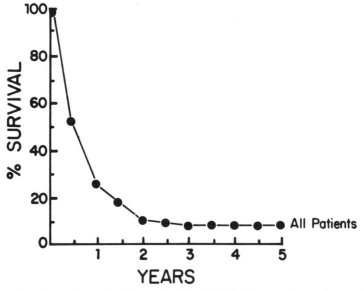

Fig. 13. *Overall survival for patients in the Washington University series.*

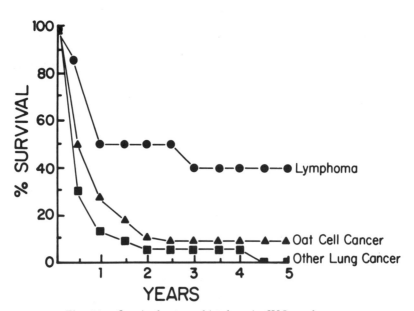

Fig. 14. *Survival rate vs histology in SVC syndrome.*

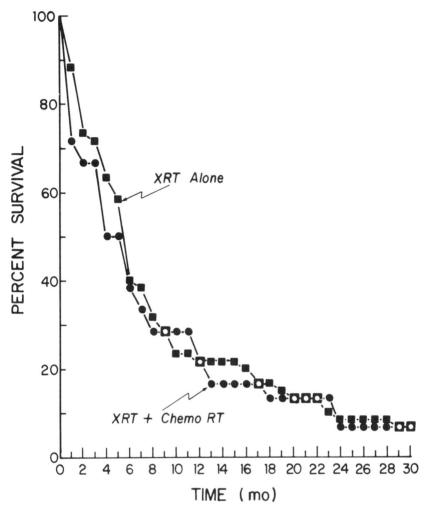

Fig. 15. *Survival rates for patients with SVC treated with radiation alone or radiation plus chemotherapy.*

was not diminished by the concurrent use of chemotherapy. Five of 13 evaluable patients who were followed long term relapsed after combination therapy (38 percent), versus 8 of 38 evaluable patients (21 percent) following radiation therapy alone. Similarly, survival time was not modified by the addition of chemotherapy to radiation therapy in patients with bronchogenic carcinoma. The over-all survival following either radiation therapy or combination therapy was 25 percent at 1 year and 10 percent at 2 years (Fig. 15).

In our series, patients treated for superior vena cava syndrome associated with lymphoma all received chemotherapy immediately following radiation therapy. Therefore, a comparison could not be made of radiation therpay alone versus simultaneous radiation therapy versus chemotherapy. Excellent or good results from radiation therapy followed by chemotherapy were obtained in 80 percent of patients with malignant lymphoma. There were no recurrences of superior vena cava syndrome in the 14 lymphoma patients.

Side Effects and Complications

Radiation Therapy

Radiation therapy for superior vena cava obstruction causes certain predictable side effects. The most common symptoms are dysphagia and odynophagia, secondary to radiation esophagitis. Such symptoms usually begin to occur at about 2000 rad and may occasionally be severe enough to preclude adequate oral intake for 1 or 2 weeks. The symptoms usually subside within 2 weeks following completion of therapy but may be exacerbated by adriamycin given concurrently or in close temporal relationship.[13] Radiation pneumonitis, pericarditis and myelitis are also possible but seldom seen.

Major complications or serious long-term sequelae are rare in most series, possibly due to the brief survival time of patients with this syndrome. We observed no late complications in our patients, of whom 20 were at risk for ≥ 18 months.

Combined Therapy

Combination therapy is frequently associated with increased morbidity. In the Washington University series, the addition of chemotherapy to radiation therapy increased the prevalence of dysphagia and leukopenia. Seventy-eight percent of patients with combined therapy experienced dysphagia, compared to only 21 percent of patients treated with radiation therapy alone. Thirty-two percent of patients treated with combined therapy experienced significant leukopenia, compared to only 2 percent of patients following radiation therapy alone. Other side effects were not appreciably increased by the addition of chemotherapy. Nausea and vomiting were present in 17 percent of patients following chemotherapy plus radiation therapy, compared to 8 percent of patients receiving radiation therapy alone. Cutaneous erythema or esophagitis were each noted in only 6 percent of patients with either combined therapy or radiation therapy alone. No major complications or serious long-term sequelae of combined therapy were observed.

Discussion

Despite the passionate plea[9] and search for chemotherapeutic programs that produce symptomatic relief in superior vena cava obstruction, the best management of patients who have the syndrome due to bronchogenic carcinoma of epidermoid, adeno, or large-cell undifferentiated subtypes remains radiation therapy alone. In the Washington University series, the incidence of favorable responses, time to onset of response, rate of recurrence, and survival were not increased by the addition of nitrogen mustard therapy. Dysphagia and leukopenia were more frequent with combination therapy. These results are similar to those observed by Levitt et al.[17] In comparing 13 patients treated with radiation therapy to 15 treated with radiation plus nitrogen mustard, those authors demonstrated a similar time to decrease in venous pressure and an equivalent median survival (7.5 months). The time to onset of symptomatic improvement was 6 days in the radiation-alone group and 5 days in the combination therapy group. Chemotherapy increased the incidence of myelosuppression. Our results are also comparable to those reported by Salsali et al.[30] in a study in which 193 patients were treated with radiation therapy, either alone or with nitrogen mustard. The median survival (8.3 months) was similar in patients who received radiation therapy alone or radiation plus chemotherapy.

In our prior publication summarizing the results of the Washington University experience,[23] we stated that "in oat cell carcinoma of the lung . . . the primary method of treatment should be radiation therapy, and . . . chemotherapy should be withheld until radiotherapeutic management of superior vena cava syndrome has been completed." Since the time of preparation of that manuscript, three publications have appeared which suggest that chemotherapy alone (or followed in several weeks by radiation therapy) can produce similar degrees of palliative relief of superior vena cava syndrome in patients with small-cell carcinoma.

In a study by Dombernowsky,[4] 26 consecutive patients with small-cell carcinoma of the lung were treated with chemotherapy consisting of cyclophosphamide, methotrexate, and CCNU with or without vincristine. In patients with limited disease, this was followed 6 weeks later by radiation therapy. No patients routinely received anticoagulation, diuretics, or corticosteroids. Of 22 patients who received only chemotherapy, or chemotherapy followed in 6 weeks by radiation therapy, all showed a partial response of superior vena cava syndrome 3–27 days after initiation of therapy (median 7 days), and 21 of 22 patients showed a complete response to therapy in 5 of 22 days (median 14 days). Of 4 patients receiving chemotherapy with simultaneous radiation therapy, 3 showed complete clinical regression of superior vena cava syndrome at 10, 13, and 20 days. The other patient had progression of disease with death due to pancytopenia. Four of 15 patients with limited-stage disease recurred at 174, 224, 255, and 316 days after chemotherapy. Four of 11 patients with extensive disease (who did not receive radiation therapy) recurred at 65, 99, 187, and 203 days. The median survival of all patients was 7.6 months. The mean white blood count nadir was 2,800, and the only death was in the patient who developed severe leukopenia following chemotherapy plus radiation therapy. Of importance is that in no patient in this study was superior vena cava syndrome noted to transiently worsen prior to showing a response. Furthermore, the prognosis for patients with superior vena cava syndrome was compared to the prognosis of patients with similar extent of disease without the syndrome, who received similar chemotherapy. There was no difference in survival.

A second study by Kane et al.[16] reported 8 patients with small-cell carcinoma of the lung who received chemotherapy with cyclophosphamide and methotrexate plus CCNU. One patient had radiation therapy followed by chemotherapy, and the remaining 7 patients had chemotherapy alone for 3 weeks. All 7 of those patients had complete responses to chemotherapy alone occurring between 5 and 15 days after chemotherapy. Two of those patients have since shown recurrence of their disease.

Finally, Valdevieso et al.[35] treated 5 patients with small-cell carcinoma of the lung with epipodophyllotoxin VP-16, cyclophosphamide, and adriamycin, plus vincristine. Four patients achieved complete remission. The time to complete remission was not mentioned in their brief report.

It seems reasonable, therefore, to consider either radiation therapy or chemotherapy as initial treatment for patients with small-cell undifferentiated carcinoma of the lung and superior vena cava syndrome. The choice should be based upon future plans for therapy. If it is intended to treat the patient with chemotherapy subsequently, this modality ought to be the initial mode of therapy, reserving irradiation for patients who fail to respond, or for those with recurrences. If it is intended to irradiate the primary tumor and mediastinum as the primary mode of management of the tumor, then superior vena cava syndrome should respond to such therapy as well, and chemotherapy might be delayed until the clinician sees an indication for such management. The wide-spread nature of small-cell undifferentiated carcinoma of the lung would suggest that the former method of management, chemotherapy alone or followed by radiation therapy, should be the preferred treatment.

The results of treatment in the Washington University series for patients with malignant lymphoma were satisfactory. Fifty percent of such patients remained alive 30 months after treatment and 43 percent survived for more than 5 years even though half of the patients were Stages III and IV. No patients suffered a recurrence of superior vena cava syndrome. These results were achieved by the initial administration of radiation therapy, followed by chemotherapy.

Combination chemotherapy has been highly effective in producing durable remissions and probably cures in some patients with non-Hodgkin's lymphomas.[21,33] Responses have been rapidly achieved even in patients with bulky disease. It is reasonable, therefore, to expect that patients with malignant lymphoma could be treated adequately with combination chemotherapy, and in such instances where a rapid response to chemotherapy is not obtained, radiation therapy for superior vena cava syndrome could be added. However, such a treatment is not supported by published data and such reports will be necessary to assess long-term survival and recurrent rates.

Supportive therapy of patients with superior vena cava syndrome can be instituted rapidly despite the absence of a definitive diagnosis, and it can be potentially life-saving, even in patients with nonmalignant etiologies for the syndrome. In addition to an elevated position, administration of oxygen to correct hypoxia, and maintenance of a patent airway, pharmacologic measures occasionally have been effective. The use of diuretic therapy and the administration of moderate doses of corticosteroids have been associated with clinical responses even in the absence of specific antineoplastic effects. Since many patients with superior vena cava syndrome are found to have thrombosis in the region of the obstruction at post mortem examination, anticoagulants and fibrinolytic agents have also been recommended. However, their routine application is not advocated except in situations where superior cava venography demonstrates thrombosis or where a lack of therapeutic response persists despite other treatment.

Summary

✓ Superior vena cava syndrome is a relatively uncommon medical emergency which is becoming more frequent as a result of the increasing incidence of lung cancer, the single most common cause for this syndrome. In acute situations, treatment is warranted without a tissue diagnosis although one is important for additional management once the acute syndrome has been resolved. Immediate institution of supportive and definitive therapy is necessary to alleviate airway and venous obstruction as well as mediastinal compression. The diagnosis is most often a clinical one with the most important confirmatory tests being a chest x-ray and venography. Radiation therapy has been the most effective method of relieving the immediate symptoms and of providing long-term control of this syndrome. Conventional fractionation to an adequate dose appears to yield results equivalent to those obtained by initial high-dose fractions. Patients with small-cell carcinoma of the lung and perhaps malignant lymphomas may be managed adequately with chemotherapy initially, with radiotherapy withheld for refractory cases. In patients with non-small-cell bronchogenic carcinoma, chemotherapy has not significantly enhanced the results of radiation therapy in this condition.

Since the majority of patients with superior vena cava syndrome can be relieved on their symptoms, the task for the future is to improve on the long-term prognosis of such patients, particularly those with this syndrome secondary to bronchogenic carcinoma.

An important subset of patients may have SVC as a result of malignant lymphoma. In these patients, a 40-percent 5-year survival after treatment with radiation therapy and chemotherapy may be achieved.

References

1. Adar R, Rosenthal T, Mozes M: Vena caval obstructions: some epidemiological observations in 76 patients. Angiology 25:433–439, 1974
2. Davenport D, Ferree C, Blake D, et al: Response of superior vena cava syndrome to radiation therapy. Cancer 38:1577–1580, 1976
3. Davenport D, Ferree, C, Blake D, et al: Radiation therapy in the treatment of superior vena caval obstruction. Cancer 42:2600–2603, 1978
4. Dombernowsky P, Hansen HH: Combination chemotherapy in the management of superior vena caval obstruction in small cell anaplastic carcinoma of the lung. Acta Medica Scandia 204:513–516, 1978
5. Evans JT, Vincent RG, Takita H: Superior vena caval obstruction with substernal thyroid. Southern Med J 67:3, 1974
6. Fairbanks JT, Tampas JP, Longstreet G: Superior vena caval obstruction in histoplasmosis. Am J Roentgenol Radium Ther Nucl Med 115:448–494, 1972
7. Fisherman WH, Bradfield JS: Superior vena caval syndrome: response with initially high daily dose irradiation. Southern Med J 66:6 677–680, 1973

8. Gardner E, Gray DJ, O'Rahilly R: Anatomy. Philadelphia, WB Saunders, 1969
9. Geller W: The mandate for chemotherapeutic decompression in superior vena caval obstruction. Radiology 81:385–387, 1963
10. Ghosh BC, Cliffton EE: Malignant tumors with superior vena cava obstruction. NY Stage J Med 73:283–289, 1973
11. Gomes M, Hufnagel C: Superior vena cava obstruction. Ann Thoracid Surg 20:344–359, 1975
12. Gordonson J, Hufnagel C, Trachtenberg S, Sargent E: Superior vena cava obstruction due to sarcoidosis. Chest 63:292–293, 1972
13. Greco A, Brereton H, Kent C, Zimbler H, Johnson R: Adriamycin and enhanced radiation reaction in normal esophagus and skin. Ann Intern Med 85:294–298, 1976
14. Haagensen C, Feind C, Herter E, et al: The Lymphatics of Cancer. Philadelphia, WB Saunders, 1972
15. Howard N: Superior mediastinal obstruction: I. Value of phlebography, in Deeley TJ (ed): Modern Radiotherapy Carcinoma of the Bronchus. New York, Appleton-Century-Crofts, 1971, pp 267–275
16. Kane R, Cohen M, Broder L, et al: Superior vena cava obstruction due to small cell anaplastic lung carcinoma. JAMA 235:1717–1718, 1976
17. Levitt SH, Jones TK Jr, Kilpatrick SJ Jr, et al: Treatment of malignant superior vena caval obstruction. Cancer 24:451–477, 1969
18. Lokich JJ, Goodman R: Superior vena caval syndrome clinical management. JAMA 231:58–61, 1975
19. Longacre AM, Shockman AT: The superior vena cava syndrome—radiation therapy. Radiology 91:713–718, 1968
20. Maxfield WS, Mecksfroth GR: Technetium-99m and phlebography. Radiology 92:913, 1969
21. McKilvey EM, Moon TE: Curability of non-Hodgkin's lymphomas. Cancer Treat. Rep 61:1185–1190, 1977
22. Dombernowsky P, Hansen HH: Combination chemotherapy in the management of superior vena caval obstruction in small cell anaplastic carcinoma of the lung. Acta Medica Scandia 204:513–516, 1978
23. Perez CA, Presant CA, Van Amburg AL III: Management of superior vena cava syndrome. Sem Oncol 5:123–134, 1978
24. Rankin RS, Westcott JL: Superior vena cava syndrome caused by nocardia mediastinitis. Am Rev Respir Dis 108:361–363, 1973
25. Roswit B, Kaplan G, Jacobson HG: The superior vena cava obstruction syndrome in bronchogenic carcinoma. Radiology 61:722–737, 1953
26. Rubin P, Ciccio S: Superior mediastinal obstruction. II. High daily

dose for rapid decompression, in Deeley TJ (ed): Modern Radiotherapy Carcinoma of the Bronchus. New York, Appleton-Century-Crofts, 1971, pp 276–297

27. Rubin P, Green J, Holzwasser G, et al: Superior vena cava syndrome: Slow low-dose versus rapid high-dose schedules. Radiology 81:388–401, 1963

28. Salsali M, Cliffton E: Superior vena caval obstruction with carcinoma of the lung. Surg Gynecol Obstet 121:783–788, 1965

29. Salsali M, Cliffton E: Superior vena caval obstruction with lung cancer. Ann Thoracic Surg 6:437–442, 1968

30. Salsali M, Cliffton E: Superior vena caval obstruction in carcinoma of the lung. NY State J Med 69:2875–2880, 1969

31. Scarantino C, Salazar OM, Rubin P, et al: The optimum radiation schedule in treatment of superior vena caval obstruction: Importance of ^{99m}Tc Scintiangiograms. Int J Radiat Oncol Biol Phys 5:1987–1995, 1979

32. Schecter MM: The superior vena caval syndrome Am J Med Sci 227:46–56, 1954

33. Schein PS, Chabner BA, Canellos GP, et al; Potential for prolonged disease-free survival following combination chemotherapy on non-Hodgkin's lymphoma. Blood 43:2 181–189, 1974.

34. Slawson RG, Scott RM: Radiation therapy in bronchogenic carcinoma. Radiology 132:175–176, 1979

35. Valdivieso M, Cabanillas F, Bedikian AY, et al: Intensive induction chemotherapy of small-cell lung cancer with ECHO, epipodophyllotoxin VP-16, cytoxan, hydroxydaunorubicin and oncovin. Proc Am Soc Clin Oncol 20:383, 1979

36. White J, Holgersen L, Simon L, et al: Superior vena cava obstruction caused by metastatic breast carcinoma: A report of two cases. Cancer 26:935–937, 1970

4

NEUROLOGICAL COMPLICATIONS
OF SYSTEMIC CANCER

J. Gregory Cairncross
Jerome B. Posner

Central nervous system complications of systemic cancer are common and varied (Table 1). About 15–20 percent of patients hospitalized for treatment of cancer suffer significant neurological symptoms at some point during their systemic illness. Most of these neurological complications result from metastatic disease to the brain or spinal epidural space, but serious neurological symptoms may also be caused by nonneoplastic disorders, including infections, vascular disturbances, and metabolic dysfunction.

The onset of neurological complications of systemic cancer may be sudden, devastating, and irreversible. However, most serious neurological disorders begin subacutely, are heralded by warning symptoms, and are amenable to treatment. With prompt diagnosis and appropriate management, the symptoms resolve or improve in most patients. Moreover, neurological improvement is often maintained until the patient succumbs to his systemic disease. This is especially true of patients with brain metastases and epidural spinal cord compression from metastatic tumor.

Although for the most part the management of CNS metastases is palliative, the control of neurological symptoms should be approached vigorously since few symptoms are more disabling and frightening to patients and their families than neurological ones (e.g., convulsions, dementia, paralysis, incontinence), and maximum benefit demands early diagnosis and treatment.

Table 1
Neurological Complications
of Systemic Cancer

Metastatic
  Brain
  Spinal
  Leptomeningeal
  Peripheral or cranial nerves
Nonmetastatic
  Metabolic
  Infection
  Vascular
  Side effects of therapy
  Paraneoplastic syndromes

This chapter emphasizes those neurological complications of systemic cancer which require urgent attention and for which effective treatment is available. These problems include cerebral herniation(s) (from brain metastases, hemorrhage, or hydrocephalus), seizures, epidural spinal cord compression, and certain nonmetastatic neurological diseases, including meningitis and vascular disorders.

Cerebral Herniation(s)

The symptoms of brain metastasis usually begin insidiously and progress slowly over days or weeks. Consequently, the diagnosis is usually established and treatment instituted before signs of life-threatening cerebral herniation develop. However, when delays in diagnosis occur or the tumor becomes acutely symptomatic, patients may develop signs of rapidly deteriorating neurological function that require urgent attention. Minor delays in diagnosis or treatment in these situations can result in death or severe and irreversible neurological disability.

The brain is enclosed in an inelastic container, the skull, and is divided into several compartments by the relatively inelastic dura mater (Fig. 1). These compartments include the supratentorial (cerebral hemispheres) and infratentorial (cerebellum and lower brainstem) spaces, joined at the upper brainstem and separated from each other by the tentorium cerebelli. The left and right cerebral hemispheres also form separate compartments, joined at the diencephalon and separated from each other by the falx cerebri. Slowly growing intracranial mass lesions are partially accommodated by compression of blood vessels, which may lead to brain

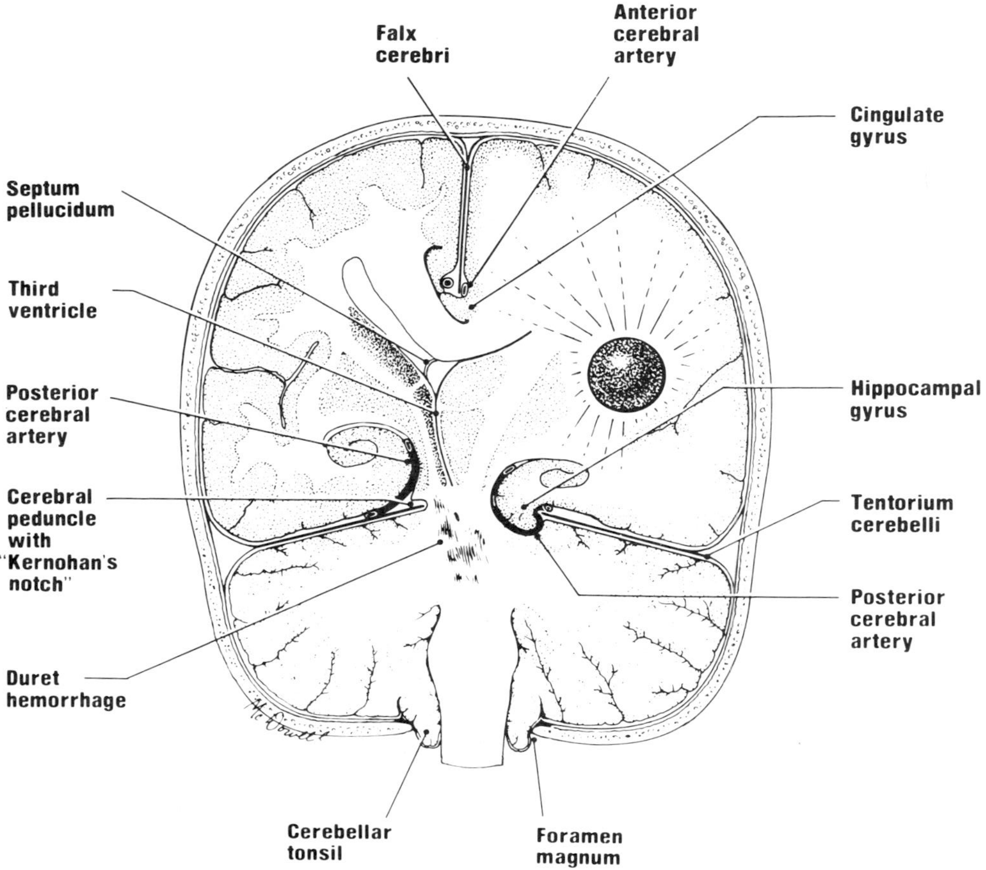

Fig. 1. A schematic representation of cerebral herniation syndromes evoked by a brain metastasis. The brain is shown in coronal section, encased in the skull. Brain metastasis and its surrounding edema have caused herniation of the cingulate gyrus under the falx cerebri, compressing the ipsilateral anterior cerebral artery. There is also herniation of the diencephalon across the midline from right to left, compressing the right lateral ventricle and producing obstruction of the left lateral ventricle, leading to hydrocephalus. The third ventricle is likewise compressed. There is herniation of the hippocampal gyrus through the tentorium cerebelli, compressing the posterior cerebral artery and pushing the brainstem from right to left, causing hemorrhage within the brainstem. There is herniation of the cerebellar tonsils through the foramen magnum, and the entire diencephalon and brainstem are shifted downward as a result of the supratentorial mass. The clinical syndromes produced by these herniations are described in the text.

Anterior cerebral artery

Cingulate gyrus

Hippocampal gyrus

Tentorium cerebelli

Posterior cerebral artery

Foramen magnum

Cerebellar tonsil

Falx cerebri

Septum pellucidum

Third ventricle

Posterior cerebral artery

Cerebral peduncle with "Kernohan's notch"

Duret hemorrhage

75

ischemia, and by increased absorption of cerebrospinal fluid if the absorptive pathways are not blocked. Eventually, as intracranial mass lesions increase in size, the brain herniates in the direction(s) of least resistance (Fig. 1), i.e., across the falx cerebri and in a rostral-caudal direction through the tentorial opening and foramen magnum.

The displacement of intracranial structures distorts and compresses both the brain and its blood vessels, thereby producing neurological signs not directly caused by the tumor. These signs and symptoms of cerebral herniation often begin abruptly because the intracranial pressure/volume curve is essentially exponential, i.e., initial increments in volume are accommodated until the tolerance of the system is reached, at which point very small increments of volume produce major changes in pressure, with their attendant brain herniation.[1]

There are three important clinical syndromes of cerebral herniation (Table 2).[2] The first two, usually caused by supratentorial masses and leading to transtentorial herniation, are termed the central and uncal syndromes. The third, usually caused by a posterior fossa mass lesion but sometimes by a cerebral hemisphere mass, is the result of herniation of

Table 2
Cerebral Herniation Syndromes

I.   Transtenorial Herniation
    A.   Uncal Herniation
        Headache
        Vomiting
        Unilateral pupillary dilatation
        Rapid progression to stupor and coma
        Decorticate and decerebrate posturing
    B.   Central Herniation
        Headache
        Progressive drowsiness
        Small reactive pupils
        Periodic respirations (Cheyne-Stokes)
        Paucity of focal motor signs
        Bilateral extensor plantar responses
II. Tonsillar (Foramen Magnum) Herniation
        Headache
        Vomiting
        Hiccoughs
        Stiff neck
        Rapid progression to stupor and coma
        Skew deviation of the eyes
        Irregular respirations
        Hypertension

---

the cerebellar tonsils through the foramen magnum and is called tonsillar or foramen magnum herniation.

The central and uncal herniation syndromes overlap considerably in their clinical signs, with the location of the lesion and its rate of growth determining the clinical picture.[2] *Uncal herniation* is characteristic of laterally positioned (e.g., temporal lobe or subdural) expanding masses. The medial surface of the temporal lobe (i.e., the uncus and hippocampal gyrus) is displaced medially and inferiorly, compressing the posterior cerebral artery, the upper brainstem, and the ipsilateral third cranial nerve, leading to ipsilateral pupillary dilatation and often ocular paralysis before consciousness is lost. There may also be an ipsilateral hemiparesis from compression of the opposite cerebral peduncle against the tentorium cerebelli (Kernohan's notch).

Central herniation is more likely to result from multifocal suprtentorial mass lesions, subacutely expanding unifocal mass lesions in the frontal or parietal areas, or hydrocephalus. The symptoms of central herniation result from lateral and downward shift of the diencephalon and upper midbrain which may culminate in buckling of the brainstem and midbrain hemorrhage (Duret hemorrhage). Herniation of the cingulate gyrus under the falx cerebri is usually asymptomatic, although the ipsilateral anterior cerebral artery may be compromised. The earliest signs of central herniation reflect symmetrical diencephalic compression and dysfunction and are characterized by a decreasing state of consciousness, small but reactive pupils, and sometimes Cheyne-Stokes respiration. Focal neurological signs such as hemiparesis may or may not be prominent. As the central herniation syndrome evolves, more prominent neurological signs, such as sustained hyperventilation, dysconjugate eye movements, pupillary fixation, and abnormal motor postures, appear. In its early stages, the central herniation syndrome is often mistaken for metabolic brain disease because it progresses slowly over many hours to several days, and because the level of consciousness is depressed, often without striking focal readings. Lumbar punctures are frequently performed because structural intracranial disease is not considered in the differential diagnosis. A history of headache or focal neurologic symptoms, or the presence of focal signs, no matter how mild, should lead one to perform a computed tomographic (CT) scan to rule out a herniating mass lesion before lumbar puncture is performed.

Tonsillar or foramen magnum herniation occurs when a large posterior fossa mass pushes the tonsils of the cerebellum through the foramen magnum, compressing the medulla. Supratentorial masses can also cause tonsillar herniation, along with transtentorial herniation (Fig. 1). Tonsillar herniation may appear suddenly following ill-advised lumbar puncture. It has a distinct and consistent clinical picture. Symptoms and signs result from both direct brainstem compression and from secondary downward compression by acutely obstructed ventricles. Alterations of consciousness accompanied by occipital headache, vomiting and stiff neck, sometimes with opisthotonus, suggest herniation from a posterior fossa mass lesion. Other signs include hiccoughs, dysconjugate eye movements, particularly skew deviation (one eye higher than the other), arterial hypertension (sometiems intermittent and imitating pheochromocytoma), orthostatic hypotension, and syncope with cough or sudden postural change. However, respiratory changes are the most serious and life-threatening sign of this disorder. A variety of irregular respiratory patterns occur,[2] and at times, particularly following lumbar puncture, sudden apnea may be the only sign of tonsillar herniation.

The major causes of cerebral herniation in patients with cancer are listed in Table 3. Brain metastases occur frequently in patients with disseminated lung cancer, breast cancer, colon cancer, renal-cell carcinoma, testicular cancer, choriocarcinoma, and melanoma. Intracerebral hemorrhage occurs in two settings: thrombocytopenic patients with acute leukemia, and patients with brain metastases from melanoma, hypernephroma, choriocarcinoma, or testicular carcinoma. Subdural hematomas develop in thrombocytopenic patients with acute leukemia. They occur occasionally in patients with other tumor types, usually in the setting of severe thrombocytopenia and dural metastases.[3] Brain abscesses complicate the leukemias, lymphomas, and head and neck malignancies. Acute hydrocephalus develops in patients with posterior fossa metastases, and pineal metastases (aqueductal obstruction), leptomeningeal metastases and, occasionally, in those with basal meningitis (e.g., cryptococcal meningitis). Radionecrosis of the brain is a rare, late complication of radiation therapy for extracranial head and neck cancers.[4] These patients present with symptoms and signs of raised intracranial pressure and focal neurological findings.

Table 3
Some Causes of
Herniation in Cancer Patients

Brain metastasis
Intracerebral hemorrhage
Subdural hematoma
Brain abscess
Acute hydrocephalus
Radiation necrosis

Table 4
Management of Acutely
Decompensating Patients

I.	Maintain the Airway
	Intubate stuporous and comatose patients and lower $PaCO_2$ to 25–30 mm Hg
II.	Mannitol
	25–100 grams IV stat (20-percent solution)
III.	Dexamethasone
	100 mg IV stat followed by 25 mg qid
IV.	Emergency CT Scan
V.	Surgical Decompression (if feasible)
VI.	Consider Intracranial Pressure Monitoring

Surgical removal of the necrotic mass may be necessary to prevent herniation.

The management of acutely decompensating patients with rapidly expanding intracranial mass lesions is summarized in Table 4.[1,2] Maintaining a clear airway is critical. Carbon dioxide retention causes cerebral vasodilatation and further increases intracranial pressure. Conversely, active or passive hyperventilation, which lowers the blood CO_2, causes cerebral vasoconstriction and decreases brain blood volume. Carbon dioxide tension should not be reduced below 20–25 mm Hg, since these levels may lead to brain acidosis and further vasodilatation. Mannitol rapidly lowers intracranial pressure by creating an osmotic gradient with higher osmolality on the blood side of the blood-brain barrier. The osmotic gradient removes water from that portion of brain having an intact blood-brain barrier (usually not from the tumor or surrounding necrotic or edematous tissue), lowering both brain volume and pressure. The effect lasts 4–6 hours. Mannitol also produces a prompt osmotic diuresis, decreasing total body water. The optimal dose of mannitol may be as low as 0.25 gm/kg,[5] but the total dose should be judged by the patient's response. Although repeated doses are often followed by severe electrolyte problems, the drug can and sometimes must be administered repeatedly. Adrenocorticosteroids (steroids) effectively reduce the edema associated with brain metastases[6] and brain abscesses.[7] It takes several hours for steroids to have full effect, even after an intravenous injection. Therefore, acutely herniating patients should be treated with hyperventilation and hyperosmolar agents along with intravenous steroids. We recommend the equivalent of 100 mg of dexamethasone as an intravenous bolus in the treatment of acutely decompensating patients. The drug appears to prevent plateau waves (intermittent sudden increases in intracranial pressure, often associated with further herniation, that accompany vasoparalysis in damaged brain) and to lower intracranial pressure.[8] A full discussion of the management of increased intracranial pressure is available elsewhere.[1,2]

Because cerebral herniation is an oncologic emergency, the treatment must begin before an etiologic diagnosis is available. Once treatment is underway, the CT scan is the diagnostic procedure of choice. If the scan reveals surgically remediable lesions, and if the patient has had an initial response to treatment, surgical evacuation should be considered. Lesions which might respond to surgery in appropriate patients include epidural and subdural hematomas, hydrocephalus, and at times solitary metastases or abscesses. These latter lesions, however, often respond to more conservative measures (radiation therapy in the former, antibiotics in the latter) once cerebral herniation is controlled by pharmacologic means.

Seizures

Seizures are often the first sign of neurological dysfunction in a patient with cancer. The major causes are listed in Table 5.

Brain metastases are a common cause of seizures. In a recent review of metastatic brain tumors at MSKCC, seizures, either focal or generalized, were the presenting symptom in 20 percent of patients.[9] An additional 10 percent developed seizures subsequently. Metastases to the calvarium or dura may cause seizures by compressing the underlying cortex. Approximately 8 percent of patients with diffuse leptomeningeal metastases present with seizures.[10]

Nonmetastatic disorders also cause seizures. Metabolic encephalopathy, particularly hyponatremia and uremia, and CNS infections are fre-

---

Table 5
Causes of Seizures in
Patients with Cancer

I. Metastatic Disorders
  Intracerebral metastases
  Calvarial and dural metastases
  Leptomeningeal metastases
II. Non-Metastatic Disorder
  Metabolic–toxic disturbances
  Vascular disorders
  Infections

Table 6
Diagnostic Evaluation
of Patients with Seizures

I.   Blood Tests
       Glucose
       BUN
       Electrolytes
       Ca^{++}
       Mg^{++}
       Liver function tests ($\pm\ NH_3$)
       Cultures
       Arterial gases
       Coagulation profile
II. Computed Tomographic (CT) Scan
III. Lumbar Puncture

quent casues. Vascular disorders, including intracerebral hemorrhage, subdural hematoma, superior sagittal sinus thrombosis (either metastatic or nonmetastatic), septic cardiac emboli, nonbacterial thrombotic endocarditis, and disseminated intravascular coagulation may present with seizures. Recently, the chemotherapeutic agent N-(phosphonacetyl)-L-aspartate (PALA)[11] has been suspected of causing seizures, and normeperidine, a metabolite of demerol, has been shown to cause an acute confusional state and seizures in patients with impaired renal function.[12]

Effective management includes treatment of both the specific cause of the seizures and the seizure itself (through the use of anticonvulsants). Seizures in and of themselves are dangerous and must be controlled. In addition to the obvious dangers of physical injury and vomiting with aspiration, seizures increase cerebral blood flow and blood volume and can cause cerebral herniation in a patient with a previously compensated mass lesion. Thus, seizures should be stopped immediately and the patient carefully observed during the postictal period for signs of cerebral herniation.

Table 6 outlines the laboratory tests and diagnostic procedures indicated in most cancer patients with seizures. A number of medications are availabe to treat seizures; the drug, dosage, and route of administration will vary with the clinical situation. For example, patients with readily correctable metabolic disturbances (e.g., hypoxia, hypoglycemia) will not require anticonvulsants. Those with single seizures from brain metastases can be treated with oral phenytoin together with adrenocorticosteroids and radiation therapy. Patients with repetitive generalized seizures (i.e.

Table 7
Use of Anticonvulsants
in Patients with Seizures

I. Seizure in Progress or Repeated Seizures Every Few Minutes
    (Status Epilepticus)
    A. Valium 3–10 mg IV, or more if required to stop
        seizure. Watch respirations and be prepared to support
        with intubation and artificial ventilation
                                then
    B. Phenytoin
        1. loading dose 1000–1500 mg IV (50 mg/min maximum)
        2. maintenance dose 300–500 mg PO/day
                                or
    C. Phenobarbital
        1. loading dose 300–400 mg IM, 100–200 mg IM q2h to a
           maximum of 800–1000 mg/24 hr[12]
        2. maintenance dose 90–180 mg PO/day
II. Single Seizure (now postictal or recovered)
    A. Phenytoin
        1. loading dose 1000 mg PO/24 hr (divided doses)
        2. maintenance dose 300–500 mg PO/day
        3. monitor phenytoin blood level

---

status epilepticus) must be treated aggressively with parenteral anticonvulsants and may require assisted ventilation. Suggestions for drug therapy are found in Table 7.

Spinal Cord Compression

Spinal cord compression is a serious and frequent complication of
systemic cancer. Early diagnosis and prompt treatment are essential in
order to preserve neurologic function. Once completely paralyzed (para-
plegic), the likelihood of meaningful recovery is small. In the cancer patient, spinal cord compression may result from epidural metastases,
intramedullary metastases, vertebral subluxation, and spinal subdural hematomas.

Metastatic tumor to the spinal epidural space is the commonest cause
of spinal cord compression in patients with cancer. The tumor reaches the
epidural space in one of several ways. The commonest is metastasis to the
vertebral bodies with invasion of the anterior epidural space. Cancers
which frequently metastasize to bone, namely carcinomas of the breast,
prostate, and lung, reach the epidural space in this manner. Paravertebral

tumors may reach the spinal canal by direct extension through the intervertebral foramina. The lymphomas frequently invade the epidural space in this manner. Hematogenous metastases to the epidural space or to the spinal cord itself are rare.

At MSKCC the commonest primary tumors causing epidural spinal cord compression are breast, lung, and prostate.[13] This is a reflection of both the prevalence of these tumor types in the patient population and the tendency for these tumors to metastasize to the spine. The lymphomas, which between 1964 and 1970 accounted for 17 percent of all cancers causing cord compression, second only to carcinoma of the breast, now account for only 5 percent of cases. The frequency of lymphoma as a cause of cord compression may be decreasing as a result of vigorous radiation of the paravertebral areas early in the course of the illness.

The interval between the diagnosis of cancer and the development of spinal cord compression is variable. Occasionally spinal cord compression is the presenting symptom in patients subsequently found to have cancer. At the other extreme, neurologic symptoms may appear 20 years after diagnosis of the primary tumor.

The spinal cord may be compressed at any level, although the thoracic region is the most common site.[13] The level of compression varies somewhat with the primary cancer. Colon cancers metastasize more frequently to the lumbosacral spine, and lung and breast tumors to the thoracic spine.

Pain, either local or radicular, is the initial symptom in 95 percent of patients with epidural metastases.[13] It precedes other symptoms by weeks to months. The location of the pain usually coincides with the level of the spinal tumor. Occasionally the site of the pain is misleading, however, being either above or below the site of cord compression. This may be true of both local or radicular pain. When pain is not a striking symptom, it may be accentuated by mechanical maneuvers, including Valsalva, spine percussion, neck flexion, and straight leg raising.

Although rarely being the initial symptoms, Gilbert et al. found weakness in 76 percent, automatic dysfunction in 57 percent, and sensory loss in 51 percent of patients at the time of diagnosis.[13] In two recent series from MSKCC, 50 percent of patients were no longer ambulatory at the time of diagnosis.[13,14] The ability to walk prior to treatment is of major prognostic importance.

The clinical diagnosis of epidural spinal cord compression is confirmed by radiographic procedures. On plain spine x-rays, Greenberg et al. noted tumor involvement of the vertebral body at the level of the cord compression in 91 percent of patients with epidural metastases.[14] Although plain films are frequently abnormal, precise localization requires myelography. This procedure is indicated in every case in which a suspicion of intraspinal disease exists. If a complete block is found from below, a lateral C_1C_2 myelogram is performed to delineate the upper level of the lesion. The contrast material is not removed so that later fluoroscopy can establish the results of therapy.

Once the diagnosis has been established, treatment must begin immediately since minor degrees of weakness may progress within hours to irreversible paraplegia. Radiation therapy is the mainstay of treatment for these patients and is delivered to a portal which extends 1–2 vertebral bodies on either side of the block. The results of studies at MSKCC indicate that radiation therapy alone is as effective as decompressive laminectomy followed by radiation.[13] In most series, only 50 percent of patients are ambulatory at the completion of treatment. However, at least 80 percent of patients ambulatory at the time of diagnosis remain so, while only 30–40 percent of patients nonambulatory when treatment begins walk again.[13,14] These figures further emphasize the necessity of early diagnosis. Although patients with radiosensitive tumors, such as lymphoma and myeloma, tend to fare better than patients with other solid tumors, Greenberg et al. have shown that good results can be anticipated following the early diagnosis and treatment of tumors generally considered to be less radiosensitive (e.g., prostate and renal carcinomas).[14] The findings on repeat myelography correlate with clinical response. Resolution of the spinal block occurs in the majority of patients ambulatory at the completion of radiation.[14] To date, different radiation doses and fractionation procedures have not been shown to make a substantial difference in outcome.[13,14]

Although radiation therapy is the treatment of choice for most patients with epidural spinal cord compression from metastatic cancer, decompressive laminectomy is indicated in certain circumstances: if tissue diagnosis is required, as when cord symptoms are the initial manifestation of the disease; if the cause of the cord compression is in doubt, as when epidural abscess or epidural hematoma are suspected; if relapse occurs in an area of prior irradiation; or if radiation is not effective and clinical deterioration continues. To date, it has *not* been possible to identify subgroups of patients (e.g., those rapidly developing neurological symptoms, those with major deficits, those with tumors less sensitive to RT, or those with involvement of the posterior vertebral elements rather than the vertebral body) who will respond better to surgery and RT than to RT alone.

Adrenocorticosteroid hormones appear to be an important adjunct to

RT in the treatment of cord compression and probably have their effect by reducing spinal cord edema.[15] Steroids (usually dexamethasone) are given prior to the first dose of radiation and are continued in a tapering fashion during the course of RT. Additionally, glucocorticoids may have oncolytic properties in a variety of human tumors, particularly the lymphomas.[16] The optimal steroid dose has yet to be determined. Greenberg et al. found that very large doses of glucocorticoids (dexamethasone 100 mg IV bolus, then 24 mg PO q6h × 2 days, then rapidly taper) were more effective than conventional doses (dexamethasone 10 mg IV bolus, then 4 mg PO q6h × 2 days, then taper) in relieving pain, but did not otherwise alter the outcome of treatment.[14] Since complications have been few and the relief of pain so dramatic, large doses of steroids continue to be used at MSKCC in the management of these patients.

Intramedullary metastases occur infrequently. Less than 4 percent of all metastatic spinal cord tumors are intramedullary.[17] Tumor cells may reach the interior of the cord by hematogenous spread, by growth along nerve roots from paravertebral tumor masses, or by invasion from the Virchow-Robin spaces in patients with leptomeningeal metastases. Neither symptoms nor signs distinguish intramedullary from the more common extradural metastases. The diagnosis of not difficult in patients with local or radicular pain, progressive paraparesis, normal spine x-rays, and an expanded spinal cord on myelography. However, in many instances the myelogram is either normal or not characteristic of an intramedullary lesion.[17] Radiation therapy is the treatment of choice.

Atlantoaxial subluxation is a potentially fatal complication of metastatic tumor to the cervical spine. Metastases to the axis lead to pathological fractures of the odontoid process and subsequent anterior dislocation of the atlas (C_1) on the axis (C_2). Upper cervical spinal cord compression and respiratory arrest may result. Myelography reveals shortening of the sagittal diameter of the spinal canal. The cord is further compromised, in many instances, by an anterior extradural mass.

Pain is the presenting complaint in the majority of patients with upper cervical spine metastases.[18] The pain is usually unilateral, high in the neck, aggravated by lateral rotation of the head, and may radiate to the shoulder or occiput. Neck pain, paraspinal muscle spasm, and limitation of movement are constant findings at the time of diagnosis. Leg weakness, gain unsteadiness, incontinence, vertigo, dysarthria, and swallowing difficulty may be prominent signs and symptoms in patients with advanced local disease.

In a recent review of 18 patients with this disorder seen at MSKCC over a 6-year period, breast carcinoma was the primary tumor in most instances (12 of 18).[18] All patients had widespread bony metastases, but other parenchymal lesions were uncommon. The observation that many of these patients had limited, and perhaps controllable, systemic disease emphasized the need for both effective short-term and long-term treatment.

The diagnosis is established by lateral x-rays of the cervical spine and an open-mouth view of the odontoid process. Tomography may be useful in the detection of early non-subluxed lesions. Myelography is not necessary in most instances.

Early lesions without major subluxation can be safely and effectively treated with a soft cervical collar and radiation therapy. Management is more difficult once major subluxation has occurred. Reduction by cervical traction followed by posterior cervical fusion and RT is the treatment of choice in patients whose general condition permits surgery.[18] Those who are not surgical candidates can be managed conservatively with good results in most cases. Support of the head and neck in a Philadelphia collar, followed by steroids and RT, is sufficient. These patients should be ambulated to tolerance as soon as they are free of pain. The steroids can be tapered and stopped, but the collar should be worn indefinitely. The wide sagittal diameter of the spinal canal at this level, the splinting properties of cervical muscles, and apparent fusion in the subluxed portion after RT are factors which permit the non-surgical management of atlantoaxial subluxation in a select group of patients. The majority of patients treated in this manner die of systemic disease without recurrence of neurologic symptoms. Whether reduction of the dislocation should be attempted in non-surgical patients prior to RT is an unanswered question. Our experience suggests that it is not essential. Special care must be taken in the movement and positioning of these patients, particularly before treatment or at any time when heavily sedated or anesthetized.

Spinal subdural hematoma is a recognized complication of lumbar puncture in thrombocytopenic cancer patients,[19] particularly patients with acute leukemias. Back pain and rapidly progressive paraparesis within 24 hours of a lumbar puncture (especiallly if a difficult or traumatic tap) in a patient with fewer than 20,000 platelets or a rapidly falling platelet count suggest this diagnosis. If the patient's general condition and platelet count permit, an emergency myelogram followed by surgical decompression are indicated. Unfortunately, the severe thrombocytopenia which led to the spinal subdural hematoma almost always precludes that approach. Likewise, attempted drainage of the subdural hematoma by needle aspiration is likely only to produce more bleeding and not relieve symptomatology. We recommend that such patients be given additional platelet transfusions and be started on high-dose steroids (beginning at 100 mg dexamethasone). While the therapeutic efficacy of such treatment has not been proved, some patients so treated have recovered neurologic function.

Central Nervous System Infections

Central nervous system infections in patients with cancer are uncommon but serious. Early and accurate diagnosis and prompt treatment are essential to prevent death or permanent disability. CNS infections include meningitis, brain abscess, and encephalitis. The organisms responsible for infections in the cancer patient are different from those encountered in the general population. In addition, the spectrum of causative organisms varies with the underlying disease. The importance of these disorders is further emphasized by the observation that CNS infections are an increasing problem. Chernik et al. reported a tenfold increase in the incidence of intracranial infections over a 15-year period.[20]

Patients with cancer are susceptible to CNS infections for many reasons. Steroids, chemotherapy, splenectomy, irradiation, and (in some instances) the underlying disease all impair immune mechanisms. These considerations are particularly important in patients with lymphoma. Patients with head and neck or spine tumors are susceptible to CNS infections because surgical defects or fistulae from progressive erosion by tumor permit organisms to gain access to the parameningeal or subarachnoid spaces.

The majority of infections occur in patients with lymphoma, leukemia, and head and spine tumors. At MSKCC, 33 percent of CNS infections in cancer patients are in those with lymphoma, 30 percent in those with head and spine tumors, and 20 percent occur in patients with leukemia. Only 18 percent of infections are found in patients with other primary tumors.[20]

Acute Meningitis

Headache, fever, and obtundation are the hallmarks of meningitis. Delays in diagnosis occur in cancer patients because headache is often attributed to brain metastasis, fever to systemic infection, and drowsiness to medications or metabolic disturbances. A lumbar puncture is indicated in all cancer patients with fever and depressed level of consciousness. An emergency CT scan prior to lumbar puncture may be necessary for pa-

Table 8
Organisms Causing Meningitis in Different Neoplastic Diseases

Primary Tumor		Organism	
		WBC > 2,700/mm³	WBC < 2,700/mm³
Lymphoma		*Listeria monocytogenes* *Diplococcus pneumoniae* *Cryptococcus neoformans*	Gram-negative rods
Leukemia	*Acute*		Gram-negative rods, esp. *Pseudomonas aeruginosa*
	Chronic	*Cryptococcus neoformans*	
Head/Spine		*Staphylococcus aureus* Gram-negative rods	
Others		*Listerial monocytogenes* *Diplococcus pneumoniae*	Gram-negative rods

tients in whom an intracranial mass lesion is suspected. Certainly patients with headache and obtundation, but no fever, should be scanned before the CSF is examined. Following careful placement of the spinal needle, the opening pressure is recorded and fluid removed for cell count and differential, Gram stain, india ink preparation, sugar and protein determinations, bacterial and fungal cultures, cryptococcal antigen measurement, and cytologic examination.

The absence of white cells in the spinal fluid does not exclude the diagnosis of bacterial meningitis, and the centrifuged sediment must be examined for oganisms. *Listeria monocytogenes,* because of its staining characteristics, is frequently misidentified as a Gram-negative rod. Lymphoma patients with meningitis, normal peripheral white counts, and small Gram-negative rods in the CSF should receive antibiotic coverage for Listeria infection while awaiting the results of cultures. Finally, in order to establish a diagnosis of fungal meningitis, it may be necessary to perform several lumbar punctures and to send large volumes of spinal fluid (20–60 cc) for staining and culture. Table 8 lists the malignancies frequently complicated by meningitis and some of the responsible organisms for each tumor type.

Knowledge of the underlying disease and the peripheral white count usually permit an accurate prediction of the offending organism, thereby guiding initial therapy.[20] Patients with lymphomas and normal white cells are susceptible to infection by *Listeria monocytogenes, Diplococcus pneumoniae* or *Cryptococcus neoformans. Hemophilus influenzae* and *Neisseria meningitidis*, common causes of meningitis in the general population, are rarely encountered. The Gram-negative organisms, including *Pseudomonas aeruginosa, Escherichia coli,* and *Proteus mirabilis* are the usual causes of meningitis in lymphoma patients with depressed white counts. With the exception of *Cryptococcus neoformans*, meningitis rarely complicates chronic leukemia. However, patients with acute leukemia and depressed white cell counts are vulnerable to CNS infections by Gram-negative rods (especially *Pseudomonas aeruginosa*), fungi other than *Cryptococcus neoformans*, and occasionally *Listeria monocytogenes*. In patients with head and spine cancers, *Staphyloccus aureus* (coagulase positive) is the most frequent cause of meningitis. Streptococci and Gram-negative rods are other causes of meningitis in this group. Many of these infections are acquired in the hospital during the postoperative period. *Listeria* and fungal infections do not occur in patients with head and spine tumors largely because they are not immunosuppressed hosts. CNS infections in other cancer patients are infrequent, but with a spectrum similar to that for lymphomas. *Listeria monocytogenes, Diplococcus pneumoniae* and *Cryptococcus neoformans* infect patients with normal white counts and the Gram-negative organisms those with low white counts.

Specific and effective antimicrobial therapy is available to treat the majority of cancer patients with meningitis. Three groups of patients deserve further mention: those with Gram-negative meningitis, those with cryptococcal meningitis, and those with shunt or reservoir infections. The treatment of Gram-negative meningitis is complicated by the frequent resistance of the infecting organism to multiple antibiotics and by the failure of the aminoglycosides to cross the blood–brain barrier. The combination of intravenous and intrathecal (i.e. lumbar) antibiotics is usually effective therapy.[21] However, intraventricular therapy may be necessary for those patients in whom parenteral plus intralumbar aminoglycoside has resulted in failure or relapse.[22] The inability to deliver drug to the ventricles in high concentration after lumbar instillation appears to explain the treatment failures. On the other hand, drug placed in the ventricle reaches the entire CSF space in effective concentrations.[22]

Cryptococcal meningitis presents similar difficulties. Although two-thirds of patients respond to a combination of parenteral flucytosine and amphotericin B, treatment failures are frequent.[23] This group of resistant patients appears to benefit from intraventricular drug administration through a reservoir system.

The increased use of shunts and reservoirs in the management of cancer patients with hydrocelphalus, leptomeningeal tumor, and CNS infections has led to an increase in catheter-related infections. These infections are usually caused by an indolent organism such as *Staphylococcus epidermidis*.[24] The infections can frequently be cleared by antibiotic treatment delivered both intravenously and into the reservoir, without removal of the shunt or reservoir.

Brain Abscess

Brain abscesses constitute nearly 30 percent of intracranial infections in cancer patients. Approximately 60 percent of these are found in patients with leukemia or head and spine tumors.[20] The Gram-negative bacilli, *Escherichia coli, Pseudomonas aeruginosa* and *Proteus mirabilis*, the fungi, *Aspergillus* and *Phycomycetes*, and the parasite *Toxoplasma gondii* are the usual offending organisms. *Toxoplasma* abscesses are found almost exclusively in patients with lymphoma. Many brain abscesses are found only at postmortem examination, having developed during overwhelming fatal bacterial and fungal septicemias. This is especially true of the leukemias. Those occurring in patients with head and spine tumors are usually diagnosed antemortem.[20]

Brain abscess should be suspected in patients with symptoms and signs of raised intracranial prsssure (i.e., headache, vomiting, papilledema), focal neurological findings (i.e., focal seizures, hemiparesis), and a potential source of infection. CSF examination is rarely helpful in establishing the diagnosis and may precipitate herniation in patients with large intracranial mass lesions. The CT scan is most helpful. Early in the evolution of the abscess, the CT scan demonstrates an ill-defined, nonenhancing, low-density lesion with mass effect. Subsequently a discrete mass lesion with a low-density core and a contrast-enhancing rim appears. Characteristically, extensive edema surrounds the abscess and contributes to its mass effect.[25]

Classically, the treatment of brain abscess has consisted of steroids to decrease edema, high doses of intravenous antibiotics, and surgical removal of the abscess at the earliest possible time. With the advent of CT scanning, which allows one to follow the progress of antibiotic treatment of abscesses, more and more reports are appearing about such lesions cured by the use of antibiotics alone.[26] Therefore, all patients whose clinical state allows should be treated with appropriate intravenous antibiotics in high doses over several weeks, and the size of the abscess followed by serial CT scanning. Such treatment will often abolish the lesion, thereby precluding surgery. Patients with incipient herniation are treated with hyperosmolar agents, steroids, and immediate surgical decompression.

Encephalitis

Viral encephalitis is not a common problem in the cancer population, representing only 3 percent of intracranial infections at MSKCC.[20] Viral encephalitis is, for the most part, a disease of patients with lymphoma and is usually due to *Herpes zoster*.[20] Although adenine arabinoside[27] and interferon[28] reduce the incidence of dissemination of *zoster* infections in immunosuppressed hosts, it remains to be seen whether these agents are effective in treating or preventing *Herpes zoster* encephalitis. *Herpes simplex* encephalitis does not appear to occur with increased frequency in cancer patients.

In the cancer population, intracranial infections with *Toxoplasma gondii* are found almost exclusively in patients with lymphoma. Toxoplasmosis is a potentially fatal CNS infection for which effective treatment exists. Cerebral toxoplasmosis may present clinically as a diffuse encephalopathy with or without seizures, as a meningoencephalitis, or as single or multiple progressive mass lesions.[29] In adults, the serological confirmation of acute infection is hampered by the widespread prevalence of anti-toxoplasma antibodies in the normal population. However, a very high dye test or immunofluorescent antibody test titer (16,000 or greater) in the presence of a high IgM fluorescent antibody test titer (160 or greater) is probably diagnostic of active infection.[30] Nevertheless, brain biopsy is frequently necessary in order to establish the diagnosis. Marked clinical improvement or complete remission of symptoms and signs has been reported to occur in 80 percent of patients treated with the combination of sulfonamides and pyrimethamine.[30]

Vascular Disorders

Patients with systemic cancer are susceptible to a spectrum of CNS vascular disturbances not seen in the general population. These disorders are listed in Table 9. Thromboembolic strokes secondary to atheromatous disease of the great vessels and hypertensive intracerebral hemorrhages, so common in general neurological practice, are uncommon in patients with cancer.[3,31]

Three disorders (disseminated intravascular coagulation, nonbacterial thrombotic endocarditis, sagittal sinus thrombosis) are considered further. The pathophysiology of these disturbances is not known with certainty. It is generally believed that they result from an ill-defined "hypercoagulable state" associated with cancer.

Table 9
Vascular Disorders in Cancer Patients

1. Intracerebral Hemorrhage
   Thrombocytopenia-associated (esp. acute leukemia)
   Tumor-associated (esp. melanoma)
2. Subdural Hematoma
   Thrombocytopenia-associated (esp. acute leukemia)
3. Septic Emboli (SBE)
4. Nonbacterial Thrombotic Endocarditis (NBTE)
5. Disseminated Intravascular Coagulation (DIC)
6. Superior Sagittal Sinus Thrombosis
   Metastatic
   Nonmetastatic
7. Hyperviscosity Syndromes (esp. myeloma)
8. Spinal Subdural Hematoma

Collins et al. have drawn attention to the neurologic syndrome associated with disseminated intravascular coagulation.[32] The clinical manifestations of this disorder, which occurs most commonly in patients with leukemia and lymphoma, include evidence of diffuse cerebral dysfunction in all patients and superimposed focal brain disease in half the cases. Agitation, confusion, seizures, lethargy, and stupor are common, suggesting a diagnosis of metabolic encephalopathy. Focal seizures, hemiparesis, aphasia, and cortical blindness are among the focal deficits observed. The neurologic illness progresses in a subacute fashion to stupor, coma, and death in most instances. Importantly, the neurologic symptoms and signs may appear before other systemic signs or before routine laboratory tests establish the coagulation abnormalities. Anticoagulants have been suggested as treatment for this disorder, but it is not clear that they are helpful.

Multiple systemic arterial emboli are the cardinal manifestations of nonbacterial thrombotic (marantic) endocarditis (NBTE). The underlying malignancy is frequently a bronchiolar or adenocarcinoma of the lung. Cerebral infarction is the commonest cause of death in these patients.[33] The diagnosis should be suspected when multiple stroke-like episodes occur in cancer patients, especially if accompanied by evidence of embolism to other organs and negative blood cultures. Cardiac murmurs are heard in one third of patients with NBTE.[33] Echocardiography is rarely helpful in demonstrating these small vegetations. The diagnosis is strongly suggested by the demonstration of multiple peripheral arterial occlusions on cerebral angiography. Heparin appears to be of benefit in the treatment of some, but not all, patients with this disorder.[34] Unfortunately, in those patients in whom heparin is effective, symptoms frequently recur when it is discontinued. Oral anticoagulants are largely ineffective[34] and there is little experience in the use of antiplatelet agents. If therapy is available for the underlying malignancy, the coagulopathy may remit.

Sagittal sinus thrombosis is an increasingly recognized disorder in the cancer population. It is known to occur in two groups of patients, those with leukemic or solid-tumor infiltration of the dura with resultant invasion or compression of the sagittal sinus, and those in whom the disorder represents a nonmetastatic or "remote effect" of malignancy. Sigsbee et al. have reported 7 patients with nonmetastatic sagittal sinus thrombosis.[35] Two different clinical presentations were noted. Five patients with hematologic malignancies presented with acute neurologic symptoms and signs (e.g., headache, seizures, obtundation, hemiparesis) early in the course of their illness, shortly after the induction of chemotherapy. Four of the 5 patients recovered with minimal residua; the fifth died as a direct result of the sinus thrombosis. None were treated with anticoagulants. A second and distinct presentation occurred in 2 patients with advanced disease (lymphoma and breast cancer). A subacute course with a progressive decline in the level of consciousness without seizures or focal signs characterized this group. Both patients died. The diagnosis was made postmortem. Antemortem, the diagnosis of sagittal sinus thrombosis can only be established with confidence by high-resolution arteriography, and only then by reviewing venous as well as arterial phase films. The treatment of sagittal sinus occlusion is controversial.[36-38] For patients with known metastatic involvement of the sinus, radiation therapy is indicated. The major issue however, is whether or not to use anticoagulants. Venous infarctions are frequently hemorrhagic, and fatal bleeding may complicate heparinization. The experience at MSKCC would suggest that most patients can be treated conservatively (i.e. without heparin) with excellent results.[35] However, those patients who deteriorate (massive cerebral edema) despite steroids and hyperosmolar agents, and who have no evidence of hemorrhage on CT scan, may benefit from anticoagulation. At the present time, the optimal management of this disorder remains uncertain.

References

1.   Rottenberg DA, Posner JB: Intracranial pressure, in Cottrell JE, Turndorf H (eds): Anesthesia and Neurosurgery. St Louis, CV Mosby Co, 1979

2. Plum F, Posner JB: Diagnosis of Stupor and Coma. Philadelphia, FA Davis Co, 1972, pp 63–139
3. Collins RC, Chernik NL, Posner JB: CNS vascular disease in patients with cancer. Trans Am Neurol Assoc 99:203–205, 1974
4. Rottenberg DA, Chernik NL, Deck MDF, et al: Cerebral necrosis following radiotherapy of extracranial neoplasms. Ann Neurol 1:339–357, 1977
5. Marshall LF, Smith RW, Rauscher LA, et al; Mannitol dose requirements in brain-injured patients. J Neurosurg 48:169–172, 1978
6. Renaudin J, Fewla D, Wilson CB, et al: Dose-dependency of Decadron in patients harboring brain metastases. J Neurosurg 39:302–305, 1973
7. Maxwell RE, Long DM, French LA: The effects of a synthetic glucocorticoid used for brain edema in the practice of neurosurgery, in Reulen HJ, Schurmann K (eds): Steroids and Brain Edema. New York, Springer-Verlag, 1972, pp 219–232
8. Kullberg G, West KA: Influence of corticosteroids on the ventricular fluid pressure. Acta Neurol Scand 41 (Suppl 13, part II):445–452, 1965
9. Cairncross JG, Kim J-H, Posner JB: Radiation therapy of brain metastases. Ann Neurol 7:529–541, 1980
10. Olson ME, Chernik NL, Posner JB: Infiltration of the leptomeninges by systemic cancer: A clinical and pathologic study. Arch Neurol 30:122–137, 1974
11. Wiley R, Posner JB (personal communication)
12. Szeto HH, Inturrisi CE, House R, et al: Accumulation of normeperidine, an active metabolte of meperidine, in patients with renal failure or cancer. Ann Int Med 86:738–741, 1977
13. Gilbert RW, Kim J-H, Posner JB: Epidural spinal cord compression from metastatic tumor: Diagnosis and treatment. Ann Neurol 3:40–51, 1978
14. Greenberg HS, Kim J-H, Posner JB: Epidural spinal cord compression from metastatic tumor: Results from a new treatment protocol. Ann Neurol (in press)
15. Ushio Y, Posner R, Kim J-H, et al: Treatment of experimental spinal cord compression caused by extradural neoplasms. J Neurosurg 47:380–390, 19777
16. Posner JB, Howieson J, Cvitkovic E: "Disappearing" spinal cord compression: Oncolytic effects of glucocorticoids (and other chemotherapeutic agents) on epidural metastases. Ann Neurol 2:409–413, 1977
17. Edelson RN, Deck MDF, Posner JB: Intramedullary spinal cord me-

tastases: Clinical and radiographic finidngs in nine cases. Neurology 22:1222–1231, 1972

18. Sundaresan N, Galicich JH, Greenberg HS, et al: Treatment of odontoid fractures in cancer patients. J Neurosurg (in press)

19. Edelson RN, Chernik NL, Posner JB: Spinal subudral hematomas complicating lumbar puncture: Occurrence in thrombocytopenic patients. Arch Neurol 31:134–137, 1974

20. Chernik NL, Armstrong D, Posner JB, et al: Central nervous system infections in patients with cancer. Medicine 52:563–581, 1973

21. Rahal JJ, Hyams PJ, Simberkoff MS, et al: Combined intrathecal and intramuscular Gentamicin for Gram-negative meningitis: Pharmacologic study of 21 patients. New Eng J Med 290:1394–1398, 1974

22. Kaiser AB, McGee ZA: Aminoglycoside therapy of Gram-negative bacillary meningitis. New Eng J Med 293:1215–1220, 1975

23. Bennett JE, Dismukes WE, Duma RJ, et al: A comparison of amphotericin B alone and combined with flucytosine in the treatment of cryptococcal meningitis. New Eng J Med 301:126–131, 1979

24. Diamond RD, Bennett JE: A subcutaneous reservoir for intrathecal therapy of fungal meningitis. New Eng J Med 288:186–188, 1973

25. Kessler JA, Messina A: The diagnosis of brain abscess by computed tomographic scanning. Neurology 27:387, 1977

26. Berg B, Franklin G, Cuneo R, et al: Nonsurgical cure of brain abscess: Early diagnosis and follow-up with computerized tomography. Ann Neurol 3:474–478, 1978

27. Whitley RJ, Ch'ien LT, Dolin R, et al: Adenine arabinoside therpay of herpes zoster in the immunosuppressed NIAID collaborative antiviral study. New Eng J Med 294:1193–1199, 1976

28. Merigan TC, Rand KH, Pollard RB, et al: Human leukocyte interferon for the treatment of herpes zoster in patients with cancer. New Eng J Med 298:981–987, 1978

29. Townsend JJ, Wolinsky JS, Baringer JR, et al: Acquired toxoplasmosis: A neglected cause of treatable nervous system disease. Arch Neurol 32:335–343, 1975

30. Ruskin J, Remington JS: Toxoplasmosis in the compromised host. Ann Int Med 84:193–199, 1976

31. Chernik NL, Loewenson RB, Posner JB, et al: Cerebral atherosclerosis and stroke in cancer patients. Neurology 28:350, 1978

32. Collins RC, Al-Mondhiry H, Chernik NL, et al: Neurologic manifestations of intravascular coagulation in patients with cancer: A clinicopathologic analysis of 12 cases. Neurology 25:795–806, 1975

33. Rosen P, Armstrong D: Non-bacterial thrombotic endocarditis in patients with malignant neoplastic disease. Am J Med 54:23–29, 1973
34. Sack GH, Lewin J, Bell WR: Trousseau's syndrome and other manifestations of chronic disseminated coagulopathy in patients with neoplasms: Clinical, pathophysiologic, and therapeutic features. Medicine 56:1–37, 1977
35. Sigsbee B, Deck MDF, Posner JB: Non-metastatic superior sagittal sinus thrombosis complicating systemic cancer. Neurology 29:139–146, 1979
36. Averback P: Primary cerebral venous thrombosis in young adults: The diverse manifestations of an unrecognized disease. Ann Neurol 3:81–86, 1978
37. Gettelfinger DM, Kokmem E: Superior sagittal sinus thrombosis. Arch Neurol 34:2–6, 1977
38. Castaigne P, Laplane D, Bousser MG: Superior sagittal sinus thrombosis. Arch Neurol 34:788–789, 1977

5

OBSTRUCTION DUE TO MALIGNANT TUMORS*

James G. Sise
Robert W. Crichlow

The growth of a malignant tumor is often heralded by obstruction of a major organ system. The dramatic clinical pictures resulting from cardiac tamponade, the superior vena cava syndrome, and intracranial or spinal cord compression are described elsewhere. Here the focus is on obstruction, by primary and secondary neoplasms of the respiratory, gastrointestinal, and genitourinary systems.

Clinical pictures and therapeutic responses vary widely with the nature of the tumor and the site and degree of obstruction. While an exophytic tumor in the capacious and distensible cecum may reach considerable size before producing obstructive symptoms, a small endobronchial lesion can cause collapse of the entire distal lung, and small areas of recurrent cervical carcinoma can produce total ureteral obstruction. The urgency for relief of obstruction varies with the location; threat to life can be far more immediate with obstruction of the airway than of the biliary tree, and distress to the patient can be greater with intestinal obstruction than ureteral compression. The usefulness of radiation therapy or chemotherapy varies with the sensitivity of the particular tumor, the extent of previous use, and the rapidity of response required. In the case of surgery technical factors are of importance, such as the difference in ease of de-

Supported in part by funds from the Sidney R. Rosenau Foundation.
*Reprinted from *Seminars in Oncology* 5(2):213–224, 1978.

compression of the biliary tree obstructed at the ampulla of Vater and that within the substance of the liver, or relief of intestinal obstruction due to a single primary tumor compared to widespread loss of peristaltic capacity with disseminated serosal metastases.

In many of the circumstances discussed herein, the aim will be palliation, not cure. Nonetheless, an aggressive approach will often be suggested as it is the obstruction per se that so frequently produces major degrees of morbidity and whose correction is of greatest palliative benefit to the patient.

Upper Respiratory Tract

Trachea

Tumors of the upper respiratory tract producing obstruction are far advanced and fortunately uncommon. Those arising in the hypopharynx or larynx seldom have airway obstruction as a significant symptom, presenting instead with a variety of other complaints. The trachea is also an unusual site of obstruction due to malignancy, both because of the low incidence of primary tumors and also because of the apparent resistance of the trachea to invasion by adjacent malignancies. Neoplasm accounts for only 16 percent of all tracheal obstruction not due to aspiration, the vast majority being caused by benign strictures following tracheal intubation.[1]

Primary tumors of the trachea affect males twice as often as females, and over 90 percent are of the squamous-cell or adenocarcinoma varieties, in about a 2:1 proportion.[2,3] Malignant tumors in the larynx and hypopharynx are almost always squamous-cell carcinomas. Lymphomas of sufficient size to produce airway problems are extremely rare.

Secondary tumors, although also an infrequent cause of obstruction of this portion of the respiratory tract, are most likely to affect the upper trachea. The most common responsible sites—lung, esophagus, and thyroid—may produce encroachment or invasion by the primary tumor or its metastases. More distant sites, such as the breast, are less often implicated.

Shortness of breath, especially with exertion, is an early symptom of airway obstruction. Wheezing, stridor, and orthopnea appear with progressive narrowing of the lumen. Though hoarseness is generally limited to laryngeal involvement, cough is common with all sites. Hemoptysis is variable. Upper-airway obstruction from tumor encroachment is gradual in onset, partly because patients accommodate to a smaller lumen than would be possible with acute narrowing. Sudden decompensation requiring emergent treatment is uncommon. In such circumstances, however, endoscopy with an eye to intubation is unlikely to be successful, and manipulation may in fact worsen the situation. A low tracheostomy is preferable, employing a transverse incision so as not to interfere with subsequent surgical fields.

In the usual situation of gradually increasing obstruction, evaluation should begin with soft-tissue radiography. Lateral views of the neck will best delineate the upper third of the trachea; swallowing views will bring slightly more tracheal shadow out of the chest and into view. Bilateral oblique views through the chest give full-length tracheal contours. While the use of a grid in the anteroposterior (AP) view will improve definition of the entire tracheal shadow, tomograms at specific levels are more informative. Bronchoscopy and biopsy are definitive but must be undertaken with care in advanced lesions for fear of precipitating complete obstruction.

Curative therapy of tumors of the hypopharynx and larynx sufficiently advanced to cause significant obstruction is seldom possible.[4] Close coordination of the medical, surgical, and radiation oncologists is necessary to provide optimal palliation. Tracheal tumors, even in their early stages, have been more difficult to approach successfully than those more proximal in the respiratory tract, although recent technical advances may have widened the opportunities for and safety of resection. Approximately 50–60 percent of the ordinary 11-cm human trachea can be resected with primary reanastomosis; of 29 patients with tracheal tumors reported by Grillo,[1] 11 proved resectable and 9 of these remained free of recurrence at follow-up intervals as long as 11 years. Secondary involvement of the trachea by neoplasm is rarely susceptible to surgical resection, and such an aggressive approach has been reserved only for slow-growing thyroid tumors, either at initial thyroidectomy or for a later recurrence.[2]

Lung

Bronchial obstruction is a relatively common complication of bronchogenic carcinoma, the most frequent cancer in American males. However, because the obstruction is gradual and distal, symptoms are not dramatic. Dyspnea occurs in at least half of the cases; misdiagnosis as a respiratory illness is common, but as frank pneumonia rare.[5] The responsible tumor is almost always a primary squamous-cell carcinoma of the bronchus, because of its relative frequency and location. Obstruction at this level due to metastases in adjacent pulmonary parenchyma or lymph nodes is a far less frequent complication of a variety of other less common tumors.

In the presence of bronchial obstruction from tumor, an ordinary chest x-ray is highly suggestive in over three fourths of cases, and discloses some abnormality in almost all. Obstruction can be evidenced by segmental consolidation, a triangular density based at the pleura, or less often by segmental or lobar emphysema. Tomograms or expiratory films can be of additional help. The diagnosis is usually established by bronchoscopy, needle biopsy, or sputum cytology. Except for treatment of frank pneumonia or the rare instance of empyema, therapy is aimed at control of the responsible tumor. Resection is possible in only a quarter of all bronchogenic carcinomas, the remainder relying principally upon radiation or chemotherapy for palliation.

Gastrointestinal Tract

Esophagus

With rare exceptions, obstruction of the esophagus by malignant neoplasms is due to a primary rather than a secondary tumor. The principle primary neoplasms, squamous-cell carcinoma and adenocarcinoma, show markedly different distributions among the esophagus (Table 1). While the squamous-cell variety predominates in the proximal thoracic portion, adenocarcinomas occur almost exclusively in the most distal esophagus at the gastroesophageal junction, arguing for their origin in the gastric rather than the esophageal mucosa. Of the occasional metastatic tumors, breast carcinoma, melanoma, oat-cell tumors of the lung, and lymphoma are most often described.[6]

Primary esophageal carcinoma usually occurs in the elderly male; the peak incidence is in the 8th decade with a male-to-female preponderance on the order of 4:1. Obstruction is a cardinal symptom, but unfortunately a late one. Being a hollow muscular tube, the esophagus is relatively distensible and therefore accommodates small lesions. Dysphagia of all degrees is evident; from very subtle early symptoms there is progressive dysphagia to solid foods, to liquids, and finally even to saliva. A necessary result of this progression is significant weight loss and the sequelae of aspiration: cough, pneumonia, and lung abscess. Patient delay in seeking

Table 1
Location and Cell Type in Carcinoma of the Esophagus*

Esophageal Level	Percentage of Total	Proportion of Cell Type at Each Level (%)		
		Squamous Cell	Adeno-carcinoma	Unclassified
Cervical	8	97	1.5	1.5
Proximal thoracic	25	94	5	1
Distal thoracic	17	87	9	4
Gastroesophageal junction	50	10	87	3

*Adapted from Gunnlaugsson et al.[7]

medical attention is common through the early and less severe degrees of dysphagia.

The diagnosis, once suspected, is usually established by a barium swallow radiograph, though a very small lesion may require in addition fluroscopy or cine-study. Esophagoscopy with biopsy is positive in 90 percent of esophageal carcinomas, and the use of brush cytology may add an additional 5–8 percent.[6] In difficult situations, blind aspiration via Levin tube for cytology may be of help.

Treatment of esophageal cancer is generally so ineffective that it is almost exclusively palliative. While groups with a large experience in esophageal cancer claim 5-year survival rates of 14 percent, 19 percent, and even 37.5 percent with various therapeutic modalities, most institutions have less success.[7–9] There is still debate about the individual and complementary roles of resection and radiation therapy for carcinomas at different levels. As yet, no prospective, randomized study has compared these two treatment modalities.

Operability may be as high as 67 percent but only 45 percent prove resectable, and 5-year survivals average 11–14 percent.[7,10] Factors that favorably influence prognosis include small size, squamous-cell carcinoma rather than adenocarcinoma, negative lymph nodes, and location in distal esophagus. Thus the rare squamous-cell carcinoma of the cardia without lymph-node metastases has a 5-year survival rate after resection of 55 percent, and the more common proximal lesions 42 percent below the aortic arch but only 19 percent above. With lymph-node involvement, survival drops to 15 percent at the cardia and 22 percent below the aortic arch. Comparable figures for adenocarcinoma at the cardia are 27 percent node negative, and 8 percent node positive.[7]

Radiation alone in curative doses has been proposed for all squamous-cell carcinomas, regardless of location.[11] It would appear that the more proximal the tumor the more favorable the response. Five-year survival rates of 30 percent and 16 percent respectively are reported for cervical and proximal thoracic esophagus,[9] but further trials are needed to confirm these data. Morbidity from this level of radiation is significant. The combined approach with surgery and pre- or postoperative radiation has been favorably reported with improved survival over either treatment alone.[9] Nakayama[10] has achieved a 5-year survival rate of 37.5 percent in selected patients by a combined modality approach, but it remains to be seen if this can be reproduced elsewhere.

Among the unresectable carcinomas, and in that larger number that show recurrence, esophageal obstruction is again and again a dominant issue. Palliation of obstructive symptoms is all-important. The patient once given or denied surgery or radiation therapy will receive little benefit short of dilatation and intubation of the strictured esophagus. Gastrostomy and/or jejunostomy for feeding purposes do not prevent the distress and morbidity of aspiration. On the other hand, intubation across the tumor with a suitable prosthesis may restore adequate swallowing capacity. Esophageal intubation can be accomplished in three ways: by traction technique (Celestin or Mousseau-Barbin), by pulsion (Souttar, Hearing, or Proctor-Livingston), or by esophagotomy with direct placement (Mackler), a technique which has been virtually abandoned. All methods require prior dilatation of the strictured area. Lesions of the cervical esophagus are generally not amenable to intubation because of subsequent pressure on the trachea, and at least a 5-cm margin below the cricopharyngeus muscle is required.

Traction tubes are directed into position after dilatation, laparotomy, and gastrotomy by pulling them over a guide through the involved area and into the stomach. This approach allows suture fixation of the tube, limiting migration. Further, tumors at the gastroesophageal junction can be dilated under direct vision, an improvement in safety. Palliation in up to 73 percent with operative mortality of less than 10 percent has been reported.[12] However, in another reported series, operative mortality was 23 percent, and survival averaged only 3.5 months.[13]

Pulsion tubes are directed into position perorally following dilatation and require no abdominal surgery. Although not sutured in place, pulsion tubes infrequently migrate. However, risk of esophageal perforation during dilatation or tube placement may be somewhat higher, and placement at the gastroesophageal junction more difficult than in the traction technique.

Stomach and Duodenum

Obstruction produces very similar clinical pictures in the stomach and first portion of the duodenum and is most commonly the result of benign peptic ulceration. When the cause is malignant neoplasm, gastric obstruction is usually from a primary carcinoma, and duodenal obstruction from an extrinsic tumor. Of all gastric carcinomas, 20 percent present with features of obstruction, and many more will eventually develop such symptoms. The mean age for detection of gastric cancer is 55 years, and males predominate over females by 2 to 1. Intrinsic tumors of the first portion of the duodenum are a rarity, and involvement by tumor here is most commonly secondary to carcinoma in the pancreas, although other sites contribute, such as the colon, liver, gallbladder, kidney, adrenal, spleen, and retroperitoneum.

Symptoms of incomplete obstruction at this level include postprandial pain due to vigorous peristalsis, and epigastric fullness. The vomiting that occurs with more complete obstruction typically follows large meals by 8–12 hours, is nonbilious, and is composed of undigested and recognizable food particles. Dehydration is inevitable. Other complications can include mucosal erosion or diffuse gastritis.

On physical examination, a palpable mass or a succussion splash can be demonstrated in nearly one third of cases. Gastric aspiration provides evidence of stasis when greater than 500 ml of fluid, or long-retained food particles, can be aspirated from a fasting patient. Achlorhydria is present in 60 percent of those with gastric carcinoma, and is helpful then in the differential diagnosis of gastric outlet obstruction. The addition of careful cytologic study is useful. Upper-gastrointestinal barium contrast radiography is best performed after lavage of the stomach to remove retained food and secretions, and will demonstrate gastric enlargement, delay, or failure in emptying, and can be highly accurate, at least in advanced lesions. Gastroscopy is particularly helpful in early lesions and in differentiating malignant from benign ulcers.

As significant obstructive symptoms are a relatively late manifestation of primary gastric carcinomas or secondary duodenal tumors, only a small percentage will be candidates for curative resection. However, for those not curable, a palliative resection with reconstitution of gastrointestinal continuity has proved a most satisfactory approach when technically feasible. Diversion alone by gastroenterostomy is a less desirable alternative that sometimes functions poorly. Gastrostomy alone probably has no role.[14]

Small Intestine

Although small-bowel obstruction is a common entity, only 10–20 percent of cases are related to a malignant neoplasm.[15-17] Primary tumors of the small intestine, representing only 1–3 percent of gastrointestinal tumors, include carcinoid, adenocarcinoma, sarcoma, lymphoma, and melanoma. Carcinoid tumors are particularly prone to cause obstruction. They tend to spread submucosally, to produce fibrosis and contraction, and to result in traction on the muscularis,[18] kinking of the bowel, and obstruction even with comparatively small and even nonpalpable tumors. The other primary carcinomas of the small intestine may produce obstruction by intussusception of an exophytic tumor mass, or by encirclement and progressive narrowing of the lumen.

The majority of obstructing tumors in the small bowel are metastatic from other sites, usually from the colorectum (44.8 percent) and less often from ovary (16.8 percent), cervix (14.6 percent), or other sites (23.8 percent).[19] Small-bowel involvement results either from a direct extension of an adjacent primary tumor, or as a result of intra-abdominal carcinomatosis, the latter a considerably less favorable presentation yielding a life expectancy of 4–11 months.[19]

Symptoms of incomplete obstruction are often vague and protracted, consisting of crampy abdominal pain and abdominal distention. As the obstruction grows more complete, nausea, vomiting, and obstipation become increasingly promiment. Physical examination yields the classic signs of intestinal obstruction, including distention, tympany, and hyperactive high-pitched peristalsis. Erect and supine films of the abdomen should establish the diagnosis and should be supplemented with a barium enema to assess the function of the distal large intestine. Upper-gastrointestinal contrast studies may verify obstruction but are often difficult to interpret. Localized study of the small bowel through a long intestinal tube better delineates the nature, location, and degree of obstruction of the small bowel.

Resection and reestablishment of small-bowel continuity is indicated for primary small-intestinal malignancies. When the obstruction is known to be due to metastatic tumor within the abdominal cavity, a choice must be made between resection and a trial of nonoperative therapy. A significant number of patients may respond to intravenous fluids and decompression of the small intestine with a long tube. Significant improvement was reported by Glass[19] using such a conservative program in 30 percent of patients with carcinomatosis and small-bowel obstruction, although half of the patients subsequently redeveloped symptoms of obstruction.

Surgical intervention of obstruction is then usually necessary. Unfortunately for this group of patients, operative mortality is in the range of 25 percent.[20] the following guidelines have been offered:[21] (1) defer colostomy as long as possible (in mixed large- and small-bowel involvement); (2) preserve maximal length of small intestine (especially ileum); (3) avoid sacrifice of the ileocecal valve; and (4) rather than dissect free individual loops, bypass areas of obstruction employing multiple side-by-side enteroenterostomies if necessary.

Patients with known carcinoma who develop intestinal obstruction must not be assumed to have incurable recurrence. In a series of such patients studied by Ketcham[20] fully one fourth were found to have either no residual carcinoma or a new primary as the cause of obstruction, and of these 40 percent achieved a long-term survival following surgery.

For those with metastic tumors as the cause of small-bowel obstruction, survival after surgery averages no longer than 11 months. Prognosis is better for those with primary malignancy. Wide excision of the involved small intestine results in average 5-year survival rates of 15 percent, and up to 45 percent with carcinoid tumors.

Colon

Obstruction occurs in the colon and rectum with about half the frequency seen in the small intestine. In contrast, however, malignant neoplasms outnumber all other causes of large-bowel obstruction by almost 4:1, and are almost exclusively adenocarcinoma. Some element of obstruction is a significant feature in the history of about 20 percent of those with colon carcinoma, and in half of these obstruction is severe or total.[22] Seventy-five percent of obstructing lesions are distal to the splenic flexure, and 30 percent lie within reach of a sigmoidoscope.[23] Noncolonic tumors that produce large-bowel obstruction tend to be of pelvic origin, such as ovary or cervix, and less often from other intra-abdominal origins or lymphoma.

Symptoms of colonic obstruction are insidious, averaging 3 months in duration, and include, in order of decreasing frequency, abdominal pain, vomiting, obstipation, weight loss, and rectal bleeding. Total obstruction in those with a competent ileocecal valve produces a closed-loop obstruction, clinically manifested by increasing pain and abdominal distention. Perforation occurs in as many as 20 percent of these patients,[22-24] is most likely to occur in the cecum, and should be anticiapted with cecal dilatation greater than 12–14 cm as measured on a plain film of the abdomen.

A mass may be palpated in nearly half of patients with obstructing carcinoma of the colorectum, by rectal or abdominal palpation equally.[23] Supine and erect or decubitus radiographs of the abdomen define the extent and also at times the location of the obstruction, as one observes the distal limit of air in the colon. A picture of small-bowel obstruction as well may be suggested in about 40 percent and may appear as the only abnormality in 5 percent.[22] A barium enema is then the key in localizing the level of obstruction as well as providing a probable diagnosis. Complete retrograde block to the barium column is not a reliable reflection of the degree of antegrade obstruction. Of 44 patients demonstrating complete retrograde block, only one half had any clinical evidence of antegrade obstruction.[25] Sigmoidoscopy will visualize the responsible tumor in approximately 30 percent of patients with intrinsic obstruction. The role of colonoscopy in the evalaution of colonic obstruction is yet to be well defined and may be limited by the technical problems of achieving satisfactory bowel preparation and the risk of further distention of colon proximal to the obstruction.

Treatment of colonic obstruction is surgical. For severe obstructions laparotomy should be delayed only for fluid and electrolyte resuscitation, since perforation is related to delay and carries a mortality approaching 50 percent. For less-severe degrees of obstruction operation is preceded by nasogastric intubation to prevent vomiting and further small-bowel distention, and by correction of fluid and electrolyte abnormalities, anemia, and whatever unassociated problems may coexist. It must be understood that no tube passed through the upper alimentary tract will ever succeed in decompressing an obstructed colon, and that surgical therapy is delayed only to allow optimal resuscitation and diagnostic studies.

For carcinomas of the right colon, a single-stage resection and primary anastomosis is advocated.[24] On the contrary, one-state procedures for obstructing carcinomas of the left colon are inordinately hazardous, and preliminary diversion followed by adequate preparation of the colon and then resection and restoration of bowel continuity are recommended. Colostomy is a more effective and safer means of decompression of the colon than cecostomy.[24] Five-year survival rates and operative mortality figures from selected series are shown in Table 2. In general, 50 percent of obstructing colon carcinomas appear to be curable at time of resection, but 5-year survival rates approximate 20 percent.

For extrinsic tumors producing colonic obstruction, a careful evaluation must be undertaken to identify the few patients who may deserve attempts at radical surgery, such as pelvic exenteration. Permanent diversion by colostomy or bypass by colocolostomy or enterocolostomy can of-

Table 2
Experience With Obstructing Carcinoma of the Colon*

Source	Total Patients	Obstructed (%)	Resected for Cure (%)	Operative Mortality (%)	5-yr Survival (%)
Goligher[48]	1664	17.6	44.1	34.1	—
Ulin[49]	1005	22.6	69.6	22.0	—
Welch[50]	1836	3.8	—	17.0	33.0
Floyd[51]	1741	14.0	47.6	24.0	15.0
Ragland[52]	1137	20.0	47.8	18.3	15.1
Glenn[53]	1815	11.6	47.6	12.4	19.5
Welch[24]	1566	8.0	—	9.0	32.1

Adopted from Glenn et al.[23]

ten be safely accomplished with satisfactory resolution of obstruction, allowing more effective use of adjunctive chemotherapy or radiation therapy.

Biliary

Biliary obstruction can result from a wide variety of extrinsic and intrinsic tumors, all of which carry an unfavorable prognosis, in part from their tendency to metastasize before producing biliary obstruction, and in part due to the proximity of vital structures limiting extirpative surgery.

Obstructing biliary tumors are best categorized as intra- and extrahepatic. Primary intrahepatic tumors account for less than 3 percent of biliary obstruction due to malignancy.[26] Of this small number the most common are the bile duct carcinomas, 10 percent of which arise within the confines of the liver; when lying at the bifurcation of the hepatic duct or when slightly proximal, they frequently produce bile duct obstruction.

Hepatoma so infrequently presents with a picture of extrahepatic biliary obstruction that the coincidence should be investigated carefully with an eye to relief by intubation and/or choledochoenterostomy. Kuroyanagi and colleagues[27] were able to collect 18 instances, in addition to two of their own, in which the hepatic and common bile ducts were obstructed by the products of a hepatoma that had invaded a major hepatic duct. They point out that such a tumor may be impossible to palpate because of its necessarily deep and central location. This same phenomenon has been reported with metastatic tumors in the liver.[28]

Extrahepatic biliary tract obstruction is far more common, and tends to occur in the periampullary region. Of malignant tumors causing jaundice, 15 percent arise in bile ducts,[26] three quarters of these are located along the common hepatic or common bile duct, but half are quite proximal and thus relatively inaccessible.[29] Carcinoma of the gallbladder occurs from 2 to 5 times as often as carcinoma of the bile duct.[29] However, less than one third present with jaundice, and of all tumors responsible for biliary obstruction, the gallbladder is the primary site in only 8 percent.[26] This particularly lethal tumor is found predominantly in females with average age greater than 60 years, and correlates well with the presence of calculous disease of the biliary tract. In patients over 65 years of age undergoing cholecystectomy for supposed benign biliary tract disease, 5–10 percent can be expected to have carcinoma of the gallbladder.[30,31]

At least three fourths of all patients with extrahepatic biliary obstruction due to malignancy have tumors in the region of the ampulla of Vater. More than 80 percent of these are carcinomas of the head of the pancreas, tumors predominating in males with an average age of 60 years, and presenting at a time when regional metastases will already have occurred in 80–90 percent.[32] Thus, jaundice, though commmonly the initial symptom, is often a late finding. Conversely, the closer the tumor lies to the bile duct, the earlier in its course will obstruction result and the more favorable the prognosis.

Some 10 percent of periampullary tumors arise in the ampulla itself.[32] Again there is predominance of males with an average age in the 6th–7th decade. Jaundice may occur early but is frequently intermittent. The remainder of periampullary tumors are divided between carcinomas of the duodenum and of the distal bile ducts. Duodenal tumors producing bile duct obstruction may be clinically indistinguishable from ampullary carcinomas. Carcinomas in the distal bile duct are difficult to biopsy and may be mistaken for strictures.

Malignant tumors of or involving the biliary tract present with a combination of three symptoms: jaundice, pain, and weight loss (Table 3). The degree of jaundice mirrors to some extent the completeness of ductal obstruction. As the obstruction increases, stools become acholic and bile acids accumulate in the skin, producing pruritus, often the most distressing of all symptoms. Unlike that due to choledocholithiasis, this form of jaundice is infrequently complicated by colangitis.

The maxim that jaundice due to malignant tumors is painless is incorrect, for the second major symptom of this group of tumors is pain. While pain is not generally acute, colicky, or severe, it is a very frequent complaint in all except ampullary tumors, and tends to be epigastric, cosntant, and to radiate to the back. Weight loss is the third major symptom of

Table 3
Findings in Obstructive Jaundice Due to Malignant Tumors in Collected Series*

Tumor Site	Jaundice (%)	Pain (%)	Weight Loss (%)	Hepatomegoly (%)	Palpable Gallbladder (%)	Abdominal Mass (%)
Duodenum, pancreas[32]	75	80	90	50–70	25–50	—
Ampulla of Vater[39]	84	24	55	50	13	—
Bile ducts[38]	93	67	67	80	—	40
Gallbladder[30]	46	79	61	36	—	30

*Series include Keil et al.,[30] Warren,[32] Yarborough,[38] and Makipour et al.[39]

tumors obstructing the biliary system, and results not only from the digestive disorders and anorexia resulting from biliary obstruction, but also from pain and the poorly understood effects of malignancy on nutrition. Pertinent physical findings in addition to jaundice and wasting most often involve a right-upper-quadrant mass, whether it be the primary tumor or a dilated gallbladder or enlarged liver. The so-called Courvoisier gallbladder (palpable, accompanying painless jaundice) is a bit of surgical lore seldom clearly demonstrable.

Thorough evaluation of jaundice is often rewarding. Total bilirubin rarely exceeds 15–25 mg/100 ml in pure obstructive jaundice. Serum transaminases are generally normal or minimally elevated, but alkaline phosphatase values show an early and sharp rise followed by increase in gamma-glutamyl transpeptidase levels. Detection of occult blood in the stool is important in detecting lesions within or eroding into the bowel lumen.

Proper radiologic study is critical.[33] Plain films generally have little to offer, and oral or intravenous cholecystography or cholangiography are unrewarding in the presence of significant jaundice. Upper-gastrointestinal barium-contrast radiography may be combined with hypotonic duodenography for delineation of the periampullary area, and is abnormal in up to 60 percent of patients with tumors of this region. Various radioactive scans may be of considerable use: conventional technetium-99 scans of the liver can reveal dilated ducts and metastatic disease if present; iodine-131 Rose-Bengall is a fairly specific means of separating obstructive jaundice frm hepatocellular disease but will add little more specificity regarding cause of obstruction. Celiac angiography may contribute to the diagnosis in up to 85 percent of cases, particularly with tumors of the pancreas.[32] Angiography of the portal venous system can also be accomplished and while adding little diagnostically, can be helpful for planning surgical therapy.

Percutaneous transhepatic cholangiography offers the most accurate and specific information for possible surgical decompression. In addition, morbidity has been substantially reduced by the "skinny" (Chiba) needle technique. Furthermore, temporary drainage of an obstructed biliary tree may be achieved by percutaneous catheter placement over a wire guide. An innovative extension of this technique has been described whereby a permanent indwelling stint is guided into position through the obstructed common duct via a percutaneous approach, thereby obviating surgery.[34]

Ebdoscopic retrograde cholangiopancreatography has developed as a reliable and accurate procedure that may be less hazardous than transhepatic cholangiography. In addition, direct visualization of the duodenum and ampulla add further useful information. Published studies of jaundiced patients have demonstrated that duodenoscopy is possible in 99 percent, cannulation of the ampulla in 80 percent, cholangiography in 69 percent, and definitive diagnosis in 76 percent.[35] The direct inspection and manipulation made possible by this technique may well supplant other less specific and inexact studies such as duodenal cytology or hypotonic duodenography.

Operative assessment should include cholangiography. In some cases a choledochoscope will allow direct visualization and directed biopsy of otherwise inaccessible lesions. The choledochoscope has been particularly valuable in assessing bile duct carcinomas, which are frequently multifocal.[36]

The treatment of biliary obstruction due to malignant tumor is surgical whenever possible. For the majority, cure will be impossible and for some a very aggressive surgical approach will be necessary to achieve palliation. The alternative, however, is a life span diminished in length and quality by liver failure, with irreversible hepatic changes beginning with 3 or 4 weeks of total obstruction, occasionally accelerated by cholangitis. For the few primary intrahepatic ductal lesions, resection may be technically impossible, and bile duct diversion may require intrahepatic cholangiojejunostomy or a permanently indwelling stint.[36,37] A number of techniques have been described, including use of replaceable U- or Y-shaped tubes brought out through the abdominal wall or a permanent indwelling straight tube. With biliary decompression of unresectable tumors, an average survival of 8–12 months is achieved.

Hepatomas are seldom discovered while still resectable by even extended hepatic lobectomy, and cure is rare. However, intubation and/or choledochoenterostomy can relieve premature liver failure in those with ductal obstruction from tumor products.[27] This syndrome should be suspected when obstructive jaundice accompanies what otherwise would appear to be an early stage of disease.

Among the extrahepatic nonperiampullary lesions prognosis is quite poor. Even of the primary bile duct carcinomas amenable to resection, the 3-year survival rate is only 4 percent. Those not resectable have an average survival of less than 12 months following bypass with choledochojejunostomy.[38]

The average survival of patients with carcinoma of the gallbladder is 3 months,[31] and those tumors presenting with obstructive jaundice are not likely to be resectable.

The only lesions causing obstructive jaundice likely to be substantially benefited by radical surgery are those in the periampullary region

Table 4
Survival After Pancreaticoduodenectomy*

Site of Primary Tumor	Survival Rate (%)		
	1 yr	5 yr	15 yr
Pancreas	46.6 (56)†	12.5 (13)	3.5 (2)
Ampulla of Vater	83.2 (79)	32.0 (26)	23.6 (9)
Common bile duct	76.3 (29)	25.0 (8)	38.4 (5)
Duodenum	93.5 (29)	41.3 (12)	18.1 (2)

*Adapted from Warren et al.[40]
†Numbers in parentheses represent number of patients.

(Table 4). In general, resectability rates range from 3 to 52 percent with an average of 15 percent.[39,40] Radical pancreaticoduodenectomy is the standard against which other procedures are judged. Tumors of the duodenum and ampulla carry the most favorable prognosis and those of the pancreas the worst. The use of such radical surgery in the face of disappointing overall results remains controversial. In the hands of those who practice radical pancreaticoduodenectomy frequently, operative mortality rates are acceptably low, and even in the case of those not cured superior palliation is afforded.[40]

Genitourinary

Consideration of obstruction of urinary flow due to malignant tumors is facilitated by separately examining those causes found above and below the bladder. For example, urethral obstruction is almost always related to prostatic carcinoma and thus predominates in males. On the other hand, ureteral obstruction is usually due to extensive local growth of cervical, ovarian, and colonic carcinoma, therefore tending to occur in females.

Ureter

Obstruction of the upper urinary tract by malignant neoplasm may follow direct extension of tumor, growth of endogenous neoplasms, or direct metastases from distant tumors. The commonest cause of ureteral obstruction is direct involvement by adjacent tumors. Carcinoma of the cervix is the most frequent offender, and is followed in frequency by tumors of the ovary, colon, prostate, and bladder, and finally the retroperitoneal neoplasms. In this group, obstruction is generally caused by compression of the ureter without actual invasion of the entire wall.

All points of the utereropelvocalyceal system are subject to neoplastic obstruction; a relatively narrow lumen makes this a relatively frequent and early phenomenon in the ureter.[41] However, primary ureteral tumors are rare and comprise only 1 percent of neoplasms of the upper tract, while those arising in the renal pelvis are somewhat more common (12 percent). These sites are best considered together, for in each site squamous and transitional cell types predominate and lesions are often multifocal, usually on the same side. Men outnumber women by as much as 4:1 and the median age at diagnosis is in the 6th decade.

Metastases from a variety of primary tumors, including breast, colon, and others, as well as lymphoma, may involve a ureter with a single discrete tumor nodule. In this rare circumstance, the tumor grows within the ureteral wall or in the periureteral lymphatics or lymph nodes. Substantial metastatic disease elsewhere is the rule, and the vast majority of patients are so symptomatic from metastases elsewhere that symptoms of ureteral obstruction pass unnoticed.[42,43] In one third to one half of cases, the metastatic ureteral involvement is bilateral.[43,44]

The most frequent symptoms of ureteral obstruction from malignant tumors are bleeding (70 percent) and pain (50 percent).[44] Pain is usually a dull ache in the flank but may be acute and colicky, as when the passage of bloodclots down the ureter mimics ureteral lithiasis. Bleeding is typically intermittent and gross, and may be detectable only by microscopic examination of the urine. Nonspecific symptoms such as weight loss and anorexia are common, and in 25 percent of cases an abdominal mass is palpable.

The presence of gross or microscopic hematuria indicates the need for evaluation of the urinary tract. An intravenous urogram may not show small ureteral tumors, but can detect early evidence of obstruction. Cystoscopy and retrograde studies are necessary to define the level of ureteral lesions and to identify tumors. Arteriography or radiographs with retroperitoneal air insufflation are occasionally helpful. Computerized axial tomography is emerging as a valuable tool in evaluation of retroperitoneal masses, and is useful in the identification of ureteral obstruction from malignant neoplasms.

Therapy depends upon the extent, location, and origin of the malignant tumor responsible for ureteral obstruction. The involvement by direct extension to the ureter is a very late and grave sign of pelvic or retroperitoneal neoplasm. In a series of 47 patients undergoing ileal-loop diversion for bilateral ureteral obstruction from pelvic tumor, 59 percent left the hospital, only 50 percent survived 3 months and 22.7 percent 6 months, with beneficiaries largely those with prostatic carcinoma.[45] Nephrostomy offers no better survival. An alternative to be considered is ureteral stint, although in one third or more of patients this may be technically impossible.[46] For primary ureteral tumors, resection by total nephroureterectomy is the treatment of choice, and provides a 4-year survival rate of approximately 20 percent.[41,44] For the rare metastatic lesions to the ureter, conservative therapy is indicated, as the overwhelming majority have sufficient metastatic disease elsewhere to severely limit survival.

Urethra

Urethral neoplasms are rare; the most frequent are squamous-cell carcinomas (65–75 percent) followed by transitional-cell carcinomas and the very infrequent adenocarcinomas. Secondary involvement of the urethra by carcinoma of the bladder is an uncommon manifestation of far-advanced tumors, and in women encroachment by other extrinsic tumors is extremely rare. In men, however, urethral obstruction by prostatic carcinomas is often seen, as the tumor is common and frequently compresses the urethra. Unfortunately, when symptoms of outlet obstruction from prostatic carcinoma develop, the tumor is in a relatively late stage.

Symptoms of urethral obstruction are decreased caliber of urinary stream, frequent voiding with small volume and sensation of incomplete emptying, and with the evolution of complete obstruction the distress of acute bladder distention.

The diagnosis of malignant tumors obstructing the urethra is established by digital rectal examination, cystoscopy, and biopsy through the cystoscope or directly into the prostate through the perineum or rectal wall. Intravenous urography is helpful in evaluating bladder changes including muscular hypertrophy and postvoiding residual. A voiding cystourethrogram is useful in delineating urethral lesions radiographically.

Immediate symptomatic relief for severe or complete obstruction is achieved with catheter decompression of the bladder, which may require the use of a Coude tip or filiform catheter with follower, but only infrequently suprapubic cystostomy. The definitive therapy of prostatic carcinoma is radical surgical removal, appropriate in only 5–10 percent of patients with symptoms of outlet obstruction because of advanced stage of disease.[47] Excellent palliation can be obtained with radiation and hormonal therapy, combined with transurethral resection of prostatic tissue for relief of outlet obstruction when necessary. For primary urethral tumor penile resection with reconstruction must be considered.

Summary

An overview of the causes, the clinical pictures, and the management of obstruction in three major organ systems due to primary and secondary malignant neoplasms has been presented. Such obstruction often produces dramatic clinical pictures that require careful, appropriate, and often aggressive therapy if patients are to receive the quality of palliation they deserve or the attendant improvement in survival that may result.

References

1. Grillo HC: Obstructing lesions of the trachea. Ann Otol Rhinol Laryngol 82:770, 1973
2. Grillo HC: Surgery of the trachea. Curr Prob Surg 7(7):5, 1970
3. Houston HE, Payne WS, Harrison EG, et al: Primary cancers of the trachea. Arch Surg 99:132, 1969
4. Silver CE: Surgical management of neoplasms of the larynx, hypopharynx and cervical esophagus. Curr Prob Surg 14(12):9, 1977
5. Adkins PC: Neoplasms of the lung, in Sabiston DC, Spencer FC (eds): Gibbon's Surgery of the Chest. Philadelphia, Saunders, 1976, p 443
6. Nelson RS: Tumors of the esophagus, in Bockus RL (ed): Gastroenterology. Philadelphia, Saunders, 1976, p 295
7. Gunnlaugsson GH, Wychulis AR, Roland C, et al: Analysis of the records of 1,657 patients with cancer of the esophagus and cardia of the stomach. Surg Gynecol Obstet 130:997, 1970
8. Nakayama K: Surgical treatment combined with preoperative concentrated irradiation for esophageal cancer. Cancer 20:778, 1967
9. Rubin P, Gooder JT, Nakayama K, et al: Cancer of the gastrointestinal tract. II Esophagus: treatment—localized and advanced. JAMA 227:175, 1974
10. Nakayama K: Statistical review of five year survivals after surgery for carcinoma of the esophagus and cardiac portion of the stomach. Surgery 45:883, 1959
11. Pearson JG: The value of radiotherapy in the management of esophageal cancer. Am J Roentgenol Radium Ther Nucl Med 105:500, 1969
12. Duvoisin GE, Ellis FH, Payne WS: The value of palliative prostheses in malignant lesions of the esophagus. Surg Clin North Am 47:827, 1967
13. Thomas AN: Treatment of malignant esophageal obstruction by endoesophageal intubation. Am J Surg 128:306, 1974

14. Palmer WL: Carcinoma of the stomach, in Bockus HL (ed). Gastroenterology. Philadelphia, Saunders, 1976, p 949
15. Davis SE, Sperling L: Obstruction of the small intestine. Arch Surg 99:424, 1969
16. Lo AM, Evans WE, Carey LC: Review of small bowel obstruction at Milwaukee County General Hospital. Am J Surg 111:884, 1966
17. Mauer HG: Small bowel obstruction in a community hospital. Minn Med 60:273, 1977
18. McNeil JE: Mechanism of obstruction in carcinoid tumors of the small intestine. Am J Clin Pathol 56:452, 1971
19. Glass RL LeDuc RJ: Small intestinal obstruction from peritoneal carcinomatosis. Am J Surg 125:316, 1973
20. Ketcham AS, Hoye RC, Pilch Y, et al: Delayed intestinal obstruction following treatment for cancer. Cancer 25:406, 1970
21. Barnett WO: Problems in abdominal surgery. VI. Intestinal obstruction fromperitoneal carcinomatosis. J Miss State Med Assoc 17:325, 1976
22. Ulin AW, Declement FA, James PM: Large bowel obstruction due to carcinoma. Am Fam Physician 3:79, 1971
23. Glenn F, McSherry CK: Obstruction and perforation of colorectal cancer. Ann Surg 173:938, 1971
24. Welch JP, Donaldson, GA: Management of severe obstruction of the large bowel due to malignant disease. Am J Surg 127:492, 1974
25. Faulconer HT, Ferguson JA, Van Zwalenburg BR: The surgical significance of complete retrograde obstruction of the colon. Dis Colon Rectum 14:428, 1971
26. Williams RD, Elliott DW, Zollinger RW: Surgery for malignant jaundice. Arch Surg 80:992, 1960
27. Kuroyanagi Y, Sawada M, Hidemura R, et al: Common bile duct obstruction by hepatoma. Am J Surg 133:233, 1977
28. Takasan H, Kitamura O, Ozawa K, et al: Metastatic carcinoma of the liver resulting in obstruction of the extrahepatic bile duct. Am J Surg 125:782, 1973
29. Orloff MJ, Charters HC: Tumors of the gall bladder and bile ducts, in Bockus HL (ed): Gastroenterology. Philadelphia, Saunders, 1976, p 831
30. Keil RH, Deweese MS: Primary carcinoma of the gallbladder. Am J Surg 125:726, 1973
31. Piehler JM, Crichlow RW: Primary carcinoma of the gallbladder. Arch Surg 112:26, 1977

32. Warren KW: Surgical aspects of exocrine tumors, in Bokus HL (ed): Gastroenterology. Philadelphia, Saunders, 1976, p 1122

33. Agee OF, Kaude JV: A radiologic approach to obstructive jaundice and disease in the region of the pancreas. Surg Gynecol Obstet 132:614, 1971

34. Viamonte M: Exhibit at Radiologic Society of North America, Chicago, 1977

35. Blumgart LH, Salmon PR: Endoscopy and retrograde choledochopancreatography in the diagnosis of the patient with jaundice. Surg Gynecol Obstet 138:565, 1974

36. Longmire WP: The diverse causes of biliary obstruction and their remedies. Curr Prob Surg 14(7):29, 1977

37. Niloff PH: A prosthesis for palliative treatment of obstructive jaundice due to cholangiocarcinoma. Surg Gynecol Obstet 135:611, 1972

38. Yarborough DR: Primary carcinoma of the extrahepatic bile ducts. Am J Surg 125:723, 1973

39. Makipour H, Cooperman A, Danzi JT, et al: Carcinoma of the ampulla of Vater—Review of 38 cases with emphasis on treatment and prognostic factors. Ann Surg 183:341, 1976

40. Warren KA, Cloe DS, Plaza J, et al: Results of radical resection for periampullary cancer. Ann Surg 181:534, 1975

41. Scott WW: Tumors of the ureter, in Campbell MF, Harrison JH (eds): Urology (ed 3). Philadelphia, Saunders, 1970, p 977

42. Alexander S, Kim K, Pinck ED, et al: Metastatic ureteral tumors. J Urol 110:288, 1973

43. Cohen WM, Freed SZ, Hasson J: Metastatic cancer to the ureter: A Review of the literature and case presentations. J Urol 112:188, 1974

44. Bergman H: Ureteral tumors, in Bergman H (ed): The Ureter. New York, Harper & Row, 1967, p 439

45. Brin EN, Schiff M, Weiss RM: Palliative urinary diversion for pelvic malignancy. J Urol 113:619, 1975

46. Gibbons RP, Mason JT, Correa RJ: Experience with indwelling rubber ureteral catheters. J Urol 111:594, 1974

47. Scott WW: Carcinoma of the prostate, in Campbell MF, Harrison JF (eds): Urology (ed 3). Philadelphia, Saunders, 1970, p 1143

48. Goligher JC, Smiddy FG: The treatment of acute obstruction or performation with carcinoma of the colon and rectum. Br J Surg 45:270, 1957

49. Ulin AW, Ehrlich EW, Schoemaker WC, et al: A study of 227 patients with acute large bowel obstruciton due to carcinoma of the colon. Surg Gynecol Obstet 108:267, 1959

50. Welch CE, Burke JF: Carcinoma of the colon and rectum. N Engl J Med 266:211, 1962
51. Floyd CE, Cohn J Jr: Obstruction in cancer in the colon. Ann Surg 165:721, 1967
52. Ragland JJ, Londe AM, Spratt JS: Correlaiton of the prognosis of obstructing colorectal carcinoma and pathologic variable. Am J Surg 121:552, 1971
53. Glenn F. McSherry CK: Carcinoma of the distal large bowel. Ann Surg 163:838, 1966

6

SERIOUS TOXICITIES ASSOCIATED WITH CHEMOTHERAPY

Michael A. Friedman
Stephen K. Carter

Ideally, cancer chemotherapy is directed to the selective destruction of neoplastic cells. Unfortunately, the selectivity factor is imperfect and the drugs currently available frequently damage normal cells as well. All chemotherapeutic agents cause substantial toxicity whether or not they effect any concurrent benefit, and this unfortunate fact is recognized by both medical oncologists and their patients. An evalaution of the worth of any chemotherapeutic regimen must be viewed as a cost-versus-benefit analysis in which the cost is host toxicity and the benefit is tumor regression. Currently, more than 30 drugs that are effective in treating at least one kind of human malignancy are available to the clinical oncologist. Since cancer chemotherapy is based upon the cell-kill hypothesis and the concept of the first-order kinetics of tumor-cell kill, these drugs are usually given in the largest doses patients can possibly tolerate. It is assumed that the larger the dose given, the greater the fraction of tumor cells that will be destroyed and the greater the chance that the patient will have his tumor completely eradicated. Properly administered, all cancer drugs must by definition cause some degree of toxicity. The experienced oncologist learns to titrate his drug doses to achieve both maximal tumor-cell kill and tolerable toxicity.

Because of the increase in both the number of chemotherapeutic

---

This work was supported in part by Cancer Education Grant CA 17995-03.

119

drugs and of patients being treated, many publications concerning clinical drug toxicity have appeared in which drug toxicities are described and classified in different ways. It has been convenient and useful for us to classify these toxicities by two criteria: predictability and frequency of occurrence. Some toxicities occur commonly and frequently and will consistently increase in specific situations, e.g., in combination with certain drugs or in patients having determinate preexisting conditions. Other toxicities occur uncommonly and unexpectedly. A representation of the classification scheme is outlined below:

I. Predictable toxicity
   A. Drug–drug interactions. These interactions have been particularly well reviewed by Chabner and Oliverio.[1]
      1. 6-Mercaptopurine + allopurinol = impaired detoxification mechanism resulting in increased myelosuppression
      2. Methotrexate + salicylates (or sulfa or probenecid) = modified renal excretion resulting in increased mucositis and myelosuppression
   B. Patient–drug interactions
      1. Preexisting or coexisting patient conditions
         a) Advanced age
            (1) Myelotoxic drug + poor marrow reserves = increased myelotoxicity
         b) Malnutrition
            (1) Many drugs + severe malnutrition = increased general morbidity
         c) Infection
            (1) Myelotoxic drug + infection = increased infectious morbidity
      2. Preexisting or coexisting specific patient conditions
         a) Co-morbid medical conditions
            (1) Bleomycin + chronic pulmonary disease = increased pulmonary toxicity
            (2) Platinum + renal insufficiency = increased renal toxicity
            (3) Androgen (or estrogen) + congestive heart failure = fluid retention in compromised host resulting in cardiovascular embarrassment

        (4) L-Asparaginase + liver disease = hepatocellular necrosis resulting in increased hepatic toxicity

        (5) Methotrexate + effusions = prolonged release of drug resulting in increased myelosuppression

    b) Conditions resulting from previous antitumor therapy

        (1) Adriamycin + radiation to mediastinum = increased cardiotoxicity

        (2) Myelotoxic drug + previously irradiated bone marrow = increased myelosuppression

II. Unpredictable toxicity

  A. Effects of radiation

    1. Skin toxicity

      a) Actinomycin D or Adriamycin + previous radiation = recall skin toxicity

      b) 5FU + sunlight = enhanced photosensitivity

  B. Idiosyncratic effects of drugs

    1. Anaphylactic reaction

      a) Bleomycin

      b) L-Asparaginase   .

Patients treated with a commonly accepted, usually tolerable ("proper") drug dose and schedule of delivery may evidence toxicity expected to be produced by the drug, but its severity may be uncommonly severe; or they may suffer from an unexpected side effect, rarer in described incidence and unpredictable in occurrence. For example, a certain dose of bleomycin is expected to cause pulmonary fibrosis; however, a similar dose may cause a life-threatening anaphylactic episode that was not expected. Moreover, combinations of drugs may yield unusual toxic situations; e.g., bleomycin plus methotrexate may cause unexpectedly severe mucositis.

Of course, medical emergencies such as life-threatening infection associated with leukopenia, bleeding associated with thrombocytopenia, and electrolyte and fluid disorders may attend any chemotherapeutic treatment. These subjects are dealt with in other chapters of this book. Other distressing side effects such as skin vessication from drug extravasation, alopecia, and pigmentation will not be specifically discussed. Rather than comprehensively catalogue all described potential drug toxicities, we will focus only on those that are infrequent in occurrence or severe in degree, some of them predictable and some not.

Adriamycin and Daunomycin

Among drugs which cause cardiac toxicity the anthracyclines are the most conspicuous. Adriamycin and Daunomycin are related anthracycline antibiotics isolated from *Streptomyces* species which share common mechanisms and action (DNA intercalation) and common toxicities. Cardiotoxicity is the unique harmful effect of these drugs and causes the greatest problem in long-term administration. This toxicity may manifest itself in transient electrocardiogram (ECG) abnormalities, definitive cardiomyopathy, or both.

ECG changes associated with Adriamycin therapy have been reported in 2–30 percent of the treated patients. These abnormalities include supraventricular tachycardias, arterial and ventricular extrasystoles, and ST-T wave changes. The changes usually are transient and occur most frequently in the first few days after drug infusion. Reduction in the R-wave voltage may occur and is usually irreversible; in the series by Cortes et al.[2] it was seen in all patients before Adriamycin-induced congestive heart failure developed. The transient ECG changes apparently are not of clinical significance, since no significant morbidity or mortality has been reported. These changes are at present not considered contraindications for continuance of Adriamycin therapy.

In contrast to transient changes, the chronic toxicity of drug-induced cardiomyopathy produces both morbidity and mortality to a significant degree. This congestive heart failure is dose dependent, and there is some relationship to certain preexisting cardiac conditions (such as mediastinal irradiation). Clinical presentation of the cardiac damage of Adriamycin is indistinguishable from that of other cardiomyopathies.

Although the tempo of the clinical course varies, it is usually a rapidly progressing syndrome of congestive heart failure and cardiovascular decompensation including dilatation of the heart, pleural effusion, and venous congestion. Reversibility of the heart failure is unpredictable. Gilladoga et al.[3] reported that Adriamycin cardiomyopathy may be reversed by conventional medical management, but this is unpredictable.

Macroscopic examination in such cases reveals the heart to be enlarged, pale, and flabby, with ventricular dilatation and hypertrophy. Pericardial effusions may be present. Mural thrombi associated with multiple pulmonary or systemic emboli are occasionally present. The coronary

Table 1
Correlation of Cardiomyopathy and the Total Dose of Adriamycin in Adults*

Investigator	Adriamycin (mg/m²)	No. of Patients At Risk	Patients with Cardiomyopathy Nonfatal	Fatal	Frequency (%)
Lefrak	<450	663	0	0	0
Cortes	<400	75	0	0	0
Lefrak	451–500	23	0	0	0
Cortes	400–499	11	1	0	9
Lefrak	501–550	31	0	1	3
Lefrak	551–600	14	1	2	21
Cortes	500–599	4	1	0	25
Lefrak	>600	27	7	6	48
Cortes	>600	10	5	2	70

*Taken from the data of Lefrak[4] and Cortes.[5]

arteries and cardiac valves are usually normal. Light microscopy shows edema between myocardial fibers, myocytolysis, disruption of sarcoplasm with vacuole formation, and myocardial fibrosis. Electron microscopy shows a marked decrease in the number of myocardial fibrils, accompanied by mitochrondrial changes, nuclear degeneration, disorganization of sarcoplasmic reticulum, and depletion of glycogen granules in the severe late presentation. These changes are nonspecific and have been described in other types of cardiomyopathy. In the early stages, these changes are probably specific for anthracycline injury.

The overall incidence of congestive heart failure caused by the toxicity is related to the total dose administered. If the total dose is kept below 450 mg/m², cardiomyopathy is only occasionally observed (Table 1). Unfortunately, this limits the amount and duration of drug therapy. The frequency of cardiomyopathy is markedly increased at total doses above 550 mg/m², so that a clinician who exceeds those dose levels must be aware of this mounting risk and balance it against the risk of malignant disease progression when therapy is discontinued.

Von Hoff[6] reviewed a total of 5,613 patients who received Daunomycin in the last 10 years (4,760 in cooperative group studies, 394 treated by independent investigators reported to the NCI, and 459 patients reported in the literature). Most of these patients had acute lymphocytic or myelocytic leukemia and received Daunomycin alone or in combination with other antileukemic agents. Eighty-two cases of congestive heart failure were reported in the 5,613 patients reviewed, or an overall incidence of 1.46 percent. There were 59 cases in children (2–20 years of age) and 23 cases in adults (over 20 years of age).

Von Hoff et al.[7] has also analyzed 4,018 patients treated with Adriamycin in the United States cooperative groups between March 1970 and March 1977. A range of variables were recorded for all patients. These totaled 67 and included age, sex, race, performance status, tumor type, prior cardiac disease, prior anticancer treatment and concomitant treatment with other drugs. Ten specific parameters were looked at in relation to the development of congestive heart failure caused by Adriamycin. These consisted of total dose and schedule of drug administration, concomitant chemotherapy, prior radiotherapy to the mediastinum, prior cardiac disease, age, sex, race, type of tumor, and performance status.

In this analysis, Adriamycin-induced CHF occurred in 88 cases (2.2 percent). This was observed at intervals ranging from 0 to 231 days with a median of 23 days, following the last administration of the drug. The mean and median total dosage of the anthracycline received by the patient with CHF was 364 and 390 mg/m^2 respectively. Death occurred within 70 days after the diagnosis of CHF in 63 of the 88 patients. In only 38 of the 63 was death attributed to the CHF. In the others it was attributed to progressive disease. In these latter 25 cases, the CHF was stable but unresolved in 12, partially resolved in 8, and totally resolved in 5.

In this analysis, the total dose of Adriamycin was related strongly to the development of CHF. The cumulative probability of developing drug-induced CHF was 0.3 at 400 mg/m^2, 0.7 at 550 mg/m^2, and 0.18 at 700 mg/m^2. When the schedules were examined, the weekly schedule had the lowest incidence of CHF at 0.8 percent (8/967); the single dose every 3 weeks was 2.9 percent (66/2262), and the three consecutive daily doses repeated every 3 weeks was 2.5 percent (14/576).

The use of transjugular right ventricular endomyocardial biopsy has been described by Friedman et al.[8] and Billingham et al.[9] as a technique for detecting early cardiac toxicity in the absence of echocardiographic changes. Apparently the majority of patients receiving these anthracycline antibiotics sustain microscopic cardiac damage.

Bristow et al.[10] have reported on studies in 33 patients treated with Adriamycin. Studies included phonocardiograms, percutaneous right ventricular endomyocardial biopsy, and cardiac catheterization. These studies indicate that the myocardial degenerative process begins before any functional abnormality can be detected, and that overt heart failure occurs only after a critical amount of morphologic damage has occurred. The pathologic damage observed with the biopsies was clearly dose related, and 27 of 29 patients biopsied at doses of $\geq$240 mg/m^2 had degenerative changes. The preejection period to left ventricular ejection time ratio (PEP/LVET) showed a threshold phenomenon and did not begin to increase until a dose of 400 mg/m^2 had been reached. In this series 7 patients had clinical evidence of cardiomyopathy as evidenced by heart failure. The heart failure occurred at total doses from 330 to 545 mg/m^2. The 3 patients with heart failure at the lowest doses (330, 395, and 445 mg/m^2) all had previous radiation to the mediastinum. It would appear that previous mediastinal radiation is a risk factor for both the myocardial degenerative process and for heart failure. It has been shown that mediastinal radiation that delivers < 600 rads to the apex has not been shown to potentiate Adriamycin cardiac toxicity.

Rinehart,[11] who used preejection period to left ventricular ejection time ratios (PEP/LVET) to estimate left ventricular function, reported that 7 of 8 adult patients receiving Adriamycin (300–525 mg/m^2) had a significant increase in the PEP/LVET ratio. In contrast, only 1 of 8 patients receiving less than 200 mg/m^2 developed prolongation of the PEP/LVET ratio. It appears that the systolic time interval as a noninvasive test may have some sensitivity in predicting cardiotoxicity, although this requires confirmation.

Jones et al.[12] has reported data which supports the usefulness of echocardiography in the detection of Adriamycin-induced heart disease. They performed echoanalyses (with calculation of the ejection fraction) of 54 cancer patients being treated with Adriamycin. Only 1 of 43 (2 percent) who received less than 400 mg/m^2 of Adriamycin had an ejection fraction of less than 0.43, whereas 6 of 13 (46 percent) who received more than this dose had an ejection fraction of less than 0.43 ($P < 0.001$). Only 2 of these patients had clinical findings of congestive heart failure; this increase indicates a subclinical damage due to Adriamycin.

Bleomycin

Bleomycin sulfate is one of a group of antibiotics originally isolated in Japan by Umezawa, from *Streptomyces verticillus*. Although the exact mechanism of the action of bleomycin is unknown, available evidence indicates that it primarily inhibits DNA synthesis and, to a lesser degree, RNA and protein synthesis.

The clinical toxicity of bleomycin in over 1,700 cases from worldwide sources is outlined in Table 2. Bleomycin is noteworthy among antineoplastic drugs because it does not produce appreciable bone marrow toxicity, and this has made the drug highly attractive for use in combination with other drugs. Cutaneous reactions are the most common toxic effects and are seen in about half of the patients. These can occur as mouth ulcers,

Table 2
Common Manifestations of Bleomycin Toxicity

Manifestation	United States (808 patients)	Japan (540 patients)
Mucositis	22%	—
Alopecia	13%	29%
Pigmentation	8%	20%
Pyrexia	26%	36%
Anorexia	17%	32%
Nausea	14%	42%*
Vomiting	10%	—
Pulmonary toxicity	10%	9%†

*In 72 evaluated patients.
†In 468 evaluated patients.

alopecia, hyperpigmentation, thickening, ulceration, redness, hyperkeratosis, nail changes, rash vesiculation, tenderness, pruritis, hyperesthesia, peeling, stria, and bleeding. In only 0.2 percent of treated patients has it been necessary to discontinue bleomycin therapy because of skin toxicity.

The most serious side effect of bleomycin is pulmonary toxicity. Its precise characterization has been extremely difficult. No pathognomonic sign, symptom, x-ray finding, or pathologic change has been established. The most frequent manifestation is pneumonitis, occasionally progressing to a fatal pulmonary fibrosis. Bleomycin-induced pneumonitis apparently produces dyspnea and fine rales which are in no way different from those caused by infectious pneumonias. On x-ray, it produces patchy opacities, usually of the lower lung fields.

In a study of Blum et al.,[13] several pulmonary function tests in 156 patients receiving bleomycin revealed abnormalities in 20 percent consisting mostly of decreases in total lung volume and a decrease in vital capacity. No predictive correlation between these changes and the development of pulmonary fibrosis could be ascertained.

Pathologic pulmonary changes due to bleomycin have been well described by Luna et al.,[14] DeLena et al.,[15] and Roujeau et al.[16] The electron-microscopic changes due to bleomycin have also been described by Bedrossian et al.[17] The general view is that the histopathologic changes due to bleomycin are nonspecific in nature and are consistent with a diagnosis of interstitial pneumonia or pulmonary fibrosis, and similar if not identical to those produced by other noxious agents such as radiation therapy, oxygen therapy, certain infections such as *Pneumocystis carinii* and drugs such as busulfan.[13] Rudders and Hensley[18] and others point out that the nature of bleomycin pulmonary toxicity is consistent with a direct toxicity rather than a hypersensitivity reaction.

The incidence of bleomycin toxicity varies according to the criteria used for definition. The incidence in reported series ranges from 0 to 40 percent. Crooke and Bradner, in a recent review, have tabulated the results of 14 studies which involved a total of 1,890 patients.[19] The overall morbidity from bleomycin therapy occurred in 11 percent of the reported cases. Deaths due to bleomycin-induced pulmonary toxicity occurred in 0–6 percent of these cases. Examination of the dose-level correlation shows that the incidence is low and is consistent with doses of 100–500 units of bleomycin. There does appear to be a significant increase in the incidence when doses in excess of 500 units are given. Thus the pulmonary toxicity of this drug is unpredictable and not dose-related with total doses ranging from 100 to 500 units. With doses of above 500 mg a threshold appears to be exceeded, and the incidence increases significantly. The findings of a comparable proportion of patients with unexpected autopsy findings indicates that subclinical pulmonary toxicity that can be documented histopathologically occurs, with at least the same frequency as clinically significant toxicity.

Several studies are available in which the relationship between bleomycin therapy and changes in pulmonary function tests is evaluated. The tests used most often have included the forced vital capacity (FVC), forced expiratory volume in 1 second (FEV$_1$), and 1-minute single-breath or steady-state carbon monoxide diffusion capacity (DL$_{CO}$). Few studies have evaluated systematic serial determinations or have clearly defined the exact timing of pulmonary function tests relative to the total dose of drug given by the cessation point of therapy. The studies have shown definite changes in TLC, FVC, and DL$_{CO}$ after bleomycin administration. These changes have revealed no consistent relationships between total bleomycin dose and changes in pulmonary function.[20–22]

Recently Izbicki and Baker[23] and Comis et al.[24] have reported the results of serial studies on FVC, FEV, and DL$_{CO}$. The preliminary results of both studies show a linear fall in DL$_{CO}$ with increasing total doses of bleomycin. Neither study showed a consistent relationship between FVC and FEV determination and total bleomycin dose.

Unfortunately, the absolute diagnosis of pulmonary toxicity is complicated because of the lack of specificity of clinical symptoms, x-ray signs, and even histopathologic changes. Therefore, the incidence figures quoted cannot be precise. The difficulties in implicating bleomycin, or any drug, in this type of nonspecific toxicity in patients with advanced stages of cancer have been pointed out by Blum and Carter[25] and Krous and Hamlin.[26]

Several factors are known to predispose patients to pulmonary toxicity from bleomycin. These include advanced age, high total doses of bleomycin, underlying pulmonary disease such as emphysema, and previous radiation therapy to the chest. Patients with one or more of these underlying conditions should receive bleomycin only with very careful monitoring.

The pulmonary toxicity appears to be both dose and age related; it is more common in patients over 70 years of age receiving total dosages of over 400 mg. In the review of Blum and Carter of 808 cases, the data demonstrated definite risk of pulmonary toxicity at about the same rate at all dose levels (3–5 percent) below total doses of 450 mg; however, there was a substantial increase in the overall incidence of pulmonary toxicity at total doses greater than 450 mg. Similarly, the incidence of toxicity was relatively constant as a function of age up to 70 years (2–6 percent) when it increased to 15 percent (9/61) in patients older than 70 years.

Patients with pulmonary toxicity secondary to bleomycin treatment should, of course, receive no further bleomycin therapy. Corticosteroids in large doses (prednisone 100 mg/day) have been tried with some success in the treatment of pulmonary toxicity,[22] but not all patients respond.

Androgens and Estrogens

These sex steroids are frequently used in the common malignant diseases breast cancer and prostate cancer. They do not cause marrow toxicity and are often well-tolerated. However, cardiovascular and calcium metabolism complications can be associated with their usage.

Both estrogens and androgens are associated with fluid retention, presumably because they have weak mineralocorticoid properties. Often this expansion of the extracellular space is manifested only by inappreciable pedal edema, but in the patient with cardiac compromise it can lead to decompensation, overt congestive heart failure, and pulmonary edema. The patient with intrinsic cardiac disease may require concomitant diuretic therapy to prevent this toxicity.

Additionally, exogenous estrogen therapy is distinctly associated with thrombotic and phlebitic occurrences. This has been most clearly demonstrated in the Veterans Administration Cooperative Urologic Group Study of Diethylstilbestrol (DES) in patients with prostatic cancer.

In this group, a high rate of mortality from myocardial infarction and cerebrovascular accident was evident in patients receiving 5 mg/day of DES compared to those receiving 1 mg/day.[27,28] Nevertheless, even at low doses, probably all patients receiving estrogens are at some increased risk of cardiac, cerebral, or pulmonary vascular accidents. Thus, care in the selection of patients for treatment is well advised; those with preexisting vascular disease should be excluded.[29]

In patients with metastatic breast cancer, the use of both androgens and estrogens has been linked to hypercalcemia. The recognition of this electrolyte disturbance and its treatment are dealt with elsewhere in this book. But it should be recalled that about 10 percent of patients with metastatic breast cancer treated with androgens and a smaller fraction treated with estrogens have hypercalcemia.[30]

L-Asparaginase

L-Asparaginase is an enzyme which effectively depletes the amino acid L-asparaginase. This action leads to inhibition of protein synthesis in the liver, pancreas, brain, and kidney, and results in a variety of predictable dysfunctions of these organs. Although L-asparaginase does not cause myelotoxicity (the common side effect of most antineoplastics), its use results in other toxicities.

Hepatotoxicity is a common side effect which is most often reversible and does not clearly result in chronic hepatic fibrosis. Perhaps 30–50 percent of patients show defects in both hepatic detoxification function (increased serum bilirubin and hyperammonemia) and hepatic synthetic function (decreased serum albumin, cholesterol, and fibrinogen).[31,32] Pancreatic toxicity is commonly expressed as glucose intolerance (from mild hyperglycemia to dehydrating glycosuria) or infrequently (5 percent) as frank pancreatitis.[31] Likewise, nephrotoxicity with proteinuria or cylindruria is infrequently observed (15-percent incidence).[31–33]

Neurologic abnormality is the other common toxicity associated with this agent. Estimates of the frequency of cerebral dysfunction range from 20 to 60 percent, and the dysfunction is characterized by mental status changes (from minor somnolence to coma) closely coincident with the starting and stopping of therapy. Less frequently, an organic syndrome develops 7 or more days after therapy is initiated.[34] It is critically important to identify the cause of any neurologic abnormality in a leukemia patient treated with L-asparaginase, since the differential diagnoses include CNS leukemia, infective meningitis, overt metabolic encephalopathy (hyperosmolar, uremic, or hepatic coma), and drug effect. Great caution must be exercised in using this drug in patients with preexisting hepatic dysfunction.

Finally, because this enzyme is a large foreign protein (usually obtained from *E. coli*) it is a potent antigen. Allergic reactions ranging from mild hypersensitivity to anaphylaxis occur in 5–20 percent of patients.[35]

Cyclophosphamide

Of all the alkylating agents, cyclophosphamide probably has the broadest impact in terms of clinical toxicity because of its frequent usage and its wide variety of side effects. Its toxicity affects the urinary, pulmonary, and hepatic organ system and, of course, causes bone marrow dysfunction.

The most common urinary tract toxicity is a bacteriologically sterile hemorrhagic cystitis, which may range from microscopic hematuria to exsanguinating bladder bleeding. Various estimates of the incidence of this finding range from 4 to 35 percent.[36] The mechanism of this toxicity is thought to be a direct toxic effect of cyclophosphamide metabolites in the urine on the bladder mucosa. Therefore, efforts to decrease the urinary concentration of these offending products or their exposure time to the sensitive surface are effective. Vigorous hydration and frequent voiding are useful in preventing this toxicity, and preexisting thrombocytopenia or coagulopathy obviously exaggerate this side effect. Careful replacement of appropriate blood products is occasionally necessary. Once severe bleeding is encountered, aggressive therapy with intravesicular formalin instillation or fulguration may be attempted. If unsuccessful, diverting the urine from the bladder (cannulation of the ureter or ureteral surgical diversion) has been effective.[36] Once obvious toxicity is noted, cyclophosphamide should be discontinued and reintroduced at a later time, only after careful consideration of alternative therapies. Clearly, this toxicity is best prevented, rather than treated when apparent. In children, prolonged therapy with cyclophosphamide sometimes causes chronic bladder injury with fibrosis.

Higher doses of cyclophosphamide (50 mg/kg) frequently are associated with diminished free-water excretion. This syndrome of inappropriate antidiuretic hormone action is characterized by urine hyperosmolality and serum hyposmolality which can lead to hyponatremic central nervous system dysfunction. The recognition of this syndrome is important since patients are urged to drink large volumes of fluid which could result in water intoxication.

Rarely, prolonged cyclophosphamide therapy is associated with chronic fibrotic lung disease (similar to "busulphan lung"). Beginning many months to many years after initiation of therapy (averaging 3–4 years), this syndrome is clinically defined by fever, cough, dyspnea, and radiologically by a diffuse intra-alveolar fibrosis.[37,38] Unfortunately, unlike methotrexate pulmonary disease, this side effect of alkylating agents is often progressive and nonreversible. Discontinuation of the busulphan or cyclophosphamide and administration of corticosteroids do not seem to be effective, and patients succumb to restrictive pulmonary disease, usually within 6 months.[37]

Finally, cyclophosphamide probably has a weak cardiotoxic potential. This side effect is minor unless the drug is given in combination with other more potent cardiotoxins like Adriamycin.[39]

Methotrexate

Methotrexate is the classic antifol that is of special interest because (1) its mechanism of toxicity is reasonably well understood, (2) an assessment of its serum concentration can be made, and (3) a method of ameliorating its toxicity is available. These features allow for monitoring and for active clinical therapeutic intervention unparalleled in medical oncology.

The most common side effects of methotrexate are mucositis and bone marrow suppression. These toxicities are directly influenced by how much drug is given (i.e., how high the serum concentation levels are) and how long the drug remains in the blood. Renal excretion is the one major disposal pathway for methotrexate, which undergoes little metabolic degradation and is primarily disposed of by active renal tubular excretion of unchanged drug. Therefore, in cases in which high serum levels are achieved or prolonged levels maintained, severe toxicity will result. This toxic situation may occur as a result of clinical features of the patient (e.g., concurrent dehydration with impaired excretion or preexisting renal disease), specific features of therapy (e.g., purposely administered prolonged or high doses of methotrexate), or interference with the patient's tubular excretion (e.g., concurrently administered salicylates, probenecid, sulfa drugs, or cephalothin). Additionally, exposure time to methotrexate can be prolonged not only in patients receiving continuous intravenous or oral doses, but also in those who have accumulated fluid in third spaces. Pleural and ascitic fluid collections may act as reservoirs that take up drug and release it slowly to the systemic circulation. All of the above circumstances are at least relative contraindications to routine methotrexate use.

Further, it should be noted that in the presence of high serum levels or renal insufficiency, methotrexate is itself a nephrotoxin, thus perpetuating and compounding toxic serum concentations.[40] Serum levels in excess of 5×10^{-5} m at 24 hours or 2×10^{-7} m at 72 hours after methotrexate administration are associated with severe toxicity.[41] Nonspecific measures to prevent or ameliorate this toxicity include increasing urine flow (vigorous hydration) and increasing drug solubility in urine (alkalinization with bicarbonate or acetazolamide). The specific antidote for excessive methotrexate serum levels is calcium leukovorin administered at frequent intervals (usually every 6 hours) until an acceptably safe serum level of methotrexate is noted (usually less than 1×10^{-7} m).[42] Experimentally, thymidine has also been used as an antidote.[42]

Infrequently, methotrexate-induced acute pulmonary toxicity is described. It occurs from days to months after the beginning of therapy and does not seem to be related to total dosage. It is associated with fever, cough, hypoxia, and dyspnea. Radiologically, scattered bilateral pulmonary infiltrates can be seen. These symptoms usually remit promptly when the drug is discontinued, but occasional deaths have been reported.[37] In such a clinical setting, differentiation must be made between this infrequent drug toxicity and acute opportunistic infection.

Methotrexate-associated hepatotoxicity manifests itself in reversible liver function test abnormality and, after lengthy daily administration, in architectural hepatic changes. Fibrosis has been noted in 16 percent and cirrhosis in 11 percent of patients receiving daily methotrexate for long periods of time.[36] Hepatotoxicity occurs rarely during intermittent or brief therapy.

The use of methotrexate intrathecally for the treatment of meningeal neoplasm is a common treatment approach that has both acute and chronic side effects. Acute meningeal irritation, characterized by headache, fever, nausea, lethargy, meningismus, and spinal fluid pleocytosis has been reported to occur in 10–40 percent of patients. The differentiation between active neoplasm, infection, and drug toxicity may be a difficult one. Acute paraplegia associated with intrathecal drug administration is rare (1 percent), but it is a dramatic occurrence which may be transient or permanent. The precise mechanism of this toxicity is unknown and methods to ameliorate it are unfocused, but cessation of the intrathecal administration is recommended. Finally, there is a serious progressive debilitating meningoencephalopathy that has been described in children with acute lymphoblastic leukemia created with cranial irradiation and intrathecal methotrexate. This rare toxicity appears clinically as confusion, tremor, ataxia, or dementia, and pathologically as nonspecific necrosis.[34]

Mithramycin

Mithramycin is an antibiotic produced by *Streptomyces atrollivaceus* that binds to DNA and preferentially inhibits RNA synthesis.

Although the specific antineoplastic use of mithramycin is currently limited to patients with testicular tumors (and then only rarely)[43] a larger number of patients receive this agent as therapy for refractory hypercalcemia. When used infrequently at low dosage (10–15 μg/kg) appreciable toxicity is infrequently encountered.[44] However, if larger amounts are used (35 μg/kg) or if doses are repeated frequently, the risk of severe toxicity increases. Severe bleeding can occur. This incompletely defined hemorrhagic diathesis is sometimes associated with thrombocytopenia, depleted procoagulants, or enhanced fibrinolysis,[45] but often is not clearly caused by any of these, and there is no specific therapy known. This toxicity is best avoided by monitoring platelet count, prothrombin, and bleeding times; when abnormalities are noted, therapy should be discontinued.

Hepatotoxicity is the most frequently encountered toxicity and is marked by elevation of serum lactic dehydrogenase (LDH), serum glutamic oxaloacetic transaminase (SGOT), and prothrombin time. This toxicity is noted with standard doses of 50 μg/kg daily for four days, and therapy must be interrupted.

Nitrosoureas

The nitrosoureas are a family of compounds that probably act through both aklylation and carbamylation. The three synthetic nitrosoureas in general usage, BCNU, CCNU, and Methyl CCNU, all share myelotoxicity and thrombotoxicity as their major dose-limiting side effects. The delayed nature of these toxicities (hematologic nadirs at 4–5 weeks posttherapy) are well recognized by all medical oncologists. However, it is equally important to stress the cumulative nature of this toxicity: after several apparently well-tolerated treatments, severe life-threatening toxicity may occur. Infrequently (5–25-percent incidence) reversible hepatotoxicity may appear a few days to weeks after therapy, characterized by abnormalities in the liver function tests (especially bilirubin).[46]

Two less commonly encountered toxicities have been noted in patients receiving nitrosoureas for prolonged periods. Chronic pulmonary fibrosis has been described in patients receiving BCNU that is clinically similar to "alkylator lung" syndrome of busulfan or cyclophosphamide. Estimates of its incidence range from 14 percent (in 28 patients) to 1.1 percent (in 794 patients).[47] Also, chronic renal insufficiency has been described in children receiving methyl-CCNU. Doses in excess of 1500 mg/m^2 have resulted in decreased overall renal mass and microscopic evidence of glomerulosclerosis and tubular-cell loss.[48] The implciations of this toxicity for adult patients are currently undefined, but attention to changes in kidney size (by intravenous pyelogram) may be prudent for patients receiving nitrosourea over long periods of time.

Streptozotocin is a fermentation-product nitrosourea derived from *Streptomyces pucetus* that is believed to have only minor hematologic toxicity. However, up to 20 percent of treated patients have demonstrable bone marrow depression that may be clinically important in those with poor marrow reserves.[47] More commonly, hepatic toxicity and nephrotoxicity are observed (60 percent) in treated patients. The renal tubule is particularly affected with evident proteinuria and glycosuria, and occasionally renal tubular acidosis is fully apparent. Although usually reversible, fatalities have been reported from irreversible renal failure.[47,48] Therefore, patients with any renal insufficiency should be given this drug with great caution.

CDDP

As an inorganic metal complex, cis-dichloro-diammine platinum (II), CDDP, possesses certain characteristic toxicities which could be predicted from its chemical structure. The most serious and common of these is nephrotoxicity, which is similar to that seen with use of other heavy metals. Histopathologically, this agent is associated with acute tubular necrosis,[49] which clinically is evidenced by azotemia, decreased creatinine clearance, and occasional hyperuricemia.[50,51] The severity of this toxicity appears to depend upon the glumerular filtration rate, since patients treated with CDDP alone have almost universally demonstrated renal toxicity. However, techniques increasing urine flow have resulted in a substantial decrease in nephrotoxicity without the loss of antitumor activity.[51,52] This may be accomplished by extracellular fluid expansion (intravenous saline), osmotic diuresis (mannitol), and drug-induced diuresis (furosemide). Even with these measures, up to 25 percent of patients have reversible renal function abnormalities.[53] Therefore, patients with urinary obstruction (bladder cancer patients especially), those intolerant of a volume fluid load (congestive heart failure), or those receiving concurrent nephrotoxins (amino glycoside antibiotics) should be treated with CDDP only under the most closely supervised circumstances.

While bone marrow toxicity has not been a prominent feature with CDDP therapy, approximately 20 percent of patients have leukopenia or thrombocytopenia[51] and there is some suggestion that this is worsened by prolonged duration of exposure to this drug when, for example, renal failure can occur.

A variety of neurotoxicities have also been noted in patients receiving CDDP. Again, similar to other types of heavy metal intoxication, ototoxicity and peripheral neuropathies have been noted. Damage to the VIII cranial nerve may be noted in up to 30 percent of patients and usually consists of high-frequency hearing loss. Less commonly, peripheral neuropathies (sensory or motor) may occur; and very rarely generalized seizures are noted.[54,55]

Rarely and unexpectedly, allergic reactions to CDDP have been described with classic broncospastic and cutaneous features. Immediate therapy with epinephrine and corticosteroids has proven effective.

Vinca Alkaloids

The two commercially available vinca alkaloids, vincristine and vinblastine, share the same qualitative spectrum of toxicities, but differ in their quantitative aspects. Both agents cause neurotoxicity and bone marrow suppression; vincristine results in more of the former and vinblastine the latter.

Both central and peripheral nervous system toxicity are to be expected with routine doses of vincristine and high doses of vinblastine.[34] Usually these motor, autonomic, or central neuropathies are merely troublesome; however, occasionally they may be more dramatically severe. Of the autonomic dysfunctions, instead of mere constipation, serious adynamic ileus and fecal impaction may occur.[56] Acute urinary retention resulting from bladder atony has been noted, as has orthostatic hypotension.[56,57] The central nervous system toxicities include affective changes such as depression and psychosis. Also, in rare instances the syndrome of inappropriate antidiuretic hormone occurs with vincristine usage, often without great clinical importance.[58] Occasionally, seizures have been reported with vincristine usage—some related to hyponatremia, others without clear cause.[34,59] Apparently, preexisting hepatic dysfunction is associated with more severe vinca toxicity because of impaired hepatic metabolic conversion.

Conclusion

Faced with the reality of treatment-associated toxicities, the general advice of "expect the worst with every treatment" seems prudent. The avenues for exploration in clinical oncology lead toward (1) the identification of new drugs that more specifically and selectively destroy tumor cells, and (2) the utilization of currently available drugs in new ways. Pharmacologic and kinetic data that show an increase in efficiency and a decrease in toxicity must be brought to bear to continue therapeutic advances in the treatment of common adult malignancies. The cost of toxicity once it has occurred is high; it is far better if it can be prevented.

References

1. Chabner BA, Oliverio VT: Drug interactions in cancer chemotherapy, in Farah A, Herken H, Welch AD (eds): Handbook of Experimental Pharmacology, New Series, Vol XXVIII/3. New York, Springer-Verlag, 1975, pp 325–342.
2. Cortes EP, Lutman G, Wanka J, et al: Adriamycin cardiotoxicity in adults with cancer. Clin Res 21:412, 1973
3. Gilladoga AC, Tan C, Wollner N, et al: Adriamycin cardiomyopathy: Diagnosis and management case reports. Proc Am Assoc Can Res 14:95, 1973
4. Lefrak EA, Pitha J, Rosenheim S, et al: A clinicopathologic analysis of adriamycin cardiotoxicity. Cancer 32:302–314, 1973
5. Cortes EP, Lutman G, Wanka J, et al: Adriamycin (NSC-123127) cardiotoxicity: A clincopathological correlation. Cancer Chemother Rep 6:215–225, 1975
6. Von Hoff DD, Rozencweig M, Layard M, et al: Daunomycin-induced cardiotoxicity in children and adults. A review of 110 cases. Am J Med 62:200–208, 1977
7. Von Hoff DD, Layard MW, Basa P, et al: Risk factors for doxorubicin-induced congestive heart failure Ann Int Med 91:710–717, 1979
8. Friedman MA, Bozdech MJ, Billingham ME, et al: Doxorubicin cardiotoxicity—Serial endomyocardial biopsies and systolic time intervals. JAMA 240:1603–1606, 1978

9. Billingham ME, Bristow M, Mason J, et al: Endomyocardial biopsy findings in adriamycin-treated patients. Proc Am Assoc Can Res 17:281, 1976
10. Bristow MR, Mason JW, Billingham ME, et al: Doxorubicin cardiomyopathy: Evaluation by phonocardiography, endomyocardial biopsy and cardiac catheterization. An Int Med 88:168–175, 1978
11. Rinehart JJ, Lewis RP, Balcerzak SP: Adriamycin cardiotoxicity in man. Ann Intern Med 81:475–478, 1974
12. Jones SE, Ewy GA, Groves BM: Echocardiographic detection of adriamycin heart disease. Proc Am Assoc Can Res 16:228, 1975
13. Blum RH, Carter SK, Agre K: A clinical review of bleomycin—A new antineoplastic agent. Cancer 31:903–914, 1973
14. Luna MA, Bedrossian CWM, Lithtiger B, et al: Interstitial pneumonitis associated with bleomycin therapy. Am J Clin Pathol 58:501–510, 1972
15. De Lena M, Guzzon A, Monfardini S, et al: Clinical, radiologic, and histopathologic studies on pulmonary toxicity induced by treatment with bleomycin (NSC-125066). Cancer Chemother Rep 56:343–356, 1972
16. Roujeau J, Narcy PH, Marsan C, et al: Fibrose pulmonaire et bleomycine. Sem Hosp Paris 49:1989–1994, 1973
17. Bedrossian CWM, Luna MA, Mackay B, et al: Ultrastructure of pulmonary bleomycin toxicity. Cancer 32:44–51, 1973
18. Rudders RA, Hensley GT: Bleomycin pulmonary toxicity. Chest 63:626–628, 1973
19. Comis RL: Bleomycin pulmonary toxicity, in Carter SK, Crooke ST, Umazawa H (eds): Bleomycin: Current Status and New Developments. Academic Press, New York, 1978, p 24
20. Samuels ML, Johnson DE, Holoye PY: Large-dose bleomycin therapy and pulmonary toxicity: A possible role of radiotherapy. JAMA 15:1117, 1976
21. Pascual RS, Mosher MB, Rajiner SS, et al: Effects of bleomycin on pulmonary function in man. Am Rev Respir Dis 108:211, 1975
22. Yagoda A, Mukerji B, Young C, et al: Bleomycin: An antitumor antibiotic clinical experience in 274 patients. Ann Intern Med 77:861, 1972
23. Izbicki RM, Baker LH: Prediction of early pulmonary toxicity due to bleomycin in cancer patients treated with combination therapy. Proc Am Soc Clin Oncol Am Assoc Cancer Res 18:345, 1977
24. Comis RL, Ginsberg SJ, Prestayko AW, et al: The effects of bleomycin in co-diffusion in patients with testicular carcinomas. Proc 10th International Congress of Chemotherapy, Zurich, 1977, Abstract 585

25. Blum RH, Carter SK: Pulmonary complications of cancer chemotherapy. New Engl J Med 288:266, 1973
26. Krous HF, Hamoin WB: Pulmonary toxicity due to bleomycin. Report of a case. Arch Pathol 95:407–410, 1973
27. Goodman LA, Gilman A: The Pharmacological Basis of Therapeutics, 5th ed. New York, Macmillan, 1975, p 1268
28. Blackard CE: The Veterans' Administration Cooperative Urologic Research Group Studies of Carcinoma of the Prostate: A review. Cancer Chemother Rep 59:225–227, 1975
29. Goodman LS, Gilman A: The Pharmacological Basis of Therapeutics, 5th ed. New York, Macmillan, 1975, p 1299
30. Goldenberg IS, Waters MN, Ravdin RS, et al: A Report of the cooperative breast cancer group. JAMA 223:1267–1268, 1973
31. Haskell CM, Canellos GP, Leventhal BG, et al: L-Asparaginase toxicity. Cancer Res 29:974–975, 1968
32. Oettgen HF, Stephenson PA, Schwartz MK, et al: Toxicity of E. Coli L-Asparaginase in man. Cancer 25:253–278, 1970
33. Ohnuma T, Rosner F, Levy RN, et al: Treatment of adult leukemia with L-Asparaginase (NSC 109229). Cancer Chemother Rep 55:269–275, 1971
34. Weiss HD, Walker MD, Weirnik PH: Neurotoxicity of commonly used antineoplastic agents. New Engl J Med 291:75–81, 1974
35. Goodman LS, Gilman A: The pharmacological basis of therapeutics, 5th ed. New York, Macmillan, 1975, p 1294
36. Schein PS, Winokur SH: Immunosuppressive and cytotoxic chemotherapy: Long-term complications. Ann Intern Med 82:84–95, 1975
37. Rosenow EC III: The spectrum of drug-induced pulmonary disease. Ann Int Med 77:977–991, 1972
38. Heard BE, Cooke R: Busulphan lung. Thorax 23:187–193, 1968
39. Minow RA, Benjamin RS, Gottlieb JA: Adriamycin (NSC-127) cardiomyopathy—an overview with determination of risk factors. Cancer Chemother Rep 6:195–201, 1975
40. Condit PT, Chanes RE, Joel W: Renal toxicity of methotrexate. Cancer 23:126–131, 1969
41. Frei E III: Methotrexate revisited. Med Ped Oncol 2:227–241, 1976
42. Frei E III, Jaffe N, Tattersall MHN, et al: New approaches to cancer chemotherapy with methotrexate. N Engl J Med 292:846–851, 1975
43. Kennedy BJ: Mithramycin therapy in advanced testicular neoplasms. Cancer 26:755–766, 1970
44. Perlia CP, Gubisch NJ, Wolter J, et al: Mithramycin treatment of hypercalcemia. Cancer 25:389–394, 1970
45. Monto RW, Talley RW, Caldwell MJ, et al: Observations on the

mechanism of hemorrhagic toxicity in mithramycin (NSC 24559) therapy. Can Res 29:697–704, 1969

46. Wasserman T: The nitrosoureas: An outline of clinical schedules and toxic effects. Cancer Treat Rep 60:709–711, 1976

47. Durant JR, Norgard MJ, Murad TM, et al: Pulmonary toxicity associated with bischloroethyl nitrosourea (BCNU). Ann Int Med 90:191–194, 1979

48. Harmon WE, Cohen HJ, Schuberger EE, et al: Chronic renal failure in children treated with methyl CCNU. New Engl J Med 300:1200–1203, 1979

49. Piel IJ, Perlia CP: Phase II study of cis-dichloro-diammine platinum (II) NSC 119875 in combination with cyclophosphamide (NSC 26271) in the treatment of human malignancy. Cancer Chemother Rep 59:995–999, 1975

50. Rossof AH, Slayton RE, Perlia CP: Preliminary clinical experience with cis-diamminedichloroplatinum (II) (NSC 119875 CACP). Cancer 30:1451–1456, 1972

51. Yagoda A, Watson RC, Gonzalez-Vitale JC, et al: Cisdichloro-diammine platinum (II) in advanced bladder cancer. Cancer Treat Rep 60:917–923, 1976

52. Merrin C: A new method to prevent toxicity with high doses of cis-diammine platinum (therapeutic efficacy in previously treated widespread and recurrent testicular tumors). ASCO C-26, Proc Am Assoc Can Res 17:243, 1976

53. Hayes D, Cvitkovic E, Golbey R, et al: Amelioration of renal toxicity of high-dose cis-platinum diammine dichloride (CPDD) by mannitol-induced diuresis. Proc Am Assoc Can Res 17:169, 1976

54. Rozencweig M, Von Hoff DD, Slavik M, et al: Cis-diammine-dichloroplatinum (II)/A new anticancer drug. Ann Intern Med 86:803–812, 1977

55. Einhorn LH and Williams SD: The role of cis-platinum in solid-tumor therapy. New Engl J Med 300:289–291, 1979

56. Holland JF, Scharlau C, Gailani S, et al: Vincristine treatment of advanced cancer: A cooperative study of 392 cases. Can Res 33:1258–1264, 1973

57. Gottlieb RJ, Cuttner J: Vincristine-induced bladder atony. Cancer 28:674–675, 1971

58. Carmichael SM, Eagleton L, Ayers CR, et al: Orthostatic hypotension during vincristine therapy. Arch Int Med 126:290–293, 1970

59. Fine RN, Clarke RR, Shore NA: Hyponatremia and vincristine therapy. Syndrome possibility resulting from inappropriate antidiuretic hormone secretion. Am J Dis Child 112:256–259, 1966

7

THROMBOTIC AND HEMORRHAGIC MANIFESTATIONS OF MALIGNANCY

Duane K. Hasegawa
Clara D. Bloomfield

The thrombotic and hemorrhagic manifestations associated with malignancy present an extremely challenging and complex set of clinical problems. In the patient with cancer, the changes in hemostasis may be a consequence of (1) the malignancy per se; (2) the treatment of the malignant disorder; and/or (3) factors unrelated to the malignancy. This chapter will examine each of these components separately and then describe a systematic approach to the diagnosis and management of acute thrombotic and hemorrhagic emergencies in the patient with cancer.

Hemostatic Alterations Directly Related to Malignancy

Both thrombotic and hemorrhagic complications may occur in patients with malignancy as an apparent consequence of the neoplasm itself. Since the likelihood of a given type of hemostatic complication (throm-

Supported in part by National Institutes of Health grant no. CA-19527, the Masonic Hospital Fund, Inc., the Minnesota Medical Foundation, and Minnesota Medical Foundation Research Grant SMF 241-78.

The authors are indebted to Dr. J. Roger Edson for critical review of the manuscript.

141

bosis, hemorrhage, or both) varies with the nature of the malignant disorder, we will consider separately (1) solid tumors; (2) leukemia and lymphoma; (3) the dysproteinemias; and (4) the myeloproliferative disorders.

Solid Tumors

Thrombosis as a Consequence of Solid Tumors

Although both thrombotic and hemorrhagic manifestations have been recognized as a consequence of solid tumors, the former appear to be much more common. The association of thrombosis and neoplasia was first described by Trousseau over 100 years ago.[1] Thrombotic complications have subsequently been observed in association with numerous solid tumors,[2-12] the most common being listed in Table 1. The overall incidence of thrombosis in patients with cancer is estimated to be 15 percent,[3] but is probably greater for those with carcinoma of the pancreas, stomach, and lung.[2] The thrombotic manifestations consequent to solid tumors include recurrent or migratory thrombophlebitis, arterial embolization, pulmonary embolism, and nonbacterial thrombotic endocarditis.[2] In addition, thromboembolic infarction in the central nervous system associated with nonbacterial thrombotic endocarditis[13-15] and nonmetastatic superior sagittal sinus thrombosis[16] have been documented in patients with solid tumors.

It is evident that localized thrombosis can result from the direct extension and propagation of tumor into adjacent blood vessels. Distant thrombotic complications, however, must involve hemostatic changes which are directly or indirectly related to the presence of neoplastic tissue. The exact mechanisms promoting thrombosis in patients with cancer remain poorly understood. Numerous coagulation abnormalities of mild to moderate severity have been recognized in patients with solid tumors. These laboratory abnormalities vary widely according to the type of tumor, the extent of disease, and the effect of therapy. The identification of the exact mechanism responsible for thrombosis is further compounded by the poor correlation between thrombotic events and the coagulation abnormalities collectively describing a "hypercoagulable" state.[3] Recognizing these clinical and laboratory limitations, the coagulation abnormality most frequently recognized in patients with solid tumors and thrombosis is disseminated intravascular coagulation (DIC). The pathophysiology and descriptive terminology of DIC have been the subject of extensive reviews.[17-20]

DIC. General considerations. In normal hemostasis, mild tissue or blood vessel injury activates the coagulation system. The initial hemo

Table 1
Thrombotic and Hemorrhagic Manifestations Directly Related to Malignancy

Type of Malignancy	Thrombosis	/Mechanism	Hemorrhage	/Mechanism
Solid Tumors				
Pancreas	+++	⎱ Chronic DIC	++	
Stomach	+++	⎰	++	
Lung	++++		++	⎱ Acute DIC
Colon	++++		++	⎰
Breast	+++		++	
Ovary	+++		++	
Prostate	+		+++	Acute DIC ?excessive fibrinolysis?
Lymphoma	−		++	
Acute Leukemia	−		+++	Acute DIC
Acute promyelocytic leukemia (APL)	−		++++	Thrombocytopenia
Dysproteinemias	−		++	Impaired fibrin polymerization Platelet dysfunction Secondary thrombocytopenia
Myeloproliferative Disorders (MD)	++	⎱ Chronic DIC	++	⎱ Acute DIC
Polycythemia vera (PV)	++	⎰ Platelet dysfunction	+++	⎰ Platelet dysfunction
Essential thrombocythemia	++		+++	
Chronic myelogenous leukemia (CML)	+		++	Acute DIC in blast crisis

Abbreviations: − rare; + possible; ++ to +++ likely; ++++ very likely.

143

static response is thought to be the formation of a platelet plug followed by the generation of fibrin strands at the site of injury. The activation of factor XII by collagen and factor VII by "tissue factor" are two normal mechanisms for this activation. The generation of thrombin from prothrombin results from a sequence of steps involving factors XII, IX, VIII, VII, X, and V, as well as prekallikrein, high-molecular-weight kininogen, phospholipid, and calcium. Thrombin then enzymatically generates fibrin monomers from fibrinogen. Fibrin monomers form fibrin polymers which are stabilized by cross-linkages in the presence of activated factor XIII.[21]

In DIC a primary or "trigger" event initiates an exaggerated hemostatic response to tissue injury.[18] If the cause for the activation of the coagulation system is severe or ongoing, circulating thrombin is generated and fibrin formation occurs. In DIC, four major alterations in hemostasis can occur which may have major clinical ramifications. First, as a result of platelet and fibrin deposition in small blood vessels microthrombi may develop, resulting in multiple organ dysfunction. The clinically most important and apparent consequences include hypoxia, neurologic deterioration, oliguria, and decreased cardiac output.[18] Second, secondary kinin activation and platelet damage occur which may result in metabolic acidosis and hypotension. Third, if the stimulus for DIC is acute and severe, marked consumption of platelets and plasma coagulation factors occur which may result in thrombocytopenia and depletion of coagulation factors. Clinically, a hemorrhagic diathesis may result. Fourth, the plasma fibrinolytic system is activated as a secondary response to the activation of the coagulation system; this may contribute to a hemorrhagic tendency.

The activation of the fibrinolytic system in both normal and DIC states involves the formation of the proteolytic enzyme plasmin from its inactive precursor, plasminogen. A known plasminogen activator is activated factor XII, which results from the activation of the coagulation system. The circulating plasmin degrades fibrin and fibrinogen into larger split products called X and Y fragments, and finally smaller moieties called D and E fragments.[17] These fragments are collectively referred to as fibrin–fibrinogen degradation products (FDP). The larger fragments may form complexes with fibrin monomers yielding a mixture of normal fibrin polymers and abnormal soluble fibrin monomers[17] from which friable clots may develop. Plasmin may degrade or inactivate factors V, VIII, and IX as well.[20] Inhibition of platelet function in the presence of FDP has been reported and may contribute to a hemorrhagic tendency.[22]

It is apparent that the clinical consequences of DIC include both thrombosis and hemorrhage. Three categories of DIC have been identified by Cooper et al. based on the laboratory findings: decompensated, compensated, and overcompensated forms.[23] In the decompensated form of DIC, which is analogous to acute consumption coagulopathy or DIC with hemorrhagic manifestations, hypofibrinogenemia, thrombocytopenia, and elevated FDP are present. In the compensated or overcompensated forms elevated FDP are present with normal or elevated fibrinogen levels and platelet counts. Cooper et al. concluded that the form of DIC observed depended upon the capacity of the liver to generate coagulation factors and of the bone marrow to generate platelets in response to intravascular clotting. Thrombocytosis and elevated FDP have been reported in as many as 52 percent of patients with bronchogenic carcinoma and 46 percent of patients with colon cancer, and are frequently found in patients with metastatic disease and thromboembolic complications.[24]

Chronic DIC and thrombosis. The above studies suggest that a compensated or overcompensated form of DIC, often termed chronic, low-grade intravascular coagulation, frequently exists in patients with malignancy. The stimulus for this form of DIC is not well defined but may involve the slow, continuous, or intermittent introduction of thromboplastin-like substances into the circulation as a result of tumor necrosis, or the localized ischemia caused by slowly growing tumor into surrounding tissue.[25] A compensatory increase in both synthesis and consumption of coagulation factors and platelets may then develop. Little evidence exists that increased levels of coagulation factors per se are associated with an increased risk of thrombosis.[26] Likewise, there is little evidence that thrombocytosis itself is associated with thrombosis, if splenectomized patients and those with myeloproliferative disorders are excluded.[26] However, increased platelet turnover and decreased platelet survival have been observed in patients at risk for thrombosis.[26]

The presence of a chronic form of DIC in patients with those solid tumors, which have often been associated with thrombosis, has been demonstrated in several studies. Harker and Slichter observed a threefold increased rate of platelet and fibrinogen consumption in patients with carcinoma of the prostate, lung, ovary, and testes when compared to normal subjects.[25] Increased fibrinogen turnover has been reported among patients with active Hodgkin's disease and adenocarcinoma of the stomach and colon.[27] Finally, Brain et al. showed that intravascular strands of fibrin from DIC could induce fragmention of erythrocytes (schistocytes), suggesting that DIC could result in microangiopathic hemolytic anemia (MAHA).[28] Subsequently MAHA was observed in association with mucin-forming adenocarcinoma,[29] a tumor in which the nonenzymatic activation of factor X has been reported.[30]

Table 2
Coagulation Studies in Disseminated Intravascular Coagulation (DIC)

Test	Chronic DIC*	Acute DIC
Prothrombin time (PT)	Short to normal	Normal to prolonged
Partial thromboplastin time (PTT)	Short	Usually prolonged
Thrombin clotting time (TT)	Normal to prolonged	Usually prolonged
Fibrinogen	Normal to elevated	Decreased
Factor V assay	Normal to elevated	Usually decreased
Serum fibrin-fibrinogen degradation products (FDP)	Elevated	Elevated
Platelet count	Normal to elevated	Variable

*Schistocytes may be present on peripheral blood smear.

Laboratory screening for chronic DIC. The laboratory studies capable of detecting prethrombotic or hypercoagulable states are limited in specificity.[26] No single test is specific for DIC both because of the multiple causes of the process and the numerous disorders which alter coagulation studies. Consequently the laboratory evaluation and monitoring of coagulation abnormalities in patients with malignancy must rely on a battery of coagulation screening tests. Table 2 outlines the most useful studies for the evaluation and monitoring of chronic DIC. It is not an exhaustive list of all studies which are applicable to DIC, but rather represents those tests which are reproducible, accurate, widely available, and capable of being rapidly performed.

These coagulation screening tests for the diagnosis of chronic DIC should be performed under the following clinical situations:

1. When the diagnosis of malignancy is made or suspected.
2. When tumor recurrence or progression is suspected or documented.
3. Before and after surgical procedures in patients with malignancies where significant tissue injury is anticipated.
4. Prior to and during antineoplastic therapy including surgery, chemotherapy, and radiation therapy.
5. When overt thrombotic complications develop during the disease course.

In any individual patient, both the cause or causes of and the process of DIC itself may vary with time. Therefore, sequential testing is essential. The *changes* in the coagulation screening tests are as significant as are the actual values.

The one-stage *prothrombin time* (PT) is either normal or slightly shortened in chronic DIC. Elevated factor V activity, which may shorten the PT, has been described in patients with malignancy.[4] We have observed a short PT and high factor V activity in patients with solid tumors with chronic DIC. A prolonged PT suggests additional coagulation disorders which are described later.

The *partial thromboplastin time* (PTT) is usually short in chronic DIC[4,19] which is partly explained by the elevated factor VIII activity which has been observed in patients with malignancy.[4,31]

Prolonged *thrombin clotting times* (TTs) are frequently observed in patients with malignant disorders and chronic DIC.[24,32] Prolonged TTs correlate with elevated FDP.[24] FDP may impair the rate of fibrin polymerization,[18] thus causing abnormally prolonged TTs.

Normal or elevated *fibrinogen* levels are present in low-grade DIC.[4,32-34] Hyperfibrinogenemia is thought to occur in states of intravascular clotting where the hepatic synthesis of fibrinogen "compensates" or "overcompensates" for increased fibrinogen consumption.[18] Hypofibrinogenemia is most often associated with acute DIC or liver disease,[19] both of which are discussed below.

Serum fibrin–fibrinogen degradation products (FDP) are typically elevated in chronic DIC.[24,32-34] However, elevated FDPs are not specific for DIC, and have been observed following surgery,[35] infection,[23] collagen disorders,[23] and deep venous thrombosis.[36] FDP levels are also influenced by renal function and by the ability of the reticuloendothelial system to clear FDP from the circulation.[3]

Normal-to-elevated *platelet counts* have been frequently observed in patients with solid tumors who have chronic DIC.[4,24] Automated platelet counts are reliable provided that interfering debris is absent from the specimen.

Examination of the *peripheral blood* film will aid in confirming the platelet count and demonstrate the presence of schistocytes in some cases of chronic DIC.

The so-called paracoagulation tests such as the ethanol gel[37] or protamine sulfate precipitation[38] tests are useful if available. These tests detect soluble fibrin monomer complexes in plasma, which if present suggest the generation of thrombin associated with DIC.

Hemorrhage as a Consequence of Solid Tumors
(Prostatic Carcinoma)

Although thrombosis and chronic DIC in its compensated and overcompensated forms are the most frequently encountered manifestations of abnormal hemostasis in patients with most solid tumors, hemorrhage and acute (decompensated) DIC occur as a consequence of solid tumors. The solid tumor most frequently associated with hemorrhage and acute DIC is carcinoma of the prostate. In Goodnight's review of solid tumors in which hemorrhage and abnormal coagulation studies were reported, 24 of 45 cases involved adenocarcinoma of the prostate; of the remaining 21 cases, 9 were adenocarcinoma of the stomach or pancreas.[39] The bleeding sites were similar to those reported in acute leukemia (see next section) except for less-frequent central nervous system involvement and a greater incidence of gastrointestinal hemorrhage.[39]

Two possible hemostatic abnormalities may explain the excessive bleeding accompanying prostatic carcinoma. First, hypofibrinogenemia, low factor V, and thrombocytopenia were reported in most of the cases reviewed by Goodnight.[39] This suggests acute DIC with secondary fibrinolysis. The introduction of thromboplastin-like material into the circulation is the probable trigger for acute consumption of clotting factors and platelets with secondary activation of fibrinolysis. DIC probably exists prior to therapy, and subsequent to it acutely worsens. This is suggested by the observed higher preoperative serum FDP levels and greater operative blood loss per gram of resected tissue in transurethral resection of adenocarcinoma compared to benign prostatic hyperplasia.[40] A second abnormality may be excessive fibrinolytic activity. Forty percent of the cases reviewed by Goodnight had marked shortening of the clot lysis time,[39] which is a feature of excessive fibrinolysis. It is known that normal prostatic tissue is a source of plasminogen activator.[41] In adenocarcinoma of the prostate, trauma to the prostate may result in excessive localized or more generalized primary activation of fibrinolysis if this plasminogen activator gains access into the circulation.[42]

Primary fibrinolysis can result in hemorrhage. It can be diagnosed by the presence of a shortened euglobulin clot lysis time of less than 2 hours, a normal or stable platelet count, hypofibrinogenemia, and elevated serum FDP.[41] The incidence of primary fibrinolysis consequent to malignant disorders is not known, although increased fibrinolytic activity has been found in patients with a variety of solid tumors[43,44] and acute leukemia.[45]

Acute Leukemia and Lymphoma

In contrast to the situation with solid tumors, hemorrhagic rather than thrombotic manifestations are the most common hemostatic consequences of the hematologic malignancies, especially acute leukemia. Hemorrhagic complications as a consequence of these tumors usually result from acute DIC with secondary fibrinolysis and/or thrombocytopenia.

Acute DIC with Secondary Fibrinolysis

In Goodnight's literature review, 76 of the 134 reported cases of malignancy in which both hemorrhage and laboratory evidence of DIC were present were classified as acute promyelocytic leukemia (APL).[39] Subsequent reports have confirmed the very high incidence of hemorrhage and DIC in APL.[46-48] Similar clinical and laboratory observations have been made in other foms of acute leukemia,[49] including acute monoblastic leukemia,[50] acute lymphoblastic leukemia (ALL),[51] and the blast crisis of chronic myelogenous leukemia.[52,53]

The hemorrhagic manifestations in patients with APL include petechiae, ecchymoses, hematuria, bleeding from venipuncture sites, and epistaxis.[54] Nearly half of the cases in Goodnight's review had central nervous system bleeding.[39] In APL, the activation of intravascular clotting is attributed to the procoagulant activity of the neoplastic promyelocyte, which has been shown to accelerate the recalcification and partial thromboplastin times of normal plasma.[45] Increased tissue factor activity has been observed in the granular fraction of APL cells, suggesting activation of the clotting system through the extrinsic pathway.[45] In patients with APL, acute DIC may be documented at diagnosis and is often exacerbated during induction chemotherapy; resolution of DIC generally occurs when remission is achieved.[48] This suggests that the rapid destruction of leukemic cells is associated with acute DIC.

In acute DIC, the consumption of clotting factors and platelets is clinically manifested by the presence of generalized bleeding. As previously mentioned, microthrombi from DIC may result in multiple organ system damage. In addition, DIC may result in a shock-like syndrome due to deranged circulatory dynamics or the trapping of whole blood or plasma in damaged tissue.[18]

Table 2 lists the laboratory studies which are readily available for the rapid evaluation of acute hemorrhagic episodes where the diagnosis of acute DIC is clinically suspected.

The *PT* is usually normal to prolonged in acute DIC. Prolongation of the PT usually reflects low factor V activity and hypofibrinogenemia, which are indicative of a consumptive process. In our laboratory, factor V assays[55] are routinely performed on specimens yielding a prolonged PT. If the factor V activity and fibrinogen are normal, and the PT prolonged, vitamin K deficiency or warfarin therapy should be suspected. Factor V deficiency and a prolonged PT are compatible with acute DIC, but are also found in severe liver disease.[56]

The *PTT* is usually prolonged in acute DIC due to depletion of factors V, VIII, and fibrinogen. A normal PTT may be observed in a patient with acute DIC who previously had a shortened PTT. This illustrates the necessity of sequential monitoring of the PTT in clinically suspected cases of DIC. Occasionally a short PTT or a specimen which clots prior to recalcification may be observed. This probably represents the presence of activated clotting factors in DIC.[20]

The *TT* is typically prolonged in acute DIC due to plasma fibrinogen levels of less than 0.1 g/dl and the presence of FDP.

Hypofibrinogenemia in the absence of severe liver disease is typically present in acute DIC. Normal fibrinogen level in the appropriate clinical setting may indicate that there was a preexisting compensated or overcompensated form of chronic DIC.[18]

Serum FDP are elevated in both acute and chronic DIC and must therefore be interpreted according to the changes in the PT, PTT, TT, fibrinogen, and platelet count.

Thrombocytopenia is often seen in acute DIC. The assessment of thrombocytopenia requires an accurate platelet count, especially in patients with hematologic malignancies in whom spuriously high platelet counts from automated methods due to cytoplasmic fragments have been observed.[57] Platelet counting by phase-contrast microscopy is the most reliable method in these circumstances. The consumption of platelets in DIC is suggested by the lack of a rise in the platelet count following platelet transfusions if splenic sequestration and/or immune destruction are ruled out.

Thrombocytopenia

Mechanisms. Thrombocytopenia is a major contributor to both superficial and life-threatening hemorrhagic events at diagnosis and during the course of therapy in patients with hematologic malignancies, especially those with acute leukemia. At least four causes of thrombocytopenia can be identified as a consequence of the malignancy. First, thrombocytopenia may result from extensive bone marrow involvement by tumor. This is common at diagnosis in acute leukemia, and may occur later in the course of many malignancies. Second, as previously discussed, thrombocytopenia is frequently associated with acute DIC.[39] Third, hypersplenism with splenic pooling of platelets may contribute to thrombocytopenia.[58] Fourth, on rare occasions immune thrombocytopenia has been observed in non-Hodgkin's lymphoma,[59-61] Hodgkin's disease,[61,62] ALL,[63] and chronic lymphocytic leukemia (CLL).[59] Immune thrombocytopenia has been associated with Coomb's positive hemolytic anemia in CLL[59] and with Hodgkin's disease[62]; in these diseases, there seems to be poor correlation between the disease activity and the presence of immune thrombo-cytopenia.[59,62] In addition, thrombocytopenia may result from myelosup-pressive chemotherapy as discussed in the section on Hemostatic Alterations Associated with Chemotherapy.

Evaluation. The presence of thrombocytopenia in patients with malignancies requires a systematic investigation. Bone marrow aspirates and biopsies are necessary to evaluate thrombocytopenia related to mar-row metastases and chemotherapy-induced myelosuppression. Monitor-ing for chemotherapy-related thrombocytopenia requires frequent platelet counts since both the absolute platelet count and the changes in the plate-let count are important features in evaluating hemorrhagic tendencies or symptoms. Estimation of spleen size by clinical means, or if indicated by liver–spleen scan, is necessary if hypersplenism is being considered as a cause of thrombocytopenia. Immune thrombocytopenia, particularly in lymphoproliferative disorders, should be suspected if bone marrow studies, splenomegaly, or infection do not explain the presence of throm-bocytopenia.[59]

Other abnormalities in hemostasis such as DIC, uremia, liver disease, and impaired platelet function may singly or in combination contribute to the hemorrhagic complications in thrombocytopenic patients. Conse-quently, a systematic evaluation to rule out these entities is also an inte-gral part of the evaluation and management of thrombocytopenia.

Treatment. If significant hemorrhage associated with thrombo-cytopenia from decreased platelet production or increased consumption occurs, transfusions with platelet concentrates are necessary. In our expe-rience, transfusions when the platelet count is $20-25 \times 10^9$/liter or less has minimized the frequency of hemorrhagic complications. In thrombocyto-penic patients requiring surgery, preoperative platelet transfusions to achieve a platelet count above 100×10^9/liter are essential for normal in-traoperative and postoperative hemostasis. Following initial platelet transfusions, platelet count determinations should be performed within 6 hours and subsequently on a daily basis for documenting a rise in the platelet count and for correlation with the clinical response to platelet transfusions. If long-term support with transfusions of platelet concen-trates is anticipated, the use of HLA-compatible platelets should be strongly considered.

In immune thrombocytopenia, management usually requires both treatment of the underlying malignant disorder and the use of glucocorti-coids and possibly splenectomy.[59,62-63] If splenectomy is performed platelet concentrates must be available for intraoperative and postoperative use. In our experience platelet transfusions are most effective following the ligation of the splenic blood vessels immediately prior to splenectomy. Additional platelet transfusions are frequently necessary until hemostasis is achieved postoperatively.

Dysproteinemias

Associated Hemostatic Alterations

Numerous hemostatic abnormalities have been recognized as a consequence of multiple myeloma and macroglobulinemia of Waldenstrom; these often result in a hemorrhagic tendency of mild to moderate severity.[3,64] Hemorrhagic symptoms have been observed when the circulating paraprotein concentration exceeds 5 g/dl.[65] The incidence of bleeding seems greater in patients with Waldenstrom's macroglobulinemia and IgA myeloma than in those with IgG myeloma.[66] Neither an increased bleeding tendency nor coagulation abnormalities are common in isolated light-chain disease.[67]

In patients with dysproteinemias, the laboratory evaluation of both bleeding tendencies and acute hemorrhagic events will often identify abnormalities in plasma coagulation and platelet function tests. In addition, thrombocytopenia and abnormalities in hepatic and renal function, which often complicate these disorders, may significantly alter normal hemostasis and contribute to a bleeding tendency.[3]

In patients with dysproteinemias, the most common plasma coagulation abnormality is the inhibition of fibrin monomer polymerization by the paraprotein.[3,64,67] The mechanism for this inhibition may involve the conversion of fibrinogen to fibrin monomer, the aggregation of fibrin monomers into polymers, or both.[68,69] Abnormalities in fibrin monomer polymerization can be detected by the presence of a prolonged TT, if other causes for TT abnormalities such as hypofibrinogenemia and elevated serum FDP are excluded. In patients with dysproteinemias who have normal fibrinogen and serum FDP values, a prolonged TT has been correlated with an increased bleeding tendency.[3] Frequent TT determinations are thus useful for monitoring the effect of the paraprotein on hemostasis.

Deficiencies of plasma coagulation factors II, V, VII, VIII, X, and XI have been observed in patients with dysproteinemias but with less frequency than a prolonged TT.[3,64,67] The interaction of IgA, IgG, or IgM paraproteins with one or more plasma coagulation factors is thought to account for the observed deficiency states. PT and PTT should be performed as screening procedures for the detection of these factor deficiencies. Low levels of factors II, V, VII, X, and XI occur not only in the presence of paraproteins but also with liver disease.[70] If the PT and/or PTT are prolonged, hepatic dysfunction should first be evaluated by additional laboratory studies such as serum albumin, transaminase, and bilirubin determinations. In the absence of liver dysfunction, a prolonged PT and/or PTT requires specific factor assays for detection of individual factor deficiencies. In patients with macroglobulinemia with a prolonged PTT, factor VIII assays are useful for screening for factor VIII antibodies, which have been reported with this disorder.[67,71] If the PT and PTT are normal, the likelihood of a significant factor deficiency is remote. Both the PT and PTT are useful screening tests in the long-term followup of patients with dysproteinemias in whom coagulation factor abnormalities were previously identified.

Laboratory abnormalities consistent with chronic DIC may occur in patients with dysproteinemias, although these are less common than TT abnormalities.[3] Since mildly prolonged TT may be present in chronic DIC, evaluation for DIC in these patients requires fibrinogen and serum FDP levels in addition to the PT, PTT, TT, and platelet count.

Thrombocytopenia unquestionably contributes to hemorrhagic complications in patients with dysproteinemias. The causes of decreased platelet counts in these disorders include bone marrow infiltration by tumor cells, splenic sequestration, and the suppressive effect of chemotherapy on platelet production. Documentation and recognition of the causes of thrombocytopenia are an integral part of the evaluation of a bleeding tendency in these patients.

Platelet dysfunction is a major determinant in the hemorrhagic manifestations seen in patients with dysproteinemias. Although not entirely defined, it appears that the platelet function abnormalities are associated with the coating or interaction of the platelet membrane with abnormal immunoglobulins.[67] There appears to be good correlation between the quantity of IgG myeloma proteins, in both serum and bound to platelets, with abnormalities in standard platelet function studies.[72]

As many as 70 percent of patients with multiple myeloma have been found to have abnormal platelet aggregation when tested with collagen, ADP, and epinephrine.[3] The frequency of abnormal platelet aggregation studies may, however, not correlate well with clinical bleeding.[3] Prolonged bleeding times and decreased platelet adhesiveness have also been described in patients with dysproteinemias,[65,67] and both tests appear to correlate well with hemorrhagic tendencies.[3]

To summarize, several hemostatic abnormalities may coexist in patients with dysproteinemias. A systematic screening for them should include a PT, PTT, TT, fibrinogen, serum FDP, platelet count, bleeding time, platelet adhesiveness studies, quantitation of the serum paraprotein, and studies of hepatic and renal function. These studies are clinically indicated at diagnosis, prior to surgery, and if hemorrhagic events supervene.

Plasmapheresis for Treatment of Clinical Bleeding

The treatment of bleeding in patients with dysproteinemias must take into account all potential causes for hemorrhage, including accompanying hepatic or renal disease. A major objective of treatment involves the reduction of the paraprotein levels with chemotherapy and/or radiation therapy. A higher incidence of bleeding has been reported if the total serum protein concentration exceeds 8 g/dl.[67] Following effective therapy, improvement in both platelet function and coagulation factor abnormalities can be expected in the majority of cases.

Thrombocytopenia as a result of either the presence of tumor or cytotoxic therapy may cause major bleeding problems. Platelet transfusions are unlikely to control acute bleeding episodes in thrombocytopenic patients with elevated levels of abnormal immunoglobulins and in nondialyzed uremic patients. Acute serious hemorrhagic events have been successfully managed by prompt plasmapheresis, often on a repeated basis, for the rapid lowering of the paraprotein levels.[3,64,67,68]

Plasmapheresis per se may cause significant hemostatic abnormalities. Following plasmapheresis and replacement with fluids devoid of coagulation factors, Flaum et al. documented a significant reduction in platelet count, fibrinogen, levels of factors V, VIII, VII-X complex, IX, and X, and prolongation of the PT, PTT, and TT in patients who were hemostatically normal prior to plasmapheresis.[73] The authors noted that all hemostatic abnormalities had returned to normal 24 hours after plasmapheresis and that no clinical bleeding developed incident to the procedure. Keller et al. observed prolonged PTs, PTTs, and TTs, and reduced fibrinogen levels and platelet counts in 12 patients with malignant paraproteinemia who were repeatedly treated with plasmapheresis.[74] Bleeding episodes occurred in 2 of 12 patients, both of whom were thrombocytopenic prior to plasmapheresis.

These studies suggest that plasma coagulation factor deficiency states and thrombocytopenia must be recognized prior to plasmapheresis.[73] If the fibrinogen is ≤ 0.1 g/dl or if the plasma coagulation factors are ≤ 50 percent of normal prior to plasmapheresis, replacement with fresh-frozen plasma may prevent hemorrhage. Similarly, if the preplasmapheresis platelet count is <100 × 10⁹/liter, platelet transfusion after plasmapheresis may control bleeding if it occurs.

Myeloproliferative Disorders (MDs)

Thrombohemorrhagic Complications

A thrombotic and bleeding tendency often co-exist as a consequence of myeloproliferative disorders (MDs). Thrombohemorrhagic complications have been reported to be more frequent in patients with essential thrombocythemia and polycythemia vera (PV) than in those with myelofibrosis and chronic myelogenous leukemia (CML).[75] Patients with essential thrombocythemia frequently have gastrointestinal bleeding, spontaneous bruising, and splenic vein thrombosis[76]; signs of arterial occlusion without venous thrombosis may be the presenting clinical feature.[77] Among patients with PV, thrombotic complications and consequent mortality have been reported in 26–63 percent and 20–40 percent respectively, and hemorrhagic complications and consequent mortality in 16–35 percent and 6–30 percent respectively.[78–81] In PV,[81] essential thrombocythemia,[76,77] and CML,[82] a reduction of thrombohemorrhagic complications occurs with reduction of the red cell mass and/or thrombocytosis by adequate treatment.

The incidence of postoperative thrombohemorrhagic complications in patients with MD is very high. A 45-percent incidence in 54 patients with PV in whom a variety of major surgical procedures were performed has been reported.[83] Postsplenectomy fatalities have been observed associated with hemorrhage in patients with CML and thrombosis of the renal, portal, and mesenteric veins in patients with other MDs.[84,85] It appears that the preoperative utilization of chemotherapy to normalize the hematologic status in patients with PV significantly reduces the frequency of postoperative thrombohemorrhagic complications.[83] Similarly, in patients with CML undergoing splenectomy, the preoperative reduction of the peripheral leukocyte count to normal or near normal with chemotherapy has been reported to reduce the frequency of postoperative bleeding.[85]

It is evident that some but not all patients with MDs develop thrombohemorrhagic complications and that improvement in the underlying hematologic disorder is generally associated with the development of fewer complications. The mechanisms responsible for thrombosis or hemorrhage are complex and not fully understood. In addition, the laboratory identification of high-risk patients is difficult due to the poor clinical correlation with abnormalities in plasma coagulation and platelet function.

Therefore the importance of clinical awareness of a potential co-existing thrombotic and hemorrhagic tendency cannot be overemphasized.

Hemostatic Laboratory Abnormalities

The hemostatic laboratory abnormalities typically observed in patients with MDs can be grouped into 3 categories: (1) chronic DIC; (2) abnormal platelet morphology and thrombocytosis; and (3) platelet dysfunction. Laboratory evaluation is indicated in the following clinical situations: at diagnosis or prior to therapy; prior to anticipated surgery; and if acute thrombotic or hemorrhagic complications develop.

Chronic DIC.   In patients with MDs chronic DIC is frequently seen. This has been demonstrated by increased platelet[86] and fibrinogen[87,88] turnover, the presence of soluble fibrin monomer complexes,[89] and correction of coagulation tests of DIC by a short course of heparin.[88,90] These studies suggest that patients with MDs require evaluation for chronic DIC. This should be done with the tests outlined in Table 2. If laboratory evidence of chronic DIC exists, the patient must be watched even more carefully for the development of thrombosis.

Abnormal platelet morphology and thrombocytosis.   In addition to chronic DIC, abnormalities in platelet morphology and thrombocytosis are frequently seen in patients with MDs at diagnosis and throughout the course of the disease. Examination of the peripheral blood film for platelet morphology will frequently show abnormally large hypogranular or agranular platelets, platelets without pseudopods, and platelets with abnormal blunted pseudopods.[91] The platelet count will frequently reveal thrombocytosis not only in patients with essential thrombocythemia[76] but also in those with PV, myeloid metaplasia, and CML.[75] In these patients the degree of thrombocytosis and the frequency of thrombotic and hemorrhagic complications vary widely, which suggests that thrombocytosis alone does not fully account for these events.[75]

Platelet dysfunction.   Platelet dysfunction is the most common hemostatic laboratory abnormality in patients with MDs. Template bleeding times are probably the most widely available test of platelet function for clinical purposes. Reliable results can be obtained provided that the platelet count is greater than 100×10^9/liter and that drugs known to cause prolonged bleeding times are avoided.[92] Prolonged bleeding times have frequently been observed in patients with MDs.[75,76,81,87,93–95] The result from this test alone, however, does not consistently correlate with either thrombocytosis or thrombohemorrhagic complications.

The most consistently observed abnormality in platelet function in patients with MDs is diminished platelet aggregation with adenosine diphosphate, epinephrine, and collagen. These abnormalities may be present both in patients with and without existing thrombohemorrhagic symptoms.[75,81,85,93-96] However, patients having plasma coagulation and/or platelet function abnormalities or thrombocytosis[94] should be regarded to have a thrombotic and/or hemorrhagic tendency. In patients with essential thrombocythemia, hemorrhagic symptoms can be controlled by lowering the platelet count with therapy.[76] In patients with CML antileukemic chemotherapy may result in the concomitant correction of hemorrhagic symptoms, abnormal platelet aggregation studies, and prolonged bleeding times.[93] In patients with all forms of MD, platelet transfusions may be necessary in controlling acute bleeding episodes,[93] particularly with operative procedures.

Hemostatic Alterations Associated with Chemotherapy

Chemotherapy has been associated with numerous hemostatic abnormalities including thrombocytopenia, DIC, decreased synthesis of various clotting factors, platelet dysfunction, and increased fibrinolytic activity. Thrombocytopenia and DIC are the most frequently encountered, clinically significant chemotherapy-induced hemostatic derangements, both in patients with solid tumors and in those with hematologic malignancies. In patients with solid tumors, the most frequent cause of all hemorrhagic episodes is probably chemotherapy-induced thrombocytopenia.[97] Belt et al. showed that 49 percent of the observed bleeding complications in 75 patients with solid tumors were attributable to drug-induced thrombocytopenia.[97] These authors observed that thrombocytopenia or a falling platelet count preceded hemorrhage, and that both the frequency and the amount of bleeding were related to the platelet count. In their series, the incidence of hemorrhage was 38 percent and 11.5 percent when the platelet count was less than 10×10^9/liter and 20×10^9/liter, respectively. In hematologic malignancies, thrombocytopenia secondary to myelosuppressive chemotherapy also significantly contributes to a bleeding tendency. In addition, chemotherapy may augment or induce DIC[3] in patients with solid tumors[4] and those with acute leukemia,[50,98] especially

Table 3
Antineoplastic Agents Associated with Abnormalities in Tests of Plasma Coagulation and Platelet Function

Antineoplastic Agent	Hemostatic Alteration	Clinical Consequence	Treatment if Clinical Consequence
Actinomycin D	Decreased synthesis of vitamin K dependent factors	Hemorrhage	Vitamin K, transfusions with fresh-frozen plasma
Anthracycline antibiotics	Increased fibrinolytic activity	Hemorrhage	Correct all accompanying hemostatic abnormalities, e.g., thrombocytopenia
L-Asparaginase	Hypofibrinogenemia; decreased factors IX and XI	Hemorrhage rare except with thrombocytopenia	Cryoprecipitate and/or platelets
	Antithrombin III deficiency	Thrombosis	?Fresh-frozen plasma?
Methotrexate	Chronic hepatic dysfunction	Hemorrhage	Vitamin K, fresh-frozen plasma
	Acute hepatic toxicity from high-dose methotrexate	Rare	Cryoprecipitate if hypofibrinogenemic —
Mithramycin	Platelet dysfunction, decreased factors II, V, VII-X	Hemorrhage	Platelet concentrates Vitamin K, ?fresh-frozen plasma?
Vincristine	Platelet dysfunction	Rare	—
Glucocoticoids	Elevated factors II, V, VII, VIII and X	?Thrombosis?	Anticoagulation
Estrogens	Elevated fibrinogen, factors VII, VIII, IX and X, plasminogen, decreased antithrombin III activity	Thrombosis	Anticoagulation

APL.[48] This is probably due to tumor lysis and consequent release of thromboplastin-like substances.

Although thrombocytopenia may result from most chemotherapeutic agents, abnormalities in tests of plasma coagulation and platelet function have also been identified in patients treated with certain antineoplastic agents. The chemotherapeutic agents most commonly associated with hemostatic abnormalities other than thrombocytopenia are listed in Table 3. These agents and the hemostatic alterations they induce are further discussed below.

Actinomycin-D

Actinomycin-D has been shown to antagonize vitamin K, which may result in deficiencies of factors II, VII, IX, and X.[3,99] PT and PTT determinations can identify the potential hemorrhagic side effects following its administration. If serious bleeding develops following actinomycin-D therapy, and if the PT and PTT are prolonged, vitamin K administration and transfusions with fresh-frozen plasma may be necessary.

Anthracycline Antibiotics

Both doxorubicin and daunorubicin appear to activate the fibrinolytic system. This has been suggested by both in vitro[100,101] and in vivo[100] studies. Following doxorubicin therapy, patients with solid tumors have been observed to have elevated FDP, circulating plasmin, and subungual hemorrhage.[100] Primary activation of fibrinolysis without DIC appears to occur. Useful pre- and posttreatment screening tests for primary fibrinolysis include PT, PTT, TT, fibrinogen, serum FDP, and euglobulin clot lysis time determinations. Elevated serum FDP values and a reduced euglobulin clot lysis time may indicate a potential hemorrhagic tendency from primary fibrinolysis. If prolongation of the PT and PTT accompany the above laboratory abnormalities, acute DIC with secondary fibrinolysis should be suspected.

L-Asparaginase

Plasma coagulation abnormalities, particularly hypofibrinogenemia, have been frequently observed in patients treated with L-asparaginase.[102-105] Other reported abnormalities include decreased factors IX and XI.[105] These three alterations result in prolonged PT, PTT, and TT. The fibrinogen abnormalities following L-asparaginase therapy appear to result from decreased fibrinogen synthesis.[106] Although significant hypofibrinogene-mia frequently occurs during L-asparaginase therapy, hemorrhagic com-plications are very rare[105] provided that severe thrombocytopenia does not develop.

An association between antithrombin III deficiency and L-asparagin-ase therapy has also been documented.[107] Antithrombin III, a naturally occurring protease inhibitor, inhibits activated factors XII, XI, X, IX, and thrombin and plasmin, thus providing a protective mechanism against thrombosis.[26] Inherited antithrombin III deficiency has been associated with a high incidence of thrombosis.[108] The antithrombin III deficiency observed in patients treated with L-asparaginase may result from the elab-oration of an abnormal antithrombin III protein[109] or decreased antithrom-bin synthesis. Recently, central nervous system hemorrhagic and throm-botic complications have been observed in some children with ALL within 2 weeks following the completion of L-asparaginase therapy.[110,111] Hypofibrinogenemia, antithrombin III deficiency, or both were observed prior to these complications.

These observations suggest that the potential of a hemorrhagic and thrombotic tendency co-exist after L-asparaginase therapy. In addition to close clinical monitoring, patients receiving L-asparaginase should be fol-lowed with sequential PT, PTT, TT, fibrinogen, and platelet count deter-minations. In patients at high risk for developing thrombotic complica-tions such as those with advanced age, prolonged immobilization, and a previous history of either venous thromboembolism or cerebral vascular accidents, antithrombin III assays, if abnormal, may identify patients at additional risk for thrombotic complications. In our experience, hemor-rhagic complications from L-asparaginase-induced hypofibrinogenemia have been largely associated with severe thrombocytopenia. These epi-sodes have been successfully treated with modest transfusions with cryo-precipitate and/or platelets. Little is known about the treatment of acute thrombotic events following L-asparaginase therapy; transfusions with fresh-frozen plasma may be useful.[111]

Methotrexate

The potential hemostatic derangements from methotrexate therapy, aside from thrombocytopenia from myelosuppression, appear to result from hepatic dysfunction.[112] Long-term, low-dose methotrexate adminis-tration has been associated with cirrhosis,[113] which potentially could result in prolongation of the PT and PTT due to multiple coagulation factor deficiencies. In addition, acute hepatocellular enzyme elevation, transient prolongation of the pretreatment PT, and decreased factor VII levels have been associated with high-dose methotrexate followed by citrovorum-factor rescue.[114] Before and during methotrexate administration, the PT and PTT are clinically useful tests for detecting these changes in hemostasis.

Mithramycin

Mithramycin therapy has been associated with three major hemostatic abnormalities which may result in hemorrhage: thrombocytopenia, platelet dysfunction, and decreased clotting factors. Thrombocytopenia may develop from bone marrow suppression.[115,116] Platelet function abnormalities, including prolonged bleeding times and impaired platelet aggregation, have been noted shortly after initiation of mithramycin therapy; these have resulted in mucocutaneous bleeding in patients with platelet counts greater than 100×10^9/liter.[117] Decreased levels of factors II, V, and VII-X complex after mithramycin treatment have been described.[116] These may be the result of DIC[3] or hepatic toxicity.

Because of the hemostatic abnormalities induced by mithramycin, frequent determinations of the platelet count, PT, and PTT during mithramycin therapy are useful tests in monitoring the patient for development of a bleeding tendency or episode. Early indicators of potential bleeding include a lengthening of the bleeding time, a falling platelet count, and a rising serum LDH.[115,117] In addition, fibrinogen and serum FDP determinations will aid in the detection of DIC in suspected cases. Hemorrhage may be minimized by temporary discontinuation of mithramycin therapy.[117] Platelet transfusions and correction of a prolonged PT and PTT, if present, with vitamin K administration may be necessary if severe hemorrhagic complications develop.

Vincristine

Vincristine administration frequently causes platelet dysfunction, but this rarely is associated with hemorrhage.[118] Following the administration of vincristine (1.5mg/m² per dose), absent epinephrine- or ADP-induced secondary aggregation are observed with normal bleeding times, and normal collagen-induced platelet aggregation.[118] Platelets incubated at higher doses of vincristine in vitro have been shown to have similar abnormalities in platelet aggregation.[118,119]

Glucocorticoids

Glucocorticoids appear to increase levels of factors II, V, VII, VIII, and X; the mechanism for this is unknown. In patients with nonmalignant disorders, elevated levels of these factors were observed after 3 or more days of prednisone, 60 mg daily.[120] As a result of the increase in these clotting factors, shortened PT and PTT are ordinarily found. If the pretreatment PT and PTT are shortened, such as in chronic DIC, further shortening of the PT and PTT may result following glucocorticoid therapy. Although an increased tendency to thrombosis has been described in Cushing's syndrome, its relation to the increase in levels of clotting factors remains to be established.

Estrogens

Estrogens have been firmly associated with an increased risk of venous thromboembolism.[121] The estrogen dose and risk of venous thromboembolism have been positively correlated among oral contraceptive users.[122] Estrogen therapy, particularly diethylstilbestrol[123] in patients with prostatic carcinoma, has also been associated with an increased incidence of thrombotic complications, including strokes.[124] In pregnant women and among oral contraceptive users, intimal proliferative lesions in both veins and arteries and decreased venous tone in the calf of the leg may contribute to the thrombogenic effect of estrogen.[125] In addition, numerous plasma coagulation abnormalities have been reported including increased factors VII,[126] VIII,[126] IX,[126] X,[127] and fibrinogen,[128] and increased plasminogen[129] and decreased antithrombin III activity.[129]

In patients on estrogen therapy, coagulation screening studies typically show a short-to-normal PT, short PTT, and a mildly elevated fibrinogen. Unfortunately no laboratory test, including decreased antithrombin III activity, has been highly predictive of which patients will develop thrombotic complications. Consequently, patients on estrogen therapy must be closely monitored clinically for the development of thrombosis. Patients with additional risk factors known to be associated with thrombotic complications should be especially closely monitored.

Hemostatic Alterations Unrelated to Malignancy that May Occur in Patients with Cancer

Factors Predisposing to Thrombosis

As previously discussed, thrombotic complications as a consequence of a number of malignancies occur. Moreover, treatment, e.g., estrogen therapy,[124,130] may predispose to thromoembolism. In addition, in the patient with cancer, clinical conditions unrelated to the malignancy per se or

Table 4
Conditions Predisposing to Thrombosis That May Occur
in Patients with Cancer But Are Not Directly Related
to the Malignancy or Its Treatment

Advanced age and prolonged immobilization
Previous history of venous thromboembolism
Heart disease—arrhythmias or congestive heart failure
Gram-negative infections
Obesity
Operations
    Intraabdominal including pelvic and prostate
    Lower extremity including hip

---

its treatment frequently exist which predispose to venous thromboembolism. These risk factors for the development of venous thromboembolism have been recently reviewed[125,131] and are listed in Table 4. Clinically, the magnitude of the increase in risk or the possible cumulative effect upon risk from these conditions has not been determined.[125] However, if multiple thrombotic risk factors are present, thrombotic complications are probably more likely.

The pathogenesis of venous thromboembolism is most often described in terms of Virchow's triad: (1) localized venous trauma, (2) venous stasis, and (3) alterations in blood coagulability. Although the mechanisms by which these three factors interrelate in thrombus formation have not been clearly defined, vascular injury[132] and venous stasis[125] are recognized as the most frequent causes of thrombosis. Numerous alterations in blood coagulability have been described in patients with thromboembolic disorders; however, few if any of these alterations demonstrate sufficient specificity to be considered causal in all thrombotic events.[26]

Since no single laboratory test is specific, the recognition of clinical conditions known to be associated with thrombosis will serve as a useful guide for more careful clinical monitoring of the patient.

Age and Immobilization

The prevalence of pulmonary embolism increases almost linearly with advancing age.[125] The increased frequency of pulmonary embolism after the age of 30 years has been chiefly attributed to either heart disease or malignancy.[133] Immobilization for 1 week or more is considered a high-risk factor for thrombosis[125]; this may apply to the elderly bedridden cancer patient with or without actual lower-extremity paralysis. Clinical situations in which immobilization may occur include a protracted postoperative course, congestive heart failure, severe infections, and neurologic disorders. The frequency of autopsy-proven venous thrombosis and pulmonary embolism is greater after 1 week of immobilization.[134] Within 10 days of the onset of paralytic strokes, the observed prevalence of deep venous thrombosis in the paralyzed lower extremity may approach 60 percent.[135]

Previous History of Venous Thromboembolism

A history of prior venous thromboembolism is a major risk factor for future thrombotic complications.[125] In a prospective study of 6,527 hospitalized patients, a previous history of pulmonary embolism was the single most important factor associated with the development of confirmed pulmonary embolic disease.[136] Among postoperative patients having a previous history of lower-extremity venous thrombosis, the prevalence of lower-limb deep-vein thrombosis has been reported to be 68 percent.[137]

Heart Disease

Severe heart disease, particularly congestive heart failure[125] or cardiac arrhythmias,[125,138] is a significant risk factor for venous thromboembolism. It is estimated that patients over 30 years of age with heart disease have a 3½-fold greater frequency of pulmonary embolism when compared to patients over 30 years of age without heart disease or an underlying malignancy.[138] In congestive heart failure, reduced venous return, immobilization, and decreased liver function may contribute to the thrombotic complications.[131] Impaired hepatic clearance of activated clotting factors may accompany states such as liver dysfunction associated with congestive heart failure.[131] Deep venous thrombosis has been observed in approximately one third of patients with acute myocardial infarction associated with advanced age, prior history of thromboembolism, and varicose veins.[139] The cumulative effects of high-risk factors are illustrated by the increased mortality from cardiovascular complications observed in men over 55 years of age who had both an underlying cardiovascular disorder and prostatic cancer treated with estrogen.[140-142] These findings suggest that elderly patients with underlying heart disease and cancer merit close observation for the development of thromoembolic complications.

Gram-negative Infections

As a consequence of DIC, infections with gram-negative organisms are a possible risk factor for the development of thrombotic complications.[125] Activation of the coagulation system may occur through the activation of factor XII by endotoxin,[126] or be due to vascular endothelial injury from endotoxin.[143] If shock accompanies the episode of septicemia, venous stasis may develop in patients who are immobilized or have underlying heart disease, increasing the risk of venous thromboembolism.

Obesity

Obesity, defined as greater than 20 percent over the ideal weight, is a risk factor[125] for both deep venous thrombosis[137] and pulmonary embolism.[138]

Operations

Postoperative venous thromboembolism is a well-recognized complication following abdominal, thoracic, hip, prostate, and lower-extremity surgery.[125,144,145] There is evidence to suggest that an increased risk of postoperative thrombosis may occur with increased tissue resection.[125] For example, isotopic fibrinogen scanning for deep-venous thrombosis has shown a severalfold increased incidence of thrombi following retropubic as compared to transurethral prostatic surgery.[146] In addition, venous thromboembolism is more likely to occur postoperatively if any of the additional risk factors described above are present.[125]

Factors Predisposing to Hemorrhage

Operations

In patients with cancer, major operations are associated with a hemorrhagic as well as a thrombotic tendency. Intraoperative bleeding is most commonly due to thrombocytopenia, hemodilution, acute DIC, or an underlying preoperative bleeding tendency (see Table 5).

Thrombocytopenia, defined as a preoperative platelet count of less than 100×10^9/liter, is frequently associated with increased intraoperative and postoperative bleeding.[58] Additional consumption of platelets with surgery may further lower the platelet count, especially if platelet production is impaired or if platelet consumption is increased due to preoperative DIC.[25]

Increased intraoperative and postoperative bleeding may result from hemodilutional states. Hemodilution occurs when surgical blood losses exceeding one third to one half of the total blood volume are replaced with fluids lacking plasma coagulation factors and platelets. The plasma coagulation abnormalities and thrombocytopenia seen with hemodilution are similar to those observed following plasma exchange[73] when fluid replace-

Table 5
Conditions Predisposing to Hemorrhage That May Occur in Patients with
Cancer But Are Not Directly Related to the Malignancy

Operations
   Thrombocytopenia
   Hemodilution
   Acute DIC

Drug-Induced Platelet Dysfunction
   Nonsteroidal anti-inflammatory agents
      Aspirin, indomethacin, phenylbutazone
   Antibiotics
      Carbenicillin, ticarcillin
   Miscellaneous
      Diphenhydramine, chlorpromazine, imipramine

Vitamin K Deficiency States
   Malabsorption syndromes
   Poor dietary intake and/or prolonged antibiotic therapy
   Vitamin K antagonists

Hepatic Disease

Uremia
   Platelet dysfunction

Hypothyroidism

Acute DIC
   Septicemia and shock
   Hemolytic transfusion reactions

ment lacks plasma coagulation factors and platelets. Hemodilution should be suspected if a markedly prolonged PT and PTT are associated with a normal or a slightly prolonged TT.

If DIC is present preoperatively, an increased bleeding tendency during and following surgery should be anticipated. This is particularly applicable in patients with adenocarcinoma of the prostate and gastrointestinal tract in whom substantial tissue injury may occur with surgery. If hypovolemic shock or metabolic acidosis develop, the hemorrhagic manifestations of DIC may become increasingly apparent.[18]

The potential hemorrhagic complications associated with surgery require a systematic preoperative and postoperative evaluation. Any history of a previous bleeding tendency or medications which may inhibit platelet function must be known in order to assess the relative risks of hemorrhage with surgery. Medications which inhibit platelet function should be avoided pre- and postoperatively if possible. Any evidence of hepatic, renal, and cardiovascular disease must be obtained by history, physical examination, and appropriate laboratory studies. Table 7 lists the preoperative laboratory screening studies which are useful for the evaluation of a bleeding tendency in patients with cancer. In patients with solid tumors, the plasma coagulation screening tests in Table 2 will typically show changes consistent with chronic DIC. If instead the PT and PTT are prolonged, hepatic disease, vitamin K deficiency, and acute DIC should be considered. Liver disease and acute DIC may also result in hypofibrinogenemia.

Thrombocytopenia, if present, requires a thorough evaluation for etiology prior to surgery and elimination of the underlying causes if possible. Platelet concentrates should be available for possible use if the platelet count is less than 100×10^9/liter. Intraoperative and postoperative platelet counts of less than 100×10^9/liter may occur if surgical blood losses exceed one half of the total blood volume. Transfusions with platelet concentrates may be necessary if abnormal bleeding and thrombocytopenia are present during and following surgery. Hemorrhage from hemodilution of plasma coagulation proteins may be prevented by the use of fresh-frozen plasma and packed red cells as replacement therapy when surgical blood losses exceed half of the total blood volume.

Postoperatively, in addition to clinical evaluation, the laboratory monitoring of the PT, PTT, TT, fibrinogen, and platelet count are useful in identifying abnormalities which may result in hemorrhage.

Drugs Other than Chemotherapeutic Agents

Numerous medications may cause in vitro platelet function abnormalities.[147-149] A partial list of these drugs is presented in Table 5.

Nonsteroidal anti-inflammatory agents. In patients with cancer, aspirin may increase the bleeding tendency associated with thrombocytopenia, surgery, and anticoagulation therapy with either heparin or warfarin. Aspirin ingestion results in significantly prolonged bleeding times in normal subjects; this is reflected in an increased bleeding tendency.[148,150] Aspirin and other nonsteroidal antiinflammatory agents, such as indomethacin and phenylbutazone, inhibit collagen-induced platelet aggregation and the secondary phase of ADP or epinephrine-induced aggregation.[147] Unlike other medications, aspirin exerts a permanent effect on the platelet population exposed to the drug. Abnormal aggregation may be observed for up to 7 days following the ingestion of 5 grains of aspirin.[151] The effect of other nonsteroidal anti-inflammatory drugs on platelet function is not permanent. However, prolongation of the bleeding time after multiple doses of indomethacin has been reported.[152]

Antibiotics. Following the administration of high doses of penicillin-G and ampicillin, mild platelet aggregation abnormalities and a dose-related prolongation of bleeding times have been observed.[153] The addition of high concentrations of cephalothin to platelet suspensions results in platelet aggregation abnormalities.[154] However, high-dose penicillin, ampicillin, and cephalothin therapy are associated with little if any increase in bleeding. In contrast, carbenicillin and ticarcillin therapy may be associated with a mild bleeding tendency which should be considered in the overall evaluation of hemorrhage.[155,156]

Miscellaneous drugs. A number of other drugs which are commonly used in patients with cancer, including diphenhydramine,[157] chlorpromazine,[157,158] and imipramine,[158] have been reported to cause in vitro platelet function abnormalities. Although, normal bleeding times have been observed in normal subjects after their ingestion, suggesting that these drugs may have little clinical significance,[152,159] in our experience the use of diphenhydramine in patients with thrombocytopenia has occasionally resulted in hemorrhage.

Vitamin K Deficiency States

Severe vitamin K deficiency may result in significant hemorrhage, including gastrointestinal and retroperitoneal bleeding.[160] The causes of vitamin K deficiency include poor dietary intake, antibiotic therapy, malabsorption states, or any combination of these.[160] In patients with cancer, vitamin K deficiency may occur in association with chemotherapy either directly, e.g., actinomycin D, or as a result of protracted nausea, vomiting, and poor oral intake. Vitamin K deficiency may also develop postoperatively or following broad-spectrum antibiotic therapy in infected patients.

Vitamin K deficiency should be suspected if coagulation screening studies reveal a prolonged PT and PTT, with a normal TT, fibrinogen, and serum FDP. In vitamin K deficiency, decreased factor II, VII, IX, and X assays confirm the diagnosis.[160]

Vitamin K deficiency is best managed either by its prevention or by its early recognition in clinical situations where it is likely to develop.[160] Although the minimum daily requirement for vitamin K is not known, parenteral administration of 5–10 mg of vitamin K once or twice a week should prevent hemorrhagic complications from this disorder. If significant bleeding develops in patients with vitamin K deficiency, both parenteral vitamin K (approximately 10–15 mg) and transfusions with fresh-frozen plasma may be necessary.

Hepatic Disease

The numerous coagulation abnormalities associated with liver disease have been extensively reviewed.[56,161,162] Severe liver disease may be associated with a bleeding tendency,[56] and in patients with cancer may significantly complicate the management of hemorrhagic episodes.

In severe liver disease, a hemorrhagic tendency is usually the result of one or more of the following: (1) decreased synthesis of clotting factors; (2) increased utilization of clotting factors; (3) elaboration of abnormal clotting factors; and (4) thrombocytopenia.[56]

Decreased synthesis of the vitamin K dependent factors (II, VII, IX, X), factor V, and fibrinogen[56,161] may be present and are associated with a prolonged PT, PTT, and TT.

In liver disease both DIC and excessive fibrinolysis may occur.[56,162] In acute hepatic necrosis[163] and cirrhosis,[164] acute DIC has been described. Excessive fibrinolytic activity may occur in liver disease as a result of impaired clearance of plasminogen activator.[19] Both DIC and excessive fibrinolytic activity may result in hemorrhage.

The synthesis of abnormal clotting factors, particularly abnormal fibrinogen, has been described in patients with hepatoma,[165,166] cancer metastatic to the liver,[167] and cirrhosis.[161] Dysfibrinogenemia should be suspected if a prolonged TT is found in association with normal FDP and fibrinogen levels[166] and with the absence of heparin in the specimen.

In liver disease, thrombocytopenia may be due to splenic sequestration, shortened platelet survival, and/or mildly impaired platelet production.[168]

Table 2 lists the coagulation screening tests which are useful for evaluating patients with liver disease. It is at times difficult to identify the individual contribution of each coagulation abnormality in a clinical bleeding state. Therefore the treatment of bleeding must be based upon both clinical judgement and laboratory studies. In patients with liver disease, vitamin K administration may be useful if a prolonged PT is observed in the presence of obstructive jaundice or if invasive procedures are to be performed.[56] Transfusions with fresh-frozen plasma are useful in acute bleeding states. If severe hypofibrinogenemia and bleeding occur in patients with liver disease, transfusion with cryoprecipitate, which contains both factor VIII and fibrinogen in a concentrated form,[169] may be useful. Occasionally transfusions with platelet concentrates are necessary in thrombocytopenic states; platelet counts following platelet transfusions are useful in monitoring clinical effectiveness.

Uremic Platelet Dysfunction

In uremia, hemorrhage is frequently associated with platelet function abnormalities.[148,170] Prolonged bleeding times and decreased platelet adhesiveness in association with normal platelet counts are seen and correlate well with clinical bleeding episodes.[171] Significantly decreased platelet adhesiveness has been observed when the BUN and serum creatinine exceeded 100 mg/dl and 7 mg/dl, respectively. The pathogenesis of uremic platelet dysfunction is not fully understood. Phenol, hydroxyphenolic acid, and guanidinosuccinic acid, when present in uremic plasma, may be responsible for the platelet abnormalities.[170]

Patients with malignancy and renal failure should be watched carefully for bleeding. In addition to renal function studies, a platelet count and bleeding time should be done if bleeding develops or surgery is anticipated. The optimal treatment of uremic platelet dysfunction involves the treatment of the cause of renal failure and/or dialysis. Platelet dysfunction is corrected in the majority of cases following either peritoneal dialysis or hemodialysis.[170] Hemodialysis within 24 hours prior to anticipated surgery may aid in achieving near-normal intraoperative and postoperative hemostasis.

Hypothyroidism

Occasionally patients with hypothyroidism present with bleeding. Decreased platelet adhesiveness and variably low levels of factors VII, VIII, IX, and XI have been observed in patients with hypothyroidism.[172] Improvement or total correction of the observed hemostatic abnormalities have been documented after treatment with L-thyroxine.

These studies suggest that hypothyroidism should be considered in patients with a history of a bleeding tendency. Plasma coagulation screening tests and platelet adhesiveness studies confirm any associated hemostatic abnormalities. Of the various hemostatic abnormalities in hypothyroidism, factor VIII deficiency appears to be the most clinically significant. Abnormal bleeding with surgery may result if the factor VIII activity is less than 50 percent. Serious bleeding episodes occurring in association with hypothyroidism, and factor VIII deficiency can be treated with cryoprecipitate. However, transfusion therapy should be minimized since correction of the hemostatic abnormalities occurs with appropriate thyroid hormone replacement.

Acute DIC

As previously discussed, acute DIC and bleeding may occur as a result of the malignancy per se (e.g., APL) or during antineoplastic therapy (e.g., mithramycin and surgery). There are additional causes of acute DIC which may be encountered during the management of patients with cancer. Septicemia due to both gram-negative and gram-positive bacteria may result in acute DIC.[18] Shock and metabolic acidosis, which may develop as a consequence of septicemia, are additional mechanisms for ongoing consumption of plasma coagulation factors and platelets.[173]

Acute DIC may result in hemolytic transfusion reactions.[18] This occasionally occurs in patients with cancer who are receiving blood products during surgery or supportive therapy.

Management of Thrombosis in Patients with Malignancy

General Considerations

As previously discussed, patients with malignancy are at high risk for the development of venous thromboembolism for a number of reasons. Table 6 outlines an approach to the evaluation of clinically suspected thrombosis.

The history and physical examination will enable the clinician to identify risk factors associated with thrombosis. A cumulative increased risk for thrombosis exists when multiple risk factors for thrombosis are present.[125] Table 4 summarizes the more important risk factors unrelated to malignancy or its treatment which may be present. The high incidence of thrombosis following surgery merits special clinical attention, particularly in patients with adenocarcinoma. As many as one third of patients with adenocarcinoma have been reported to develop deep-venous thrombosis following abdominothoracic surgery.[30]

In high-risk situations, or when thromboembolism is clinically suggested, additional diagnostic procedures may be warranted. When deep venous thrombosis is suspected, both invasive and noninvasive diagnostic studies are available. Technically adequate venography is considered the reference method for the diagnosis of deep-venous thrombosis; however, this invasive procedure is associated with some patient morbidity and consequently it is not an ideal screening test for subclinical throm-

Table 6
Diagnosis and Management of Acute Thrombotic Events in Patients with
Malignancies

History

  Identify conditions predisposing to thrombosis (see Table 4)
  Consider type of malignancy (see Table 1) and its status (i.e. relapse,
    remission, etc.)
  Determine current medications, including antineoplastic agents
  Review previous platelet counts and plasma coagulation studies
  Identify previous history of hepatic, renal, or cardiovascular disease

Physical Examination

  Identify signs of extremity deep-venous thrombosis
  Careful cardiopulmonary examination for pulmonary embolus, evidence of
    CHF, arrythmias, or new cardiac mummurs
  Careful neurologic examination for evidence of CVA, paralysis

Laboratory Studies

  For lower-extremity thrombosis
    Impedence plethysmography, ^{125}I-fibrinogen leg scanning, Doppler
      ultrasonography, and venography as indicated
  For pulmonary embolism
    Chest roentgenograms, ventilation-perfusion lung imaging, and pulmonary
      angiography
  Electrocardiogram and other cardiovascular studies as indicated
  Arterial pH, pCO_2, and pO_2
  Hemoglobin and leukocyte count with differential
  Platelet count and examination of the peripheral blood smear
  PT, PTT, TT, fibrinogen, and FDP
  Liver function tests: Serum bilirubin, albumin, and transaminases as
    indicated
  Renal function tests: BUN, serum creatinine, and routine urinalysis as
    indicated

Therapy

  Treat underlying cause(s) of thrombosis (including the malignancy as
    indicated) and associated complications
  Correct concomitant hemorrhagic complications if present (Table 8)
  Heparin therapy
    Dose—25–30 units/kg body weight as an initial intravenous bolus followed
      by the same dose every hour by constant infusion
    Duration—variable, approximately 7–10 days
  Laboratory monitoring of heparin therapy
    Adjust heparin dose to yield a PTT 1.5–2 times normal *or* a TT between
      30–90 seconds in a 1:4 dilution
    PTT or TT determinations every 8–12 hours
    Monitor PT, fibrinogen, platelet count, and FDP during heparin therapy
      daily or more often as indicated

---

bosis.[144] In high-risk patients,[125]I-fibrinogen leg scanning is a very useful screening test.[174] However, in patients suspected to have proximal or calf vein thrombosis, the combination of ^{125}I-fibrinogen leg scanning and impedance plethysmography is recommended.[174] Doppler ultrasonography appears to be an alternative to impedance plethysmography in institutions which have experience with this technique. If recurrent deep-venous thrombosis is suspected, both ^{125}I-fibrinogen leg scanning and venography may be necessary.[144]

In patients with suspected pulmonary embolism, routine chest radiographs and ventilation–perfusion lung imaging are important studies.[175] Pulmonary angiography is the definitive study for evaluating patients who have equivocal results with ventilation–perfusion imaging.[175]

Screening coagulation tests (PT, PTT, TT, fibrinogen, platelet count, and serum FDP) will often show changes consistent with chronic DIC.

Prophylactic Anticoagulation

The Nonsurgical Cancer Patient

In patients at high-risk for thrombosis, in addition to careful clinical and laboratory monitoring, the advantages and disadvantages of prophylactic anticoagulation therapy should be considered. The nature of the risk factors probably most significantly influences the decision regarding anticoagulation therapy.

Data are lacking on the efficacy of either oral anticoagulants or long-term heparin therapy in the prevention of thrombotic complications in nonsurgical patients with cancer with no previous history of venous thromboembolism. Warfarin prophylaxis for venous thromboembolism poses many problems which have been discussed by Zacharski et al.[176] They consider cancer patients to have relative contraindications for warfarin therapy if they have active gastrointestinal bleeding or a history of peptic ulcer disease within the prior 6 months; other sites of internal bleeding; prior intracranial bleeding; acute pancreatitis; evidence of liver disease from other than malignancy; advanced renal or cardiac disease; hypertension; platelet count less than 50×10^9/liter; or are likely not to comply. They suggest that patients who receive warfarin should have PT monitoring, maintain a constant diet, avoid excessive alcohol and avoid nonprescription medications to prevent drug interactions and consequent change in the anticoagulant effect of warfarin.[176]

The management of nonsurgical patients with cancer with recurrent thrombotic events is equally complex. A recent study, which included 13 patients with cancer, showed that warfarin therapy was more effective than low-dose subcutaneous heparin in the prevention of recurrent venous thromboembolism.[177] In this study, however, dose-adjusted warfarin therapy was associated with a significantly increased bleeding risk. In their review, Sack et al. reported that although 36 of 55 patients with malignancy, chronic DIC, and acute thrombosis were successfully treated with heparin, approximately one third of these patients had recurrent thrombotic symptoms upon discontinuation of heparin therapy.[2] It has recently been shown that antithrombin III deficiency occurs with the therapeutic use of heparin.[178] Antithrombin III deficiency may in part account for the development of new thrombotic episodes in these patients.

These observations underscore the clinical dilemma in the prevention of potentially life-threatening thrombotic complications associated with certain malignancies. No ideal anticoagulation agent or regimen yet exists for the prevention of venous thromboembolism in patients with cancer. The VA Cooperative Study of Anticoagulation[176] may provide additional data on both the efficacy and the incidence of bleeding complications with long-term warfarin therapy. Long-term low-dose subcutaneous heparin appears to be the only feasible alternative to warfarin in the prevention of recurrent venous thromboembolism. However, the relative effectiveness of long-term subcutaneous heparin compared to warfarin therapy has not yet been established.

At the present time in the nonsurgical cancer patient prophylactic anticoagulation therapy should be considered only in extremely high-risk situations. Even then, close clinical monitoring during the treatment of the underlying malignancy may aid to minimize and perhaps prevent unexpected thrombotic complications. If the decision is made to use anticoagulation therapy, a thorough evaluation for a hemorrhagic tendency should be performed prior to anticoagulation.

The Surgical Cancer Patient

In contrast with the experience in nonsurgical cancer patients, the effectiveness of low-dose heparin prophylaxis in surgical patients has been clearly demonstrated. In their review of nearly 200 surgical patients with cancer, Gallus and Hirsh noted an overall incidence of thrombosis of 12 percent in patients treated with "minidose" heparin and 38 percent in patients who were not heparinized.[144] The treated patients usually received heparin 5,000 units preoperatively and then 5,000 units every 8–12 hours for 4 or more days. The effectiveness of low-dose heparin therapy is less conclusive in patients undergoing prostatic surgery.[144,174]

Patients with the solid tumors listed in Table 1, in whom surgery is anticipated, should first undergo a systematic evaluation for thrombosis. Preoperatively, coagulation screening tests should be performed (see Table 2). If laboratory abnormalities exist, both a thrombotic and a bleeding tendency should be anticipated before surgery. Usually the causes of the coagulation screening abnormalities are identified by additional historical information and further medical evaluation. As previously discussed, patients with certain malignancies (e.g., dysproteinemia, MD) may require additional plasma coagulation and/or platelet function studies preoperatively.

In patients with malignant disorders who have one or more of the risk factors listed in Table 4, low-dose heparin therapy is recommended in conjunction with abdominal or thoracic surgery. Patients who are on or were recently on estrogen therapy probably should be included in this group. Heparin, 5,000 units, is usually recommended 2 hours before surgery and then every 12 hours until shortly before hospital discharge.[145] In patients undergoing prostatic surgery, low-dose heparin therapy may have limited effectiveness.[145,174] Consequently the prophylactic use of an intermittent lower-extremity compressive device is recommended.[145] In patients with prostatic cancer undergoing retropubic prostatectomy, both of these modalities in combination may be of benefit.

Postoperative monitoring of the PT, PTT, fibrinogen, and platelet count are useful in high-risk patients. In patients undergoing uncomplicated operations, a short PTT associated with an increase in fibrinogen, serum FDP, and platelet count are typically observed after surgery.[35] Acute DIC, with or without additional hemorrhagic abnormalities (Table 5), should be suspected if the postoperative PT and PTT are longer than normal and the fibrinogen and platelet count are falling. In addition, postoperative impedance plethysmography and ^{125}I-fibrinogen leg scanning may be useful in high-risk patients.

Heparin Therapy for Deep-Venous Thrombosis and Pulmonary Embolism

Heparin should be used for the initial management of nearly all cases of thromboembolic complications in the patient with cancer. There is no concensus concerning the recommended dose, schedule, or duration of heparin therapy. The anticoagulant effect of a given dose of heparin varies widely among patients.[179] When adjusting the heparin dose the hemorrhagic risk relative to the benefit of a given anticoagulant effect must continually be considered.[180] The hemorrhagic risk with heparin therapy cannot be overemphasized; it may be significantly increased by drug-induced platelet dysfunction, surgery, and heparin-induced thrombocytopenia.[180]

Wessler and Gitel recommend an initial heparin dose of 30,000–40,000 U.S.P. units per day administered intravenously for approximately 2 days either by a continuous infusion or as a bolus every 4 hours.[180] They recommend a heparin dose of 20,000–25,000 U.S.P. units per day after 48 hours, if there is no evidence of thrombus propagation.

At slightly higher doses, we have observed bleeding in patients with uremia or thrombocytopenia. Our current recommendation for patients with cancer and either deep-venous thrombosis or pulmonary embolism is an initial intravenous bolus of heparin of 25–30 units/kg of body weight followed by the same dose every hour by constant infusion. Lower doses probably should be used in patients with liver or renal disease and in patients who have just recently had surgery.[179] Patients with venous thromboembolic complications occurring within the first 3 days after surgery may have less bleeding if reduced doses of heparin are used.

Among the tests for the monitoring of heparin therapy, the activated PTT is the most widely used, and a PTT of 1½–2 times normal has been recommended.[179] We are currently monitoring heparin therapy with TT determinations on serial dilutions of patient and normal plasma.[172] With TT monitoring, the initial goal is to achieve a TT between 30 and 90 seconds in a 1:4 dilution. This may at first require adjustments in heparin dosage, and monitoring of the TT approximately every 8 hours is recommended. Less-frequent determinations are needed when the TTs are reasonably stable. In our experience the majority of patients demonstrate clinical improvement within a few days of heparin therapy. Some correction of the laboratory abnormalities associated with chronic DIC will often accompany clinical improvement.

The most common side effect with heparin therapy is bleeding due to its anticoagulant effect. In addition, thrombocytopenia, usually occurring within 10 days of initiation of heparin therapy, has been reported.[180,181] The incidence of heparin-induced thrombocytopenia in one study was 30 percent.[182] Recent studies suggest that in some cases, the thrombocytopenia is immune-mediated and heparin-dependent.[183,184] Clinically, thrombotic complications[185] and laboratory abnormalities consistent with DIC[186] have been associated with heparin-induced thrombocytopenia.

Following the usual short course (7–10 days) of intravenous heparin therapy, the clinician is faced with the question of continued oral anticoagulant therapy. As we have discussed above, in patients with cancer, oral anticoagulant therapy may pose significant risks.[177,179] Moreover, long-term oral anticoagulant therapy may not be effective in preventing recurrent thrombotic complications.[2] It is unknown whether long-term subcutaneous heparin therapy is effective in preventing recurrent thrombosis in patients with cancer. Control of the underlying malignancy and attempted prevention of other conditions predisposing to thrombosis is probably the best long-term approach to prevention of recurrent thromboembolic events.

Management of Acute Hemorrhagic Events in Patients with Malignancy

General Considerations

The treatment of acute hemorrhagic events in patients with cancer first requires a rapid and thorough search for the cause or causes of bleeding. Table 7 summarizes the pertinent clinical and laboratory data required to identify potential causes of bleeding.

Table 7
Evaluation of Acute Hemorrhagic Manifestations in Patients with Malignancies

History

Identify the presence of any bleeding tendency prior to or after the diagnosis of cancer, or after antineoplastic therapy
Determine current medications, including antineoplastic agents
Review previous platelet counts and plasma coagulation studies
Identify previous history of hepatic disease, uremia, or vitamin K deficiency
Review previous hepatic and renal function studies

Physical Examination

Identify site(s) of bleeding
Assess vital signs, perfusion, and cardiovascular status
Determine neurologic status

Laboratory Studies

Hemoglobin and leukocyte count with differential
Platelet count
PT, PTT, TT, fibrinogen, and FDP
Arterial pH, pCO_2, and pO_2
Electrocardiogram and chest roentgenograms as indicated
Serum bilirubin, albumin, and transaminases as indicated
BUN, serum creatinine, and routine urinalysis as indicated
Microbiological studies as indicated

A thorough history is important to identify both life-long and recent hemorrhagic symptoms. Mild or moderate bleeding tendencies may be clinically apparent only with hemostatic challenges such as operations, major injuries, or dental surgery. Menorrhagia from the time of menarche, easy bruisability, and spontaneous nosebleeds in childhood are symptoms of von Willebrand's syndrome. In inherited hemorrhagic disorders, the family history is usually, but not always, positive. Hemorrhagic symptoms of recent onset suggest causes directly related to the malignancy, its treatment, or one of the disorders listed in Table 5.

A thorough review of the patient's medications may identify the contribution to current bleeding of drug-related platelet dysfunction or previous anticoagulation therapy. Conditions predisposing to vitamin K deficiency (Table 5) may be identified by history alone. A review of previous hepatic, renal, hematologic, and coagulation studies will aid in assessing the duration of disorders associated with a bleeding tendency.

Examination of the patient will demonstrate the site or sites of bleeding and yield information on possible bleeding into vital organs, e.g., neurologic changes and retinal hemorrhages. As previously discussed, acute DIC will often result in ongoing shock and metabolic acidosis. Conversely, DIC should be suspected in unexplained shock-like syndromes.[18]

Laboratory screening studies (Table 7) for the evaluation of acute bleeding episodes include hemoglobin, leukocyte count with differential, platelet count, PT, PTT, TT, fibrinogen, and FDP. Laboratory studies of hepatic, renal, and cardiovascular function are essential (Table 7). If septicemia is suspected, either with or without DIC, appropriate microbiologic studies should be undertaken.

In patients with bleeding, all identifiable causes should be treated as promptly as possible. Table 8 outlines the most common acquired causes of bleeding and their treatment. Among patients who have a bleeding tendency due to a malignancy per se, early and successful treatment of the underlying neoplasm is crucial. Close clinical and laboratory monitoring is essential in the prevention of hemorrhagic complications from certain chemotherapeutic agents. It is necessary to anticipate and prepare for hemorrhagic complications in patients with cancer who are to have major surgery. This may require arranging for the availability of cryoprecipitate, fresh-frozen plasma, and/or platelet concentrates prior to and following surgery. Hemorrhage may be minimized by treating all potential causes of bleeding preoperatively and preventing their development after surgery.

Table 8
Management of Acute Hemorrhagic Manifestations in Patients with Malignancies

Problem to be Treated	Treatment	Pages on Which Discussed
I. Acute hemorrhagic event and its complications	Local measures Blood replacement	
II. Underlying causes		
A. Malignant disorder		
1. APL	Antineoplastic therapy *and*	
	Heparin + blood component trans- fusion therapy for acute DIC	149–150, 181–184
2. Waldenstrom's macroglobulinemia	Plasmapheresis	152–155
3. Myeloproliferative disorders	Platelet concentrates	155–157
B. Thrombocytopenia	Platelet concentrates *and*	150–152
1. Marrow replacement by tumor	Antineoplastic therapy	
2. Hypersplenism	Treat underlying cause	
3. Immune thrombocytopenia	Corticosteroids, splenectomy	
C. Antineoplastic chemotherapy	Table 3	157–162
D. Drug-induced platelet dysfunction	Platelet concentrates Stop drug if possible	167–168
E. Vitamin K deficiency	Parenteral vitamin K and fresh-frozen plasma	168
F. Hepatic disease		
1. Prolonged PT	Fresh frozen plasma *and* vitamin K	169
2. Hypofibrinogenemia	Cryoprecipitate	
G. Uremia	Dialysis	170

(continued)

179

Table 8 (*continued*)
Management of Acute Hemorrhagic Manifestations in Patients with Malignancies

Problem to be Treated	Treatment	Pages on Which Discussed
II. Underlying causes		
H. Hypothyroidism	Cryoprecipitate, thyroid hormone replacement	170
I. Acute DIC	Treat underlying cause Blood component transfusion therapy as necessary *and* fresh-frozen plasma, packed red cells	149–150, 171 181–182
1. Shock		
2. APL	Heparin	
J. Hemodilution	Fresh-frozen plasma, packed red cells, and if thrombocytopenic, platelet concentrates	154–155

Management of Acute DIC in Patients with Malignancy

General Principles

There is nearly universal agreement that the treatment of the underlying cause of the DIC is essential in controlling hemorrhage.[3,19] Complications of DIC such as shock and acidosis should be promptly corrected. Transfusions with blood components (packed red cells, fresh-frozen plasma, cryoprecipitate, and platelet concentrates) should be used if laboratory evidence of depletion of platelets and/or plasma clotting factors exists in the presence of hemorrhage. Transfusion therapy may be used in severe depletion states to prevent overt clinical bleeding. If the treatment of the underlying malignancy is expected to cause or exacerbate a preexisting depletion state, e.g., induction chemotherapy of APL, blood component therapy may prevent hemorrhage.

Additional considerations in the management of acute DIC include the correction of all other potential causes of bleeding (see Table 8). Avoidance of medications which cause platelet dysfunction is important.

Parenteral vitamin K administration will help in restoring the vitamin K dependent factors, especially in patients with compromised hepatic function. In patients with acute DIC, parenteral vitamin K should be used during broad-spectrum antibiotic therapy and during periods when the dietary intake is suboptimal for greater than 4–5 days.

Epsilon amino caproic acid (EACA), a competitive inhibitor of plasminogen activator, should almost never be used in the management of acute DIC.[56] The inhibition of the fibrinolytic system with EACA in the presence of ongoing intravascular coagulation may result in disseminated thrombosis.

If primary or excessive fibrinolysis is suspected, treatment of its underlying cause and blood component therapy should first be attempted. If these measures fail to control bleeding, the combination of EACA, intravenous heparin, and blood component therapy should be considered.

Blood Component Therapy

As discussed previously, in acute DIC elevated FDP and depletion of nearly all clotting factors occur. Platelet dysfunction may result from elevated FDP,[22] and the elimination or reduction of circulating FDP may improve hemostasis. Exchange transfusions with whole blood should largely correct the hemostatic abnormalities of acute DIC. Exchange transfusions are feasible in infants and small children if one can rapidly obtain vascular access. In older children and adults the volume of blood needed for exchange transfusions becomes prohibitive. However, a partial exchange transfusion with fresh-frozen plasma and packed red cells may still be useful if congestive heart failure exists. If poor tissue perfusion complicates acute DIC, transfusions with fresh-frozen plasma and packed red cells for volume expansion will prevent the dilution of plasma clotting proteins that occurs when protein solutions not containing clotting proteins are used. If hypofibrinogenemia (approximately $\leq$ 0.1 g/dl) is present, 1 donor unit of cryoprecipitate for every 6 kg of body weight should raise the fibrinogen concentration by approximately 0.1 g/dl.

Platelet transfusions are likely to be most beneficial in patients with acute DIC who have (1) platelet counts of less than 100×10^9/liter associated with bleeding; (2) a falling platelet count and cannot undergo exchange transfusion; and (3) an underlying disease process in which the associated DIC is not promptly reversible, e.g., APL during induction chemotherapy. The dosage of platelet concentrates should be adjusted based upon the response of the platelet count to platelet transfusions.

Heparin Therapy (Table 9)

The use of heparin therapy in acute DIC remains controversial. The need for heparin therapy in acute DIC probably continues only as long as the cause of DIC exists. In some situations, e.g., promptly treated septicemia, the cause of DIC and the consequent hemorrhage can be quickly removed, and heparin therapy is thus not indicated. Moreover, heparin therapy may have serious side effects, which include hemorrhage and heparin-induced thrombocytopenia.[180-187] The half-life of heparin varies according to the dose, and the status of both hepatic and renal function.[180] These variations in heparin half-life may pose clinical problems in deciding on the heparin dosages for a particular patient.

As a guideline, therefore, heparin therapy in the management of acute DIC should be considered under the following situations. First, heparin therapy may be useful if transfusions with blood components alone are insufficient to maintain plasma coagulation factors at levels sufficient to achieve hemostasis while the underlying cause or causes for the DIC are being treated. Second, heparin therapy may be useful if the underlying cause for acute DIC is apt to worsen or persist for more than 24–48 hours (e.g., induction therapy of APL).

If heparin therapy is required in acute DIC, we believe that the safest and most effective method of administration is by a continuous intra-

Table 9
Heparin Therapy of Acute DIC in Patients with Malignancy

Indications for Heparin Therapy
    Acute promyelocytic leukemia—in conjunction with induction chemotherapy
    When there is continuing depletion of plasma coagulation factors following
        blood component therapy in:
            Other forms of acute nonlymphoblastic leukemia
            Carcinoma of the prostate

Ancillary Therapy (Table 8)
    Treat underlying cause of DIC
    Treat causes of hemorrhage and its complications
        Blood component therapy
        Correct metabolic acidosis, shock, etc.

Heparin Therapy
    Dose—approximately 10–15 units/kg body weight by constant intravenous
        infusion
    Duration—must be individualized

Laboratory Studies
    Heparin monitoring
        TT 30–90 seconds in a 1:2 dilution approximately every 4–8 hours
    Monitor response to blood component therapy
        PT, factor V activity, PTT, fibrinogen, platelet count, and hemoglobin
            approximately every 12 hours
        FDP daily
    Serum albumin, bilirubin, and creatinine
        Lower hourly doses of heparin may be required in the presence of liver or
        renal disease

---

venous infusion. We have used an initial dose of approximately 10–15 units/kg of body weight per hour. For monitoring heparin therapy, the most widely used test is the activated PTT. If the activated PTT is used to monitor heparin therapy for acute DIC, a twice-normal activated PTT is recommended. In acute DIC, the PTT is often prolonged prior to starting heparin, which may significantly reduce its usefulness for monitoring heparin therapy. In our experience the use of TT determinations on serial dilutions of patient and normal plasma has been effective in monitoring plasma heparin concentration and thereby minimizing the hemorrhagic complications from excessive heparin.[172] During heparin therapy for acute DIC, a TT ranging between 30 and 90 seconds in a 1:2 dilution is recommended.

Within a few hours of initiation of continuous intravenous heparin therapy, TT determinations should be done to aid in adjusting the hourly heparin dose. Fairly frequent TT determinations may be necessary as the heparin requirement may rapidly decrease if the underlying causes of DIC are promptly corrected. During heparin therapy, PT, factor V, and fibrinogen determinations are useful to document the status of the depletion state and its possible improvement. In acute DIC, we usually monitor the PT, PTT, fibrinogen, and platelet counts every 12 hours to determine when and if blood component therapy is needed. In the management of the DIC associated with the treatment of APL, heparin therapy is usually required for 5–7 days.[48] In patients with other malignant disorders, the duration of heparin therapy will vary according to the cause or causes of DIC in a given individual.

Summary

Serious thrombohemorrhagic complications may develop at diagnosis and during the course of therapy in patients with malignancies. The causes of these complications are multifactorial. The malignancy per se, its treatment, and conditions unrelated to the malignancy or its management may result in thrombosis or bleeding. All these factors must be considered in the treatment of acute thrombotic or hemorrhagic events. The treatment of acute thrombohemorrhagic complications should be individualized; guidelines for the diagnosis, treatment, and the monitoring of these events have been discussed. Control of the underlying malignancy remains the most effective means of minimizing thrombotic and hemorrhagic complications in patients with cancer.

References

1. Trousseau A: Phlegmasia alba dolens. Clinique Medicale de L'Hotel Dieu de Paris 3. Ed. 2. Paris, Balliere, 1865
2. Sack GH Jr, Levin J, Bell WR: Trousseau's syndrome and other manifestations of chronic disseminated coagulopathy in patients with neoplasms: Clinical, pathophysiologic and therapeutic features. Medicine (Baltimore) 56:1–37, 1977
3. Bick RL: Alterations of hemostasis associated with malignancy: Etiology, pathophysiology, diagnosis and management. Semin Thromb Hemostas 5:1–26, 1978
4. Davis RB, Theologides A, Kennedy BJ: Comparative studies of

blood coagulation and platelet aggregation in patients with cancer and nonmalignant diseases. Ann Intern Med 71:67–80, 1969

5. Case Records of the Massachusetts General Hospital (Case 13-1978). N Engl J Med 298:786–792, 1978
6. Edwards EA: Migrating thrombophlebitis associated with carcinoma. N Engl J Med 240:1031–1035, 1949
7. Kennedy WE: The association of carcinoma in the body and tail of the pancreas with multiple venous thrombi. Surgery 14:600–609, 1943
8. Fisch C, Jones AW, Gambill WD: Acute thrombophlebitis associated with carcinoma of the stomach. Gastroenterology 18:290–295, 1951
9. Perlow S, Daniels JL: Venous thrombosis and obscure abdominal malignancy. Arch Intern Med 97:184–188, 1956
10. McKay DG, Mansell H, Hertig AT: Carcinoma of the body of the pancreas with fibrin thrombosis and fibrinogenopenia. Cancer 6:862–869, 1953
11. Sproul EF: Carcinoma and venous thrombosis: The frequency of association of carcinoma in the body or tail or the pancreas with multiple venous thrombosis. Am J Cancer 34:566–585, 1938
12. Amundsen MA, Spittell JA Jr, Thompson JH Jr, et al: Hypercoagulability associated with malignant disease and with the postoperative state. Evidence for elevated levels for anti-hemophilic globulin. Ann Intern Med 58:608–616, 1963
13. Rosen P, Armstrong D: Nonbacterial thrombotic endocarditis in patients with malignant neoplastic diseases. Am J Med 54:23–29, 1973
14. Reagan TJ, Okazaki H: The thrombotic syndrome associated with carcinoma: A clinical and neuropathologic study. Arch Neurol 31:390–395, 1974
15. Collins RC, Al-Mondhiry H, Chernik NL, et al: Neurologic manifestations of intravascular coagulation in patients with cancer: A clinicopathologic analysis of 12 cases. Neurology (Minneap) 25:795–806, 1975
16. Sigsbee B, Deck MOF, Posner JB: Nonmetastatic superior sagittal sinus thrombosis complicating systemic cancer. Neurology (Minneap) 29:139–146, 1979
17. Owen CA Jr, Bowie EJW: Chronic intravascular coagulation syndromes. A summary. Mayo Clin Proc 49:673–679, 1974
18. Sharp AA: Diagnosis and management of disseminated intravascular coagulation. Br Med Bull 33:265–272, 1977

19. Hamilton PJ, Stalker AL, Douglas AS: Disseminated intravascular coagulation: A review. J Clin Pathol 31:609–619, 1978
20. Bick RL: Disseminated intravascular coagulation and related syndromes: Etiology, pathophysiology, diagnosis, and management. Am J Hematol 5:265–282, 1978
21. Nelson JC, Lerner RG: Detection of factor XIIIa (active fibrin-stabilizing factor) in normal plasma. Blood 52:581–591, 1978
22. Mustard JF, Packham MA: Factors influencing platelet function: Adhesion, release, and aggregation. Pharmacol Rev 22:97–187, 1970
23. Cooper HA, Bowie EJW, Owen CA Jr: Evaluation of patients with increased fibrinolytic split products (FSP) in their serum. Mayo Clin Proc 49:654–657, 1974
24. Sun NCJ, McAfee WM, Hum GJ, et al: Hemostatic abnormalities in malignancy, a prospective study of 108 patients. Part I. Coagulation Studies. Am J Clin Pathol 71:10–16, 1979
25. Harker LA, Slichter SJ: Platelets and fibrinogen consumption in man. N Engl J Med 287:999–1005, 1972
26. Hirsh J: Hypercoagulability. Semin Hematol 14:409–425, 1977
27. Lyman GH, Bettigole RE, Robson E, et al: Fibrinogen kinetics in patients with neoplastic disease. Cancer 41:1113–1122, 1978
28. Brain MC, Dacie JV, O'Hourihane DO'B: Microangiopathic haemolytic anaemia: the possible role of vascular lesions in pathogenesis. Br J. Haematol 8:358–374, 1962
29. Brain MC, Azzopardi JG, Baker LRI, et al: Microangiopathic haemolytic anemia and mucin-forming adenocarcinoma. Br J Haematol 18:183–193, 1970
30. Pineo GF, Brain MC, Gallus AS, et al: Tumors, mucus production, and hypercoagulability. Ann NY Acad Sci 230:262–270, 1974
31. Losito R, Beaudry P, Valderrama JC, et al: Antithrombin III and factor VIII in patients with neoplasms. Am J Clin Pathol 68:258–262, 1977
32. Sun NCJ, Bowie EJW, Kazmier FJ, et al: Blood coagulation studies in patients with cancer. Mayo Clin Proc 49:636–641, 1974
33. Hagedorn AB, Bowie EJW, Eleback LR, et al: Coagulation abnormalities in patients with inoperable lung cancer. Mayo Clin Proc 49:647–653, 1974
34. Sufrin G, Mink I, Fitzpatrick J, et al: Coagulation factors in renal adenocarcinoma. J Urol 119:727–730, 1978
35. Egan EL, Bowie EJW, Kazmier FJ, et al: Effect of surgical operations on certain tests used to diagnose intravascular coagulation and fibrinolysis. Mayo Clin Proc 49:658–664, 1974

36. Wood EH, Prentice CRM, McNicol GP: Association of fibrinogen-fibrin related antigen (FR-antigen) with postoperative deep-vein thrombosis and systemic complications. Lancet 1:166–169, 1972
37. Breen F, Tullis S: Ethanol gel test improved. Ann Intern Med 71:433–434, 1969
38. Gurewich B, Hutchinson E: Detection of intravascular coagulation by a serial dilution protamine sulfate test. Ann Intern Med 75:895–902, 1971
39. Goodnight SH Jr: Bleeding and intravascular clotting in malignancy: A review. Ann NY Acad Sci 230:271–288, 1974
40. Mertens BF, Greene LS, Bowie EJW, et al: Fibrinolytic split products (FSP) and ethanol gelation test in preoperative evaluation of patients with prostatic disease. Mayo Clin Proc 49:642–646, 1974
41. Kwaan HC: Disorders of fibrinolysis. Med Clin North Am 56:163–176, 1972
42. Tagnon HJ, Schulman P, Whitmore WF, et al: Prostatic fibrinolysin. Study of a case illustrating role in hemorrhagic diathesis of cancer of the prostate. Am J Med 15:875–884, 1953
43. Cliffton EE, Grossi CE: Fibrinolytic activity of human tumors as measured by the fibrin-plate method. Cancer 8:1146–1154, 1955
44. Wilson EL, Dowdle E: Secretion of plasminogen activator by normal, reactive and neoplastic human tissues cultured in vitro. Int J Cancer 22:390–399, 1978
45. Gralnick HR, Abrell E: Studies of the procoagulant and fibrinolytic activity of promyelocytes in acute promyelocytic leukaemia. Br J Haematol 24:89–99, 1973
46. Drapkin RL, Gee TS, Dowling MD, et al: Prophylactic heparin therapy in acute promyelocytic leukemia. Cancer 41:2484–2490, 1978
47. Sultan C, Heilmann-Gouault M, Tulliez M: Relationship between blast cell morphology and occurrence of a syndrome of a disseminated intravascular coagulation. Br J Haematol 24:255–259, 1973
48. Collins AJ, Bloomfield CD, Peterson BA, et al: Acute promyelocytic leukemia: Management of the coagulopathy during daunorubicin–prednisone remission induction. Arch Intern Med 138:1677–1680, 1978
49. Gralnick HR, Marchesi S, Givelber H: Intravascular coagulation in acute leukemia: Clinical and subclinical abnormalities. Blood 40:709–718, 1972
50. McKenna RW, Bloomfield CD, Dick F, et al: Acute monoblastic leukemia: Diagnosis and treatment of ten cases. Blood 46:481–494, 1975
51. Champion LAA, Luddy RE, Schwartz AD: Disseminated intravas-

cular coagulation in childhood acute lymphocytic leukemia with poor prognostic features. Cancer 41:1642–1646, 1978

52. Ben-Zeev D, Schwartz SO, Friedman IA: Promyelocytic-myelocytic leukemia as a terminal manifestation of chronic granulocytic leukemia. Report of a case. Blood 27:863–870, 1966

53. Peterson LC, Bloomfield CD, Brunning RD: Blast crisis as an initial or terminal manifestation of chronic myeloid leukemia. A study of 28 patients. Am J Med 60:209–220, 1976

54. Gralnick HR, Sultan C: Acute promyelocytic leukaemia: Haemorrhagic manifestation and morphologic criteria. Br J Haematol 29:373–376, 1975

55. Edson JR, Krivit W, White JG: Kaolin partial thromboplastin time: High levels of procoagulants producing short clotting times and masking deficiencies of other procoagulants or low concentrations of anticoagulants. J Lab Clin Med 70:463–470, 1967

56. Roberts HR, Cederbaum AI: The liver and blood coagulation: Physiology and pathology. Gastroenterology 63:297–320, 1972

57. Stass SA, Holloway ML, Peterson V, et al: Cytoplasmic fragments causing spurious platelet counts in the leukemic phase of poorly differentiated lymphocytic lymphoma. Am J Clin Pathol 71:125–128, 1979

58. Slichter SJ, Harker LA: Hemostasis in malignancy. Ann NY Acad Sci 230:252–261, 1974

59. Kaden BR, Rosse WF, Hauch TW: Immune thrombocytopenia in lymphoproliferative diseases. Blood 53:545–551, 1979

60. White LA Jr, Brubaker LH, Aster RH, et al: Platelet satellitism and phagocytosis by neutrophils: Association with antiplatelet antibodies and lymphoma. Am J Hematol 4:313–323, 1978

61. Jones SE: Autoimmune disorders and malignant lymphoma. Cancer 31:1092–1098, 1973

62. Cohen JR: Idiopathic thrombocytopenic purpura in Hodgkin's disease. A rare occurrence of no prognostic significance. Cancer 41:743–746, 1978

63. Rao S, Pang EJ-M: Idiopathic thrombocytopenic purpura in acute lymphoblastic leukemia. J Pediatr 94:408–409, 1979

64. Shapiro SS, Hultin M: Acquired inhibitors to the blood coagulation factors. Semin Thromb Hemostas 1:336–385, 1975

65. Penny R, Castaldi PA, Whitsed HM: Inflammation and haemostasis in paraproteinaemias. Br J Haematol 20:35–44, 1971

66. Lackner H, Hunt V, Zucker MB, et al: Abnormal fibrin ultrastruc-

ture polymerization and clot retraction in multiple myeloma. Br J Haematol 18:625–635, 1970

67. Perkins HA, MacKenzie MR, Fudenberg HH: Hemostatic defects in dysproteinemias. Blood 35:695–707, 1970

68. Cohen I, Amir J, Ben-Shaul Y, et al: Plasma cell myeloma associated with an unusual myeloma protein causing impairment of fibrin aggregation and platelet function in a patient with multiple malignancy. Am J Med 48:766–776, 1970

69. Coleman M, Vigliano EM, Weksler ME, et al: Inhibition of fibrin polymerization by lambda myeloma globulins. Blood 39:210–223, 1972

70. Coutant G, Hamers J, Baele G, et al: Simultaneous occurrence of hypocholesterolemia, hypocalcemia and hypofibrinogenemia in a case of multiple myeloma. Acta Haematol 54:358–361, 1975

71. Brody JI, Haider ME, Rossman RE: A hemorrhagic syndrome in Waldenstrom's macroglobulinemia secondary to immunoadsorption of factor VIII. Recovery after splenectomy. N Engl J Med 300:408–410, 1979

72. McGrath KM, Stuart JJ, Richards F II: Correlation between serum IgG, platelet membrane IgG, and platelet function in hypergammaglobulinaemic states. Br J Haematol 42:585–591, 1979

73. Flaum MA, Cuneo RA, Appelbaum FR et al: The hemostatic imbalance of plasma-exchange transfusion. Blood 54:694–702, 1979

74. Keller AJ, Chirnside A, Urbaniak SJ: Coagulation abnormalities produced by plasma exchange on the cell separator with special reference to fibrinogen and platelet levels. Br J Haematol 42:593–603, 1979

75. Walsh PN, Murphy S, Barry WE: The role of platelets in the pathogenesis of thrombosis and hemorrhage in patients with thrombocytosis. Thromb Haemostas 38:1085–1096, 1977

76. Gunz FW: Hemorrhagic thrombocythemia: A critical review. Blood 15:706–723, 1960

77. Hussain S, Schwartz JM, Friedman SA, et al: Arterial thrombosis in essential thrombocythemia. Am Heart J 96:31–36, 1978

78. Videbaek A: Polycythemia vera. Course and prognosis. Acta Medica Scandia 138:179–187, 1950

79. Wasserman LR, Bassen S: Polycythemia. J Mount Sinai Hosp NY 26:1–49, 1959

80. Shievitz E, Thiede T: Complications and causes of death in polycythemia vera. Acta Medica Scandia 172:513–523, 1962

81. Berger S, Aledort LM, Gilbert HS, et al: Abnormalities of platelet function in patients with polycythemia vera. Cancer Res 33:2683–2687, 1973
82. Mason JE, DeVita VT, Canellos GP: Thrombocytosis in chronic granulocytic leukemia: Incidence and clinical significance. Blood 44:483–487, 1974
83. Wasserman LR, Gilbert HS: Surgery in polycythemia vera. N Engl J Med 269:1226–1230, 1963
84. Gordon DH, Schaffner D, Bennett JM, et al: Postsplenectomy thrombocytosis. Its association with mesenteric, portal, and/or renal vein thrombosis in patients with myeloproliferative disorders. Arch Surg 113:713–715, 1978
85. McBride CM, Hester JP: Chronic myelogenous leukemia: Management of splenectomy in a high-risk population. Cancer 39:653–658, 1977
86. Brodsky I, Kahn SB, Ross EM, et al: Platelet and fibrinogen kinetics in the chronic myeloproliferative disorders. Cancer 30:1444–1450, 1972
87. Martinez J, Shapiro SS, Holburn RR: Metabolism of human prothrombin and fibrinogen in patients with thrombocytosis secondary to myeloproliferative states. Blood 42:35–46, 1973
88. Tytgat GN, Collen D, Vermylen J: Metabolism and distribution of fibrinogen. II. Fibrinogen turnover in polycythaemia, thrombocytosis, haemophilia A, congenital afibrinogenaemia and during streptokinase therapy. Br J Haematol 22:701–717, 1972
89. Carvalho A, Ellman L: Activation of the coagulation system in polycythemia vera. Blood 47:669–698, 1976
90. German HJ, Smith JA, Lindenbaum J: Chronic intravascular coagulation associated with chronic myelocytic leukemia. Use of heparin in connection with a surgical procedure. Am J Med 61:547–552, 1976
91. Edson JR: Acquired qualitative abnormalities of platelet function, in Seligson D (ed): CRC Handbook Series in Clinical Laboratory Science, Vol. 1. Boca Raton, Florida, CRC Press, 1979, pp 463–469
92. Harker LA, Slichter SJ: The bleeding time as a screening test for evaluation of platelet function. N Engl J Med 287:155–159, 1972
93. Cardamone JM, Edson JR, McArthur JR, et al: Abnormalities of platelet. function in the myeloproliferative disorders. JAMA 221:270–273, 1972
94. Murphy S, Davis JL, Walsh PN, et al: Template bleeding time and clinical hemorrhage in myeloproliferative disease. Arch Intern Med 138:1251–1253, 1978

95. Hoagland HC, Silverstein MN: Primary thrombocythemia in the young patient. Mayo Clin Proc 53:578–580, 1978

96. Gerrard JM, Stoddard SF, Shapiro RS, et al: Platelet storage pool deficiency and prostaglandin synthesis in chronic granulocytic leukaemia. Br J Haematol 40:597–607, 1978

97. Belt RJ, Leite C, Haas CD, et al: Incidence of hemorrhagic complications in patients with cancer. JAMA 239:2571–2574, 1978

98. Smith IE, Powles R, Clink HM, et al: Early death in acute myelogenous leukemia. Cancer 39:1710–1714, 1977

99. Olson RE: Vitamin K-induced prothrombin formation antagonism by actinomycin-D. Science 145:926–928, 1964

100. Bick RL, Fekete LF, Wilson WL: Adriamycin and fibrinolysis. Thromb Res 8:467–475, 1976

101. Bick RL, Murano G, Fekete L, et al: Daunomycin and fibrinolysis. Thromb Res 9:201–203, 1976

102. Haskell CM, Canellos GP, Leventhal BG, et al: L-asparaginase: Therapeutic and toxic effects in patients with neoplastic disease. N Engl J Med 281:1028–1034, 1969

103. Oettgen HF, Stephenson PA, Schwartz MK, et al: Toxicity of E. coli L-asparaginase in man. Cancer 25:253–278, 1970

104. Whitecar JP, Bodey GP, Harris JE, et al: L-asparaginase. N Engl J Med 282:732–734, 1970

105. Ramsay NKC, Coccia PF, Krivit W, et al: The effect of L-asparaginase on plasma coagulation factors in acute lymphoblastic leukemia. Cancer 40:1398–1401, 1977

106. Bettigole RE, Himelstein ES, Oettgen HF, et al: Hypofibrinogenemia due to L-asparaginase: Studies of fibrinogen survival using autologous ^{131}I-fibrinogen. Blood 35:195–200, 1970

107. Deutsch E, Fischer M, Frischauf H, et al: Blood coagulation changes under L-asparaginase therapy, in Grundmann E, Oettgen HF (eds): Recent Results in Cancer Research, Vol. 33. New York, Springer-Verlag, 1970, pp 331–341

108. Egeberg O: Inherited antithrombin deficiency causing thrombophilia. Thromb Diath Haemmorh 13:516–530, 1965

109. Conard J, Durant G, Seger J, et al: Acquired abnormal antithrombin-III in L-asparaginase treated patients? IV International Congress On Thrombosis and Hemostasis-Abstracts, Vienna, 1973, p 228

110. Priest JR, Ramsay NKC, Coates TD, et al: Stroke syndrome complicating remission induction chemotherapy for acute lymphocytic leukemia. Proc Am Cancer Res 20:97, 1979

111. Priest JR, Ramsay NKC, Latchaw RE, et al: Thrombotic and hemor-

rhagic strokes complicating early therapy for childhood acute lymphoblastic leukemia. Cancer 46:1548–1554, 1980

112. Bleyer WA: The clinical pharmacology of methotrexate. New applications of an old drug. Cancer 41:36–51, 1978

113. Nesbit M, Krivit W, Heyn R: Acute and chronic effects of methotrexate on hepatic, pulmonary and skeletal systems. Cancer 37:1048–1054, 1976

114. Warkentin P, Hasegawa D, Nesbit M, et al: High-dose methotrexate (MTX) hepatotoxicity: significance of frequency of administration. Proc Am Assoc Cancer Res 20:98, 1979

115. Kennedy BJ: Metabolic and toxic effects of mithramycin during tumor therapy. Am J Med 49:494–503, 1969

116. Monto RW, Talley RW, Caldwell MJ, et al: Observations on the mechanism of hemorrhagic toxicity in mithramycin (NSC 24559) therapy. Cancer Res 29:697–704, 1969

117. Ahr DJ, Scialla SJ, Kimball DB Jr: Acquired platelet dysfunction following mithramycin therapy. Cancer 41:448–454, 1978

118. Steinhertz PG, Miller DR, Hilgartner MW, et al: Platelet dysfunction in vincristine treated patients. Br J Haematol 32:439–450, 1976

119. White JG: Effect of colchicine and vinca alkaloids on human platelets. III. Influence on primary internal contraction and secondary aggregation. Am J Pathol 54:467–478, 1969

120. Ozsoylu S, Strauss HS, Diamond LK: Effects of corticosteroids on coagulation of the blood. Nature 195:1214–1215, 1962

121. Vessey MP, Weatherall JAC: Venous thromboembolic disease and the use of oral contraceptives. A review of mortality statistics in England and Wales. Lancet 2:94–96, 1968

122. Inman WHW, Vessey MP, Westerholm B, et al: Thromboembolic disease and the steroidal content of oral contraceptives: A report to the Committee on Safety of Drugs. Br Med J 2:203–209, 1970

123. Morales A, Pujari B: The choice of estrogen preparations in the treatment of prostatic cancer. Can Med Assoc J 113:865–867, 1975

124. Veterans Administration Cooperative Urologic Research Group: Treatment and survival of patients with cancer of the prostate. Surg Gynecol Obstet 124:1011–1017, 1967

125. Coon WW: Epidemiology of venous thromboembolism. Am Surg 186:149–164, 1977

126. Egeberg O, Owren PA: Oral contraception and blood coagulability. Br Med J 1:220–221, 1963

127. Coope J, Thomson JM, Poller L: Effects of "natural oestrogen" replacement therapy on menopausal symptoms and blood clotting. Br Med J 4:139–143, 1975

128. Howie PW, Mallinson AC, Prentice CRM, et al: Effect of combined oestrogen–progestogen oral contraceptives, oestrogen, and progestogen on antiplasmin and antithrombin activity. Lancet 2:1329–1332, 1970

129. Peterson RA, Krull PE, Finley, et al: Changes in antithrombin III and plasminogen induced by oral contraceptives. Am J Clin Pathol 53:468–473, 1970

130. Carter AC, Sedransk N, Kelley RM, et al: Diethylstilbestrol: Recommended dosages for different categories of breast cancer patients. Report of the Cooperative Breast Cancer Group. JAMA 237:2079–2085, 1977

131. Davies GC, Salzman EW: The pathogenesis of deep vein thrombosis, in Joist JH, Sherman LA (eds): Venous and Arterial Thrombosis. Pathogenesis, Diagnosis, Prevention, and Therapy. New York, Grune & Stratton, 1979, pp 1–22

132. Wessler F: The current status of the hypercoagulable state, in Joist JH, Sherman LA (eds): Venous and Arterial Thrombosis. Pathogenesis, Diagnosis, Prevention, and Therapy. New York, Grune & Stratton, 1979, pp 23–31

133. Coon WW, Coller FA: Some epidemiologic considerations of thromboembolism. Surg Gynecol Obstet 109:487–501, 1959

134. Sevitt S, Gallagher N: Venous thrombosis and pulmonary embolism: A clinico-pathological study in injured and burned patients. Br J Surg 48:475–489, 1961

135. Warlow C, Ogston D, Douglas AS: Venous thrombosis following strokes. Lancet 1:1305–1306, 1972

136. Sigel B, Justin JR, Gibson RJ, et al: Risk assessment of pulmonary embolism by multivariate analysis. Arch Surg 114:188–192, 1979

137. Kakkar VV, Howe CT, Nicolaides AN, et al: Deep vein thrombosis of the leg. Is there a "high-risk" group? Am J Surg 120:527–530, 1970

138. Coon WW: Risk factors in pulmonary embolism. Surg Gynecol Obstet 143:385–390, 1976

139. Mauer BJ, Wray R, Shillingford JP: Frequency of deep venous thrombosis after myocardial infarction. Lancet 2:1385–1387, 1971

140. Corriere J Jr, Cornog JL, Murphy JJ: Prognosis in patients with carcinoma of the prostate. Cancer 25:911–918, 1970

141. Byar DP: Proceedings: The Veteran's Administration Cooperative Urological Reserach Group's study of cancer of the prostate. Cancer 32:1126–1130, 1973

142. Blackard CE, Doe RP, Mellinger GT, et al: Incidence of cardiovascular disease and death in patients receiving diethylstilbestrol for carcinoma of the prostate. Cancer 26:249–256, 1970

143. Richardson SGN, Matthews KB, Cruickshank JK, et al: Coagulation activation and hyperviscosity in infection. Br J Haematol 42:469–480, 1979

144. Gallus AS, Hirsh J: Prevention of venous thromboembolism. Semin Thromb Hemostas 2:232–290, 1976

145. Council on Thrombosis of the American Heart Association: Prevention of venous thromboembolism in surgical patients by low-dose heparin. Circulation 55:423A–426A, 1977

146. Kakkar VV: The diagnosis of deep vein thrombosis using the ^{125}I-fibrinogen test. Arch Surg 104:152–159, 1972

147. Packham MA, Mustard JF: Clinical pharmacology of platelets. Blood 50:555–573, 1977

148. Weiss HJ: Platelet physiology and abnormalities of platelet function. N Engl J Med 293:580–588, 1975

149. Soloway HB: Drug-induced bleeding. Am J Clin Pathol 61:622–627, 1974

150. Mielke CH Jr, Kaneshiro MM, Maher IA, et al: The standardized normal ivy bleeding time and its prolongation by aspirin. Blood 34:204–215, 1969

151. Pearson HA: Comparative effects of aspirin and acetaminophen on hemostasis. Pediatrics 62(Suppl):926–929, 1978

152. Buchanan GR, Martin V, Levine PH, et al: The effects of "anti-platelet" drugs on bleeding time and platelet aggregation in normal human subjects. Am J Clin Pathol 68:355–359, 1977

153. Brown CH III, Bradshaw MW, Natelson EA, et al: Defective platelet function following the administration of penicillin compounds. Blood 47:949–956, 1976

154. Cazenave J-P, Guccione MA, Packham MA, et al: Effects of cephalothin and penicillin G on platelet function in vitro. Br J Haematol 35:135–152, 1977

155. Brown CH III, Natelson EA, Bradshaw MW, et al: The hemostatic defect produced by carbenicillin. N Engl J Med 291:265–270, 1974

156. Johnson GJ, Rao GHR, White JG: Platelet dysfunction induced by parenteral carbenicillin and ticarcillin. Am J Pathol 91:85–106, 1978

157. Mills DCB, Roberts GCK: Membrane active drugs and the aggregation of human blood platelets. Nature (London) 213:35–38, 1967

158. Warlow C, Ogston D, Douglas AS: The effect of chloropromazine and antihistamines on human blood platelets in vitro and in vivo. Bibl Anat 12:249–253, 1973

159. Champion LAA, Schwartz AD, Luddy RE, et al: The effects of four commonly used drugs on platelet function. J Pediatr 89:653–656, 1976

160. Ansell JE, Kumar R, Deykin D: The spectrum of vitamin K deficiency. JAMA 238:40–42, 1977

161. Lechner K, Niessner H, Thaler E: Coagulation abnormalities in liver disease. Semin Thromb Hemostas 4:40–56, 1977

162. Straub PW: Diffuse intravascular coagulation in liver disease? Semin Thromb Hemostas 4:29–39, 1977

163. Rake MO, Flute PT, Pannell G, et al: Intravascular coagulation in acute hepatic necrosis. Lancet 1:533–537, 1970

164. Coleman M, Finlayson N, Bettigole RE, et al: Fibrinogen survival in cirrhosis: Improvement by "low dose" heparin. Ann Intern Med 83:79–81, 1975

165. von Felten A, Straub PW, Frick PG: Dysfibrinogenemia in a patient with primary hepatoma: First observation of an acquired abnormality of fibrin monomer aggregation. N Engl J Med 280:405–409, 1969

166. Gralnick HR, Givelber H, Abrams E: Dysfibrinogenemia associated with hepatoma. Increased carbohydrate content of the fibrinogen molecule. N Engl J Med 299:221–226, 1978

167. Morse EE: Fibrinogen and fibrinogenopathies. Ann Clin Sci 1:155–161, 1971

168. Harker LA, Finch CA: Thrombokinetics in man. J Clin Invest 48:963–974, 1969

169. Ness PM, Perkins HA: Cryoprecipitate as a reliable source of fibrinogen replacement. JAMA 241:1690–1691, 1979

170. Rabiner SF: Uremic bleeding, in Spaet TH (ed): Progress in Hemostasis and Thrombosis, Vol. 1. New York, Grune & Stratton, 1972, pp 233–250

171. Eknoyan G, Wacksman SJ, Glueck HI, et al: Platelet function in renal failure. N Engl J Med 280:677–681, 1969

172. Edson JR, Fecher DR, Doe RP: Low platelet adhesiveness and other hemostatic abnormalities in hypothyroidism. Ann Intern Med 82:342–346, 1975

173. Hardaway RM: Disseminated intravascular coagulation in experimental and clinical shock. Am J Cardiol 20:161–173, 1967

174. Hull R, Hirsh J: Diagnosis of venous thrombosis by invasive and non-invasive techniques, in Joist JH, Sherman LA (eds): Venous and Arterial Thrombosis: Pathogenesis, Diagnosis, Prevention, and Therapy. New York, Grune & Stratton, 1979, pp 33–56

175. Siegel BA, Biello DR: The diagnosis of pulmonary embolism, in Joist JH, Sherman LA (eds): Venous and Arterial Thrombosis: Pathogenesis, Diagnosis, Prevention, and Therapy. New York, Grune & Stratton, 1979, pp 81–91

176. Zacharski LR, Henderson WG, Rickles FR, et al: Rationale and ex-

perimental design for the VA Cooperative Study of anticoagulation (warfarin) in the treatment of cancer. Cancer 44:732–741, 1979

177. Hull R, Delmore S, Genton E, et al: Warfarin sodium versus low-dose heparin in the long-term treatment of venous thrombosis. N Engl J Med 301:855–858, 1979

178. Marciniak E, Gockerman JP: Heparin-induced decrease in circulating antithrombin-III. Lancet 2:581–584, 1977

179. Gallus AS, Hirsh J: Treatment of venous thromboembolic disease. Semin Thromb Hemostas 2:291–331, 1976

180. Wessler S, Gitel SN: Heparin: New concepts relevant to clinical use. Blood 53:525–544, 1979

181. Gollub S, Ulin AW: Heparin-induced thrombocytopenia in man. J Lab Clin Med 59:430–435, 1962

182. Bell WR, Tomasulo PA, Alving BM, et al: Thrombocytopenia occurring during the administration of heparin. A prospective study in 52 patients. Ann Intern Med 85:155–160, 1976

183. Babcock RB, Dumper CW, Scharfman WB: Heparin-induced immune thrombocytopenia. N Engl J Med 295:237–241, 1976

184. Trowbridge AA, Caraveo J, Green JB III, et al: Heparin-related immune thrombocytopenia. Studies of antibody–heparin specificity. Am J Med 65:277–283, 1978

185. Rhoads GR, Dixon RH, Silver D: Heparin-induced thrombocytopenia with thrombotic and hemorrhagic manifestations. Surg Gynecol Obstet 136:409–416, 1973

186. Bell WR, Anderson ND, Anderson AO: Heparin-induced coagulopathy. J Lab Clin Med 89:741–750, 1977

187. Joist JH: Laboratory control, prevention and management of complications of anticoagulant therapy, in Joist JH, Sherman LA, (ed): Venous and Arterial thrombosis: Pathogenesis, Diagnosis, Prevention, and Therapy. New York, Grune & Stratton, 1979, pp 173–189

8

HYPERCALCEMIA IN CANCER

Frances E. Bull

Hypercalcemia in patients with cancer has evoked special interest in the past decade, because of improvements in its management and because of clarification of some of its underlying mechanisms. It is a common complication of cancer: several older surveys of the causes of hypercalcemia in hospitalized patients indicated malignancy was the commonest underlying condition.[1] With the advent of the autoanalyzer in the past decade, calcium determinations are done almost routinely on outpatients as well as hospitalized patients and now mild, and sometimes even intermittent, elevations of calcium are frequently detected which are due to parathyroid adenomas.[2] This disease is substantially more common than the hypercalcemia of malignancy.[2] It remains true, however, that symptomatic hypercalcemia requiring therapy is primarily neoplastic in origin.[1]

The exact prevalence of hypercalcemia in cancer patients is not known, but it occurs most commonly in cancer of the breast where it is estimated that 10–25 percent of patients will experience it during the course of their disease.[3-5] Other tumors especially likely to produce hypercalcemia include squamous-cell cancers of the lung, head and neck, cervix, and esophagus; lymphoma, myeloma, and leukemia; and hypernephroma.[5]

For the oncologist, the appearance of hypercalcemia signifies a potentially lethal but generally reversible metabolic problem, resulting fundamentally from an uncontrolled malignancy. The triggering event may be an intercurrent illness resulting in dehydration and immobilization, the administration of a hormone to a patient with breast cancer, or the use of a thiazide diuretic.[3]

197

Clinical Aspects

The level of blood calcium is normally quite stable and reflects a balance between calcium intake, calcium turnover in bone, and calcium excretion. Hypercalcemia in neoplastic disease will result when bone resorption exceeds bone accretion and the renal calcium excretion is inadequate to handle the increased calcium load required to maintain normal blood levels. Patients may manifest this increased blood calcium with symptoms involving several organ systems, and with an intensity varying from minor feelings of fatigue to critical dehydration and coma, depending upon the speed of onset and severity of the hypercalcemia, the underlying malignancy, and their cardiac and renal status. The correlation of symptoms with levels of blood calcium, or even of ionized calcium, is imprecise; there is substantial individual variation.

Renal Effects

Although not the organ giving rise to early severe symptoms, the effect of a rising blood calcium on renal function sets in play a vicious cycle of escalating levels of calcium. Hypercalcemia itself directly reduces the glomerular filtration rate.[6] Additionally, there is a renal tubular effect with impairment of renal concentrating ability and free water loss, which leads to dehydration and a further decrease in the glomerular filtration rate.[7] All of this results in a decline in calcium excretion, and an aggravation of hypercalcemia. Phosphates are also progressively retained, and azotemia ensues. With an increase in both phosphate and calcium, in the presence of acidosis, soft-tissue calcification begins, and renal parenchymal calcinosis further damages renal function.[3,6] Nephrolithiasis is seen less commonly in the hypercalcemia of malignancy than with primary hyperparathyroidism, however.[8]

Gastrointestinal Effects

Loss of appetite, nausea, and vomiting are among the earliest symptoms of hypercalcemia, and aggravate the dehydration. Constipation may be severe due to the effect of calcium ion on smooth muscle. An increased incidence of peptic ulcer disease and pancreatitis has been noted.[6]

Central Nervous System Effects

Lethargy and weakness are common early symptoms of hypercalcemia, and may progress into stupor and coma, or into restlessness and psychosis.[3,6] Even focal symptoms have been noted, suggesting a cerebral metastasis. Electroencephalograms may show the diffuse slow waves associated with metabolic disturbances.[3,6]

Cardiovascular Effects

Calcium ions affect the contractility of cardiac and smooth muscle, and a shortened cardiac systole and shortened QT interval with ST-T wave abnormalities occur in hypercalcemia. Various arrhythmias have been recorded, and can be the cause of death at very high calcium levels. Bradycardia, tachycardia, and hypertension may occur. The potentiation of digitalis toxicity by hypercalcemia is a well-known complication.[6]

Pathogenesis of Cancer Hypercalcemia

The past decade has seen the rapid development of evidence favoring at least three humoral mechanisms for bone destruction by tumors which may lead to the production of hypercalcemia. Although most patients with

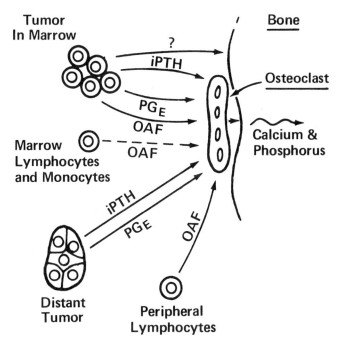

Fig. 1. *Diagramatic representation of the presently recognized mechanisms of hypercalcemia of malignancy. iPTH is parathormone-like immunoreactivity; PG_E is prostaglandin E; OAF is osteoclastic activating factor (see text).*

hypercalcemia of malignancy have metastatic disease in bone demonstrable by x-ray, scan, or biopsy, there are a few who do not, and possible humoral factors were first sought and then demonstrated in these.[5] The classic concept of how bone metastases produce bone dissolution was a physical one, i.e., that tumor growth per se lysed bone.[5] As humoral substances emerging from tumor cells and activating distant osteoclasts were defined, it became reasonable to believe similar humoral activation of osteoclasts occurred from metastatic deposits within the bone as well. Figure 1 diagrams the current concepts of bone dissolution by tumor cells.

Parathyroid Hormone

The ectopic production by tumors of a peptide immunologically similar to parathormone (iPTH) has been demonstrated repetitively in extracts of tumors,[9] by arterio-venous differences across tumor beds, by its production by tumor cells in culture,[10] and by its decrease with treatment of tumors.[5] The syndrome this substance produces is called pseudohyperparathyroidism, and it closely simulates primary hyperparathyroidism: increased bone resorption, elevation of blood calcium, depressed blood phosphorus, and increased urinary excretion of calcium, phosphorus, and urinary cyclic AMP. However, the blood chlorides tend to be normal, not elevated, and the bicarbonate elevated, not lowered, resulting in a metabolic alkalosis in pseudohyperparathyroidism.[8,11]

This ectopic iPTH has fewer COOH-terminal fragments than is present in primary hyperparathyroidism, and therefore its quantification will give lower values at a given level of blood calcium.[12] There is relatively little overlap in the values of iPTH in primary and pseudohyperparathyroidism.[12]

Lafferty also noted some clinical differences between primary and ectopic hyperparathyroidism: the latter tended to have a much shorter history of hypercalcemia symptoms, a higher blood calcium, more weight loss, more anemia, fewer kidney stones, and hand x-rays devoid of subperiosteal bone resorption.[8]

About one half of the tumors producing iPTH are hypernephromas and squamous-cell carcinomas of the lung. A wide variety of other tumors occasionally have been reported to produce this syndrome, including squamous-cell cancers of the head and neck, cervix, penis, and esophagus; lymphomas; leukemias; but rarely breast carcinoma.[6]

The coexistance of cancer and primary hyperparathyroidism has been reported repeatedly, particularly in patients with breast cancer.[5,13] Surgical correction of the parathyroid disease should benefit these patients.

Several reports have suggested the usefulness of selective catheterization of the neck veins for determination of parathormone levels as a technique of proving and localizing the adenoma.[14,15]

Prostaglandins

The prostaglandins are a family of substances consisting of 20-carbon fatty acids which exhibit an array of different physiologic activities. In vitro, prostaglandin E (PG_E) has been shown to stimulate bone resorption through osteoclastic stimulation.[16] In several transplanted animal tumors known to produce PG_E there has been demonstrated an increased number of osteoclasts adjacent to the tumor, and the production of mild increases in calcium. This effect can be blocked by either indomethacin or aspirin, substances known to block prostaglandin synthesis.[17-21] Trials of indomethacin, 75–150 mg/day, or aspirin, 1.8–4.8 g/day, in humans with hypercalcemia not due to iPTH have resulted in occasional responses, primarily in hypernephromas and squamous-cell carcinomas of the lung. Responses to indomethacin have correlated poorly with the effect on prostaglandins in the blood.[5] Seyberth et al. reported measuring the major urinary metabolite of PG_E (PGM) as an index of PG_E production in a series of patients.[22] Normal amounts of PGM were found in untreated primary hyperparathyroid patients, cancer patients with normal blood calcium, and a few with high blood calcium, but they identified a group of hypercalcemic cancer patients with elevated PGM. PGM excretion and blood calcium could be normalized in these patients by indomethacin if no bone metastases were present, and incompletely normalized if bone metastases were present, suggesting that a bulky tumor burden limited the usefulness of indomethacin.[22] Most of these patients had squamous-cell carcinomas of the lung.

Some human breast cancers contain more PG_E than benign breast lesions or normal breast tissue, and these cancers have been shown to synthesize the substance. The presence, or subsequent development, of bone metastases in these studied cases was confined to those patients whose cancers synthesized PG_E, suggesting that the bone-resorptive activity of PG_E may aid metastatic implantation in bone.[23,24] A clinical trial of indomethacin in hypercalcemic breast cancer patients did not affect the calcium, but the disease was considered to be bulky.[24]

Osteoclastic Activating Factor

A polypeptide which stimulated osteoclastic activity was first found in the supernatants of leucocyte cultures from patients with periodontal disease and bone resorption.[25] This factor, called osteoclastic activating factor (OAF), was subsequently identified in the supernatants of cultures of myeloma cells,[26] lymphoma cells,[27] Burkitt's lymphoma cells,[28] and lymphocytes obtained preoperatively from patients with breast cancer.[5] Chemical analysis of this factor has revealed two polypeptides, one larger than the other, which are fully interchangeable.[29] The production of OAF from lymphocytes has been shown to be dependent upon the presence of monocytes making PG_E.[30] Recently, corticosteroids were shown to block the response of the osteoclasts to OAF without altering its production in vitro.[31] This latter observation may explain the responses recorded from the use of glucocorticoids in the hypercalcemia of breast cancer, myeloma, and lymphomas better than the classic explanation of the antitumor effects of glucocorticoids on these tumors.

Other Factors

Although osteoclastic hypertrophy generally can be identified adjacent to metastatic disease in bone, functioning as the mediator of bone resorption in response to iPTH, PG_E, and OAF as discussed above, occasionally bulky tumor will be found surrounding atrophic bone spicules without any intervening osteoclasts.[20] Eilon studied the bone resorptive effect in vitro of the cells and the culture supernatant of four human breast cancer cell lines and noted that bone resorption occurred which could not be blocked by indomethacin, and hence was not PG_E. It also occurred when bone was devitalized, and therefore was independent of osteoclastic mediation.[32] The substance involved in this direct bone lysis is not known.

Vitamin D and its metabolites will induce active bone resorption in vitro.[33] There is no evidence as yet of ectopic production of these substances, although a cytosol receptor for 1,25-dihydroxy-vitamin D has been found in a cultured breast cancer cell line.[34] Non-vitamin D phytosterols have been found in human breast cancer tissue and in blood which have osteolytic activity in vitro, but which correlate poorly with blood calcium levels in vivo.[35]

Hormonal therapy of breast cancer, particularly in patients with osseous metastases, may induce hypercalcemia: this has been reported with androgens, estrogens, and progesterone, and generally occurs during the first few weeks of therapy. This may be a transient event prior to response, or may represent a stimulation of the tumor.[3,36,37]

Immobilization causes bone resorption to exceed bone accretion. Bone mesenchyme responds to mechanical stress with a decrease in bone resorption.[38] A patient with progressive bone pain or a pathologic fracture may aggrevate hypercalcemia by inactivity.

It is clear that the mechanism of hypercalcemia in a given patient may be multifactorial. The determination of iPTH can be accomplished in many laboratories now, but generally takes several days. The determination of PGM as a technique of determining the desirability of antiprostaglandin therapy is presently at the research level. The possible role of OAF, hormonal therapy, and immobilization can be inferred. The immediate therapeutic maneuvers, described below, do not require precision in defining the mechanisms, but this remains the ultimate goal.

Treatment of Hypercalcemia

The vigor and complexity of the treatment program must be individualized for each patient, based upon the calcium level and the clinical assessment of the patient. Table 1 provides broad guidelines for progressively more vigorous therapy.

For mild elevations of calcium in an almost asymptomatic patient, oral hydration and treatment of the underlying tumor is all that is needed, the elevated calcium being a marker of tumor activity. Most patients with co-existent cancer and primary hyperparathyroidism will be in this group, and this should be a diagnostic consideration.

Hydration

Essentially all symptomatic patients will be dehydrated. As indicated above, hypercalcemia induces free water loss by the renal tubule, resulting in polyuria which leads to a decrease in blood volume. It also causes anorexia, nausea, and vomiting, which prevents adequate oral hydration. Prompt intravenous hydration is fundamental to restoration of both the blood volume and the glomerular filtration rate, and to interrupt the cycle of progressive hypercalcemia. Normal saline should be used since it has been shown that calcium excretion parallels sodium excretion by the proximal tubule,[39] and hence calcium diuresis as well as expansion of the blood volume will ensue. The first liter or two should be administered rapidly over a few hours. If the patient is known to have underlying renal or heart disease, close monitoring of venous pressure and urinary output will be needed, and a central venous catheter may be helpful.

Diuretics

After the patient has been rehydrated, additional calcium excretion can be accomplished with furosemide, 40–100 mg every 6–12 hours, which induces a sodium diuresis by its action on the proximal convoluted

Table 1
Outline for Management of Hypercalcemia*

Acute Management
  Calcium ≤ 13 mg%; patient minimally symptomatic
  1. Oral hydration if possible
  2. Mobilize
  3. Monitor serum calcium and creatinine
  Calcium 13–15 mg%; patient moderately symptomatic
  1. Hydrate with IV normal saline 4–6 liters/24 hours
  2. Furosemide 40–100 mg every 12–24 hours. Start after blood volume is
      restored
  3. Potassium 40–80 mEq/24 hours
  4. Monitor serum calcium, creatinine, electrolytes, magnesium, intake and
      output, and daily weights
  Calcium ≥ 15 mg%; patient markedly symptomatic
  1. Hydrate with IV normal saline, 6–10 liters/24 hours. Consider
      monitoring with central venous pressure line; maintain at 10 cm
  2. Furosemide, 40–80 mg every 6 hours when CVP is 10 cm
  3. Potassium 15–20 mEq/liter of saline
  4. After 24 hours if calcium not responding satisfactorily, consider:
        a. Calcitonin 3–8 MRC units/kg IM every 6 hours, *or*
        b. Mithramycin 25 μg/kg IV
  5. Monitor calcium, creatinine, electrolytes, magnesium, intake and output
      every 12 hours
  6. If creatinine remains elevated and urine output poor at 24 hours,
      consider hemodialysis
Chronic Management
  1. Attempt definitive treatment of tumor. If carcinoma of the breast,
      multiple myeloma, or lymphoma, consider corticosteroids as part of
      chronic treatment of the tumor
  2. Oral phosphate, 2 grams per day diluted with water
  3. Consider mithramycin 25 μg/kg IV every 4–7 days if necessary
  4. Consider indomethacin 25 mg every 6–8 hours

---

*Patient management must be individualized. Please see text for discussion.

tubule and ascending loop of Henle.[40] Again, calcium excretion will parallel sodium excretion, and potassium and magnesium will be excreted.[40] If
the blood volume, and hence the glomerular filtration rate, has not been
normalized, furosemide will cause calcium reabsorption instead of excretion, defeating the purpose of the drug. The use of furosemide in the rehydrated patient adds to the safety of continued use of normal saline as well.
Thiazide diuretics should not be used since they may aggravate the hypercalcemia.

Suki's original description of the treatment of hypercalcemia with saline diuresis and furosemide[40] was more vigorous than that suggested in

Table 1. He used furosemide 80–100 mg intravenously every 1–2 hours. Serum electrolytes were obtained every 4–6 hours, and urine electrolytes were determined on pooled 4-hour urine collections. Isotonic saline with 20 mEq of potassium chloride per liter and 5-percent dextrose in water were infused simultaneously in a 4:1 proportion to replace urine losses of water and electrolytes.[40] Generally a less vigorous program suffices, and is simpler to manage on a general medical service. With either program, potassium and magnesium losses must be expected and replaced.

Dialysis

Hemodialysis is capable of lowering serum calcium well, but the effect is transitory.[41] This can be considered when the underlying malignancy is considered treatable and renal function precludes adequate forced diuresis. This is rarely indicated.

Calcitonin

Calcitonin is a polypeptide hormone, secreted by the parafollicular cells of the thyroid, that produces hypocalcemia and hypophosphatemia by inhibiting bone resorption by the osteoclasts and by increasing the renal clearance of calcium.[42] The commercially available calcitonin, synthetic salmon calcitonin, is also the most potent and longest acting. It comes in vials cotaining 400 Medical Research Council (MRC) units, and is reconstituted with the gelatin solution accompanying it. A test dose of 1 MRC unit should be injected intradermally, and the area observed for 15 minutes for erythema and wheal formation, which would indicate an allergy to the protein of the calcitonin or gelatin. The usual effective dosage for treatment of hypercalcemia is 3–8 MRC units/kg by 24-hour IV infusion, or the same dose intramuscularly every 6 hours. Calcitonin adheres to glass, so plastic bags must be used for intravenous infusion.[43] The reported nadir of the hypocalcemic effect is 4 hours (Fig. 2). Serum phosphate and magnesium also decline, and urine phosphate and magnesium increase, due to a decrease in renal tubular resorption of these ions. Several reports indicate that the hypercalcemia of malignancy, or of primary hyperparathyroidism, will be brought temporarily under control in 75–90 percent of patients.[43-45] An occasional patient experiences nausea, but serious side effects are absent. The speed of its action makes it attractive for acute use, especially in the patient with azotemia or myocardial dysfunction making intense saline diuresis difficult. Its lack of hematopoietic toxicity make it an attractive alternative to mithramycin in the thrombocyto-

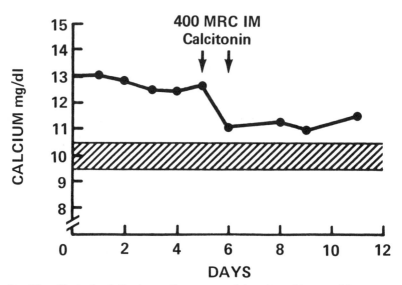

Fig. 2. *The effect of calcitonin on the serum calcium in a 54-year-old woman with carcinoma of the breast with bone metastases and thrombocytopenia. Prolonged hydration with furosemide had lowered and then stabilized calcium at a level at which she was still moderately symptomatic. Symptoms were relieved after calcitonin.*

penic patient. It has been used continuously for up to 6 or more weeks, with the dosage adjusted to the level of serum calcium, without hypersensitivity or loss of effectiveness noticed,[44] but it is an expensive medication for such use. The possibility of synergism with mithramycin resulting in symptomatic hypocalcemia has been reported recently,[42] and these medications probably should not be used together until this observation has been confirmed and explained.

Mithramycin

Mithramycin is a potent antineoplastic antibiotic which inhibits osteoclastic bone resorption at doses lower than that needed for its antitumor effect. Kinetic studies of its effect on bone demonstrate a preferential effect on bone resorption and little effect on bone formation.[46] The inhibition of bone resorption starts in 6–12 hours, lasts 4–5 days, and is reflected in a lowering of blood calcium and phosphorus, and urine calcium and hydroxyproline.[46–48] The usual pattern of response in the hypercalcemic patient is a stabilization of blood calcium by 12 hours postinjection, followed by a decrease in 36–48 hours (Fig. 3). A single injection of 25 μg/kg often suffices for lowering the calcium.[47,48] An additional injection at 48 hours may be needed for normalization. Because of the delay in its effect, repetitive daily doses may produce hypocalcemia.[49] The duration of effect of a single dose varies from 3 to 7 or more days depending upon the aggressiveness of the underlying process.

Mithramycin can be used chronically, if necessary, to palliate hypercalcemia, with intermittent doses every 3–7 days, as dictated by the serum calcium. This dosage schedule generally will not produce renal, hepatic, or hematologic toxicity although these parameters must be monitored.[49] Often the drug can be given as an IV bolus: however, this may produce nausea and vomiting in some patients which can be alleviated by changing to a 6–8-hour infusion.

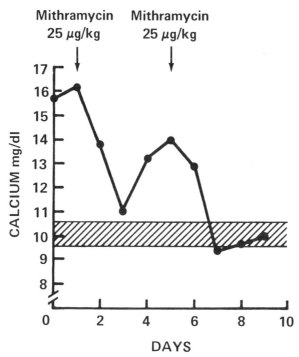

Fig. 3. *The effect of mithramycin on the serum calcium in a 69-year-old woman with carcinoma of the breast with bone metastases. Twenty-four hours of hydration with furosemide had stabilized but not lowered her calcium prior to mithramycin. Note maximal hypocalcemic effect is at 48 hours.*

Because of the 48-hour latent period for the full hypocalcemic effect, the use of mithramycin alone in a highly symptomatic patient is not wise; hydration and sodium diuresis are the mainstays of the immediate, emergent management. Nevertheless, it is a powerful tool in the overall management of the patient with hypercalcemia.

Inorganic Phosphate

The administration of inorganic phosphate will lower the serum calcium and reduce the urinary calcium.[50] Complexes of calcium phosphate presumably are formed and deposited in bone and soft tissues: there is evidence for the inhibition of bone resorption, for stimulation of bone formation, and for the soft-tissue deposition of calcium.[51] Used intravenously, inorganic phosphate usually will reduce the serum calcium within 24 hours. The effect is dose dependent and also dependent upon the degree of elevation of serum phosphate induced by the infusion. The serum phosphate generally returns to the pretreatment level 24–36 hours after the infusion.[52] Complications of the intravenous route of phosphate administration include hypotension and renal failure, possibly due to excessively large doses or excessive speed of administration.[52-54] Extraskeletal calcinosis may occur in hypercalcemic states without phosphate therapy, but there is continuing concern that phosphate therapy may induce or worsen this, producing functional impairment of vital organs.[55] Inflammation and calcification along the vein used for the infusion has occurred.[52] Symptomatic hypocalcemia may occur as well, most commonly with larger doses or in patients with renal insufficiency.[52,56]

The usual dose of intravenous phosphate is 50 mmol (1.5 grams) of phosphorus diluted in 1 liter of fluid and infused over 6–8 hours.[50] Because of concern about the complications listed above and the availability of alternate methods of treating hypercalcemia, intravenous phosphate is used infrequently, and only in patients requiring rapid reduction of their calcium level and not responding to other therapy. Those with elevated phosphorus due to renal impairment should not receive it.

Oral phosphate continues to find use in the chronic treatment of moderate hypercalcemia. Its effect is more gradual, taking several days to become evident. In addition to helping control serum calcium levels, there is one report suggesting that oral phosphates may alleviate bone pain in patients with multiple myeloma.[57] As with intravenous phosphates, normal pretreatment renal function and serum phosphorus levels are desirable.[58,59] The usual dose is 2 grams of phosphorus per day in divided doses, and diluted to minimize diarrhea. The commercially available oral phosphate preparations include sodium phosphate and biphosphate (Fleet's Phospho-Soda), 5 ml every 6 hours in water, providing about 2 grams of phosphorus; mono- and dibasic sodium and potassium phosphate (Neutra-Phos), eight 250-mg capsules in divided doses providing 2 grams of phosphorus a day.

Corticosteroids

In the 1950s, when corticosteroids were first available and used empirically in many conditions, occasional responses were noted in the hypercalcemia of malignant disease. When analyzed, the responding patients generally had carcinoma of the breast,[3,4] multiple myeloma, or lymphoma, although there were occasional examples of other tumor types.[60] Seriously ill hypercalcemic patients often did not respond regardless of tumor type.[61] Attempts to use large intravenous corticosteroid doses acutely also had minor and inconsistent effects on calcium.[52] Chronic use in these favorable tumor types, however, often had a gradual lowering effect on the calcium that was discernible within a few days to weeks.[60] Occasionally lytic bone lesions due to breast cancer would regress[4] and myeloma proteins would decrease.[60] Metabolic balance studies on patients with myeloma revealed that corticosteroids decreased bone resorption rather than altering gastrointestinal absorption or renal excretion of calcium.[61,62] The usual interpretation of all of these observations is that corticosteroids affect hypercalcemia by producing an antitumor response. As discussed in the pathogenesis section, however, corticosteroids may block the stimulatory effect of OAF on the osteoclast in addition.[31]

Antiprostaglandin Therapy

The technique of using elevated urinary metabolites of prostaglandin E to identify patients whose hypercalcemia might respond to inhibitors of prostaglandin synthesis is presently a research tool.[22] An empiric trial of indomethacin or aspirin in patients with low-bulk hypernephroma or squamous-cell carcinoma of the lung, the two tumors apparently most commonly benefited,[22] would seem reasonable.

Other Measures

Initially, a low-calcium diet of 200 mg per day is desirable. This is an unpalatable diet, and relaxation of this strict limitation should be considered when the acute metabolic problem is controlled. Mobilization of the patient is also helpful. Chelating agents and sodium sulfate are no longer used.

Once the acute metabolic derangement is corrected, attempts to control the underlying malignancy is the most important consideration. If this can be accomplished, chronic therapy aimed at control of hypercalcemia should not be necessary. If the malignancy cannot be controlled, chronic intermittent mithramycin and oral phosphates together with maximum mobilization of the patient may be used, with corticosteroids and antiprostaglandin therapy reserved for the tumor types thought to be sensitive to these medications.

References

1. McLellan G, Baird CW, Melick R: Hypercalcemia in an Australian hospital adult population. Med J Austrail 2:354–356, 1968
2. Boonstra CE, Jackson CE: Hyperparathyroidism detected by routine serum calcium analysis. Ann Intern Med 63:468–474, 1965
3. Jessiman AG, Emerson K Jr, Shah RC: Hypercalcemia in carcinoma of the breast. Ann Surg 157:377–393, 1963
4. Mannheimer I: Hypercalcemia of breast cancer: management with corticosteroids. Cancer 18:679–691, 1965
5. Myers WPL, Bockman R: Studies on the pathogenesis of cancer hypercalcemia. Trans Am Clin Climatol Assoc 88:177–190, 1976
6. Muggia FM, Heinemann HO: Hypercalcemia associated with neoplastic disease. Ann Intern Med 73:281–290, 1970
7. Zeffren JL, Heinemann HO: Reversible defect in renal concentrating mechanism in patients with hypercalcemia. Am J Med 33:54–63, 1962
8. Lafferty FW: Pseudohyperparathyroidism. Medicine 45:247–260, 1966
9. Sherwood LM, O'Riordan JLH, Aurbach GD, et al: Production of parathyroid hormone by nonparathyroid tumors. J Clin Endocrinol Metab 27:140–146, 1967
10. Besarab A, Caro JF: Mechanisms of hypercalcemia in malignancy. Cancer 41:2276–2284, 1978
11. Heinemann HO: Metabolic alkalosis in patients with hypercalcemia. Metabolism 14:1137–1152, 1965
12. Benson RC, Riggs BL, Pickard M: Immunoreactive forms of circulating parathormone in primary and ectopic hyperparathyroidism. J Clin Invest 54:175–181, 1974

13. Drezner MK, Lebovitz HE: Primary hyperparathyroidism in para-neoplastic hypercalcemia. Lancet 1:1004–1006, 1978
14. Reitz RE, Pollard JJ, Wang CA, et al: Localization of parathyroid ade-nomas by catheterization and radioimmunoassay. N Engl J Med 281:348–351, 1969
15. Samaan NA, Hickey RC, Hills CS Jr, et al: Parathyroid tumors: pre-operative localization and association with other tumors. Cancer 33:933–939, 1974
16. Klein DC, Raisz LG: Prostaglandins: stimulation of bone resorption in tissue culture. Endocrinology 86:1436–1440, 1970
17. Voelkel EF, Tashjian AH Jr, Franklin R, et al: Hypercalcemia and tu-mor-prostaglandins: the VX_2 carcinoma model in the rabbit. Metabo-lism 24:973–986, 1975
18. Tashjian AH Jr, Voelkel EF, Levine L, et al: Evidence that the bone resorption-stimulating factor produced by mouse fibrosarcoma cells is prostaglandin E_2: a new model for the hypercalcemia of cancer. J Exp Med 136:1329–1434, 1972
19. Tashjian AH Jr: Role of prostaglandins in the production of hypercal-cemia by tumors. Cancer Res 38:4138–4141, 1978
20. Glasko CSB: Mechanisms of bone destruction in the development of skeletal metastases. Nature 263:507–508, 1976
21. Galasko CSB, Bennett A: Relationship of bone destruction in skeletal metastasis to osteoclast activation and prostaglandins. Nature 263:508–510, 1976
22. Seyberth HW, Segre GV, Morgan MA, et al: Prostaglandins as medi-ators of hypercalcemia associated with certain types of cancer. N Engl J Med 293:1278–1283, 1975
23. Bennett A, McDonald AM, Simpson JS, et al: Breast cancer, pro-staglandins, and bone metastases. Lancet 1:1218–1220, 1975
24. Powles TJ: Factors influencing metastasis in bone, in Stoll BA (ed): New Aspects of Breast Cancer: Volume III, Secondary Spread in Breast Cancer. London, Heinemann Medical Books, 1977, pp 82–86
25. Horton JE, Raisz LG, Simmons HA, et al: Bone resorbing activity in supernatant fluid from cultured human peripheral blood leukocytes. Science 177:793–795, 1972
26. Mundy GR, Raisz LG, Cooper RA, et al: Evidence for the secretion of an osteoclast stimulating factor in myeloma. New Engl J Med 291:1041–1046, 1974
27. Mundy GR, Rick ME, Turcotte R, et al: Pathogenesis of hypercalce-mia in lymphosarcoma cell leukemia. Am J Med 65:600–606, 1978

28. Mundy GR, Luben RA, Raisz LG, et al: Bone-resorbing activity in supernatants from lymphoid lines. N Engl J Med 290:867–871, 1974

29. Mundy GR, Raisz LG: Big and little forms of osteoclast activating factor. J Clin Invest 60:122–128, 1977

30. Yoneda T, Mundy GR: Monocytes regulate osteoclast-activating factor production by releasing prostaglandins. J Exp Med 150:338–350, 1979

31. Strumpf M, Kowalski MA, Mundy GR: Effects of glucocorticoids on osteoclast-activating factor. J Lab Clin Med 92:772–778, 1978

32. Eilon G, Mundy GR: Direct resorption of bone by human breast cancer cells in vitro. Nature 276:726–728, 1978

33. Raisz LG, Trummel CL, Holick MF, et al: 1,25-Dihydroxycholecalciferol: a potent stimulator of bone resorption in tissue culture. Science 175:768–769, 1972

34. Eisman JA, Martin TJ, MacIntyre I, et al: 1,25-Dihydroxyvitamin-D receptor in breast cancer cells. Lancet 2:1335–1336, 1979

35. Gordon GS, Cantino TJ, Erhardt L, et al: Osteolytic sterol in human breast cancer. Science 151:1226–1228, 1966

36. Kennedy BJ, Tibbetts DM, Nathanson IT, et al: Hypercalcemia: a complication of hormone therapy of advanced disease. Cancer Res 13:445–459, 1953

37. Hall TC, Dederick MM, Nevinny HB: Prognostic value of hormonally induced hypercalcemia in breast cancer. Cancer Chemother Rep 30:21–23, 1963

38. Harris WH, Heaney RP: Skeletal renewal and metabolic bone disease. N Engl J Med 280:193–202, 253–259, 303–311, 1969

39. Walser M: Calcium clearance as a function of sodium clearance in the dog. Amer J Physiol 200:1099–1104, 1961

40. Suki WN, Yium JJ, Von Minden M, et al: Acute treatment of hypercalcemia with furosemide. N Engl J Med 283:836–840, 1970

41. Strauch BS, Ball MF: Hemodialysis in the treatment of severe hypercalcemia. JAMA 235:1347–1348, 1976

42. Caro JF, Besarb A, Glennon JA: Symptomatic hypocalcemia following combined calcitonin and mithramycin therapy for hypercalcemia due to malignancy. Cancer Treat Rep 62:1561–1563, 1978

43. Vaughn CB, Vaitkevicius VK: The effects of calcitonin in hypercalcemia in patients with malignancy. Cancer 34:1268–1271, 1974

44. Silva OL, Becker KL: Salmon calcitonin in the treatment of hypercalcemia. Arch Int Med 132:337–339, 1973

45. Sjöberg HE, Hjern B: Acute treatment with calcitonin in primary hy-

perparathyroidism and severe hypercalcemia of other origin. Acta Chir Scand 141:90–95, 1975

46. Kiang DT, Loken MK, Kennedy BJ: Mechanism of the hypocalcemic effect of mithramycin. J Clin Endocrinol Metab 48:341–344, 1979

47. Parsons DM, Baum M, Self M: Effect of mithramycin on calcium and hydroxyproline metabolism in patients with malignant disease. Br Med J 1:474–477, 1967

48. Perlia CP, Gubisch NJ, Wolter J, et al: Mithramycin treatment of hypercalcemia. Cancer 25:389–394, 1970

49. Elias EG, Evans JT: Hypercalcemic crisis in neoplastic disease: management with mithramycin. Surgery 71:631–635, 1972

50. Goldsmith RS, Ingbar SH: Inorganic phosphate treatment of hypercalcemia of diverse etiologies. N Engl J Med 274:1–7, 1966

51. Eisenberg E: Effect of intravenous phosphate on serum strontium and calcium. N Engl J Med 282:889–892, 1970

52. Fulmer, DH, Dimich AB, Rothschild EO, et al: Treatment of hypercalcemia: comparison of intravenously administered phosphate, sulfate, and hydrocortisone. Arch Intern Med 129:923–930, 1972

53. Shackney S, Hasson J: Precipitous fall in serum calcium, hypotension, and acute renal failure after intravenous phosphate therapy for hypercalcemia. Ann Intern Med 66:906–916, 1967

54. Massry SG, Mueller E, Silverman AG, et al: Inorganic phosphate treatment of hypercalcemia. Arch Intern Med 121:307–312, 1968

55. Carey RW, Schmitt GW, Kopald H, et al: Massive extraskeletal calcification during phosphate treatment of hypercalcemia. Arch Intern Med 122:150–155, 1968

56. Goldsmith RS, Ingbar SH: Hyper- to hypocalcemia. N Engl J Med 274:284, 1966

57. Goldsmith RS, Bartos J, Hulley SB, et al: Phosphate supplementation as an adjunct in the therapy of multiple myeloma. Arch Int Med 122:128–133, 1968

58. Ayala G, Chertow BS, Shah JH, et al: Acute hyperphosphatemia and acute persistant renal insufficiency induced by oral phosphate therapy. Ann Intern Med 83:520–521, 1975

59. Breuer RI, LeBauer J: Caution in the use of phosphates in the treatment of severe hypercalcemia. J Clin Endocrinol Metab 27:695–698, 1967

60. Myers WPL: Cortisone in the treatment of hypercalcemia in neoplastic disease. Cancer 11:83–88, 1958

61. Thalassinos NC, Joplin GF: Failure of corticosteroid therapy to correct the hypercalcemia of malignant disease. Lancet 2:537–539, 1970
62. Lazor MZ, Rosenberg LE: Mechanism of adrenal-steroid reversal of hypercalcemia in multiple myeloma. N Engl J Med 270:749–755, 1964
63. Bentzel CJ, Carbone PP, Rosenberg L: The effect of prednisone on calcium metabolism and ^{47}Ca kinetics in patients with multiple myeloma and hypercalcemia. J Clin Invest 43:2132–2145, 1964

9

ELECTROLYTE ABNORMALITIES IN CANCER PATIENTS

Alan S. Kliger
David H. Lovett

In man, as in all land-dwelling creatures, the internal environment is maintained constant by a delicate balance between the fluids and salts of the body. Complex systems have evolved to control the osmolality, the volume, and the concentrations of many ions within narrow limits. When these control systems or the effector organs through which they operate are impaired by tumors or the products of tumors, fluid and electrolyte disorders may result. Such abnormalities may develop slowly or rapidly, may have little consequence or may be life-threatening. Furthermore, the extracellular concentrations of fluid and electrolytes may be affected by the chemotherapy or radiation therapy used to treat cancer. This may occur by a direct toxic mechanism, such as the effect of vincristine or cyclophosphamide on water balance, or as a side effect of destroying a large mass of tumor cells. The intracellular space is rich in potassium, phosphorus, purines, and other substances which flood into the extracellular fluid when neoplastic cells are lysed. Such sudden large increases in the concentration of these molecules can exceed the body's ability to excrete them, and acute electrolyte disturbances may result. In addition, conversion of purines to uric acid and calcium phosphate deposits may impair renal function and prevent excretion of these toxic substances. Finally, tumors invading bones or producing hormones can acutely raise the plasma concentration of calcium, a potentially life-threatening metabolic disorder.

Hypercalcemia and acute renal failure are considered in detail in Chapters 8 and 10 of this text. The purpose of this chapter is to discuss the other major clinical disorders of fluid and electrolyte balance seen in patients with neoplastic diseases, and to provide a practical guide to the management of these imbalances. We consider in detail disorders of sodium, potassium, uric acid, phosphate, magnesium, and water balance.

Disorders of Water Balance

The concentration of salt and body fluids is regulated to maintain a constant osmolality between 286 and 294 mOsm/kg H_2O.[1] This steady state is maintained by a balance of fluid ingestion and urinary excretion. The first half of the control system, normal control of fluid intake, is maintained by the thirst mechanism. During water depravation, the osmolality of extracellular fluid rises, and the sensation of thirst is activated. Fluid ingestion then tends to restore the fluid balance. The thirst center is located in the hypothalamus,[2] and lesions in this part of the brain can result in loss of thirst, persistent hyperosmolality, and hypernatremia. In addition, cerebral function must be intact so that the sensation of thirst can be translated to the seeking and drinking of fluids. Thus, cerebral lesions also can result in hyperosmolality. The other half of the water balance system concerns regulation of fluid excretion by the kidney. Normal individuals drink widely varying fluid volumes, even when they are not hyperosmolar or thirsty. Any excess fluid ingested is promptly excreted by the kidneys, and the fluid balance is maintained. The finely tuned ability of the kidneys to regulate fluid excretion is governed by the neurohypophyseal release of antidiuretic hormone (ADH). Secretion of this hormone is very sensitive, responding to 1–2-percent changes of osmolality. When osmolality begins to rise, ADH is secreted and the permeability of the renal distal tubule and the collecting duct to water is increased. This enhanced reabsorption of water restores the osmolality towards normal and a concentrated urine is elaborated. When excess water intake results in a fall of serum osmolality, ADH secretion stops, the distal tubule and collecting ducts become relatively impermeable to water, a hypotonic urine is elaborated, and the excess water is excreted. Thus, the ADH–renal system and the thirst mechanism tend to maintain body fluid osmolality constant.

Several disorders in this balance system can result from tumors, either by invasion of anatomic structures or by elaboration of antidiuretic hormone-like substances. Since Na is the major extracellular cation, hyperosmolality is usually characterized by a high serum Na concentration (>150 mEq/liter), and hypo-osmolality by a low Na concentration (<135 mEq/liter). Since serum Na is measured in virtually every hospitalized patient, abnormalities of Na concentration are a commonly used shorthand to signify defects in osmolar control. When ADH is absent (central diabetes insipidus), inadequate (partial diabetes insipidus), or ineffective in the kidney (nephrogenic diabetes insipidus), polyuria results. The thirst mechanism is triggered, and large fluid volumes are ingested. Under these conditions, the serum Na concentration may be elevated if urinary water excretion exceeds intake, or normal if large fluid volumes are ingested. Therefore the three common clinical presentations of disordered water metabolism are hyponatremia, hypernatremia, and polyuria.

Hyponatremia

The normal stimulus to secretion of ADH is an increase in osmolality. When the serum osmolality is low, there should be no detectable ADH secretion. If normal subjects are given ADH and are allowed to ingest fluids freely, fluid retention and hyponatremia result.[3] Furthermore, these subjects develop a negative Na balance, excreting more Na than is present in the diet, a result of volume expansion and decreased proximal tubular Na reabsorption.[4] In clinical medicine, a similar picture can be seen, the syndrome of inappropriate secretion of ADH (SIADH). This syndrome is characterized by hypo-osmolality, normovolemia, normal renal and adrenal function, a less than maximally dilute urine, and appreciable urinary sodium excretion (Tables 1 and 2). First described in patients with bronchogenic carcinoma,[5] this syndrome also has been found in patients with carcinoma of the duodenum and pancreas,[6] thymoma,[6] carcinoma of the larynx,[7] carcinoma of the prostate with pulmonary lymphangitic carcinomatosis,[8] lymphosarcoma,[7] reticulum-cell sarcoma,[9] and Hodgkin's disease.[10] Antidiuretic activity can be detected in extracts of oat-cell carcinoma of the lung,[11] giant-cell carcinoma of the lung, bronchial carcinoid, and adenocarcinoma of the pancreas[11] and their metastases. The same clinical syndrome has also been seen in patients with mesothelioma.[12] In a group of 14 consecutive patients with acute myelogenous leukemia studied in England, 11 had serum Na < 135 mEq/liter, an increased urinary Na excretion, decreased free water clearance, and inappropriately concentrated urine. Two of these 11 patients had hyponatremia before chemotherapy and in the others the fall of serum Na coincided with a fall in the peripheral blast count following therapy with daunorubicin and cytosine arabinóside.[13] In an expanded sample of 42 patients with acute myeloid leukemia, more than 75 percent had features consistent with SIADH.

Table 1
Tumor-Related Causes of SIADH

Neoplasms
1. Carcinoma of the lung (oat cell, giant cell, other)[5,11]
2. Bronchial carcinoid[11]
3. Adenocarcinoma of the pancreas[6,11]
4. Carcinoma of the duodenum[6]
5. Thymoma[6]
6. Mesothelioma[12]
7. Carcinoma of the larynx[7]
8. Acute and chronic leukemia[13,16]
9. Hodgkin's disease[10]
10. Lymphosarcoma[7]
11. Reticulum-cell sarcoma[9]
Chemotherapeutic Agents
1. Vincristine[17,18]
2. Cyclophosphamide[19,20]

However, the plasma level of ADH was measured in three patients, and was not elevated in any.[14] Hyponatremia has also been seen in chronic lymphocytic leukemia, chronic myelogenous leukemia,[15] and in childhood leukemia.[16]

Two chemotherapeutic agents have been associated with SIADH. In several studies, children and adults receiving vincristine to treat acute lymphocytic leukemia or acute myeloid leukemia developed SIADH. In one case, urinary ADH levels measured by radioimmunoassay were elevated 8 days following vincristine administration, and remained high with repeated vincristine therapy.[17] Recurrent hyponatremia was prevented by prophylactic fluid restriction. In many cases, SIADH accompa-

Table 2
Diagnostic Criteria for SIADH*

1. Hypo-osmolality and hyponatremia of extracellular fluids
2. Urine less than maximally dilute
3. No volume depletion
4. Continued renal excretion of sodium
5. Normal renal function
6. Normal adrenal function

*Adapted from Bartter and Schwartz (Ref. 6).

nied other toxic manifestations of vincristine, including ileus, abdominal distension, and peripheral neuropathy. A proposed mechanism of vincristine-induced SIADH is a direct effect of the drug on nervous system sites of ADH formation or storage.[18]

Administration of high-dose (> 50 mg/kg) cyclophosphamide may result in impaired water excretion characterized by weight gain, hyponatremia, and inappropriately concentrated urine. This syndrome occurs 4–12 hours after cyclophosphamide administration and lasts 20–24 hours.[19] Plasma ADH levels measured in three treated patients were elevated in only one. Thus the etiology of this disorder may be a direct nephrotoxic effect of the drug, or true SIADH. As might be expected, cyclophosphamide therapy has been reported to aggravate the hyponatremia seen in a patient with oat-cell carcinoma-induced SIADH.[20]

Treatment of SIADH in this setting depends upon the clinical severity of the hyponatremia. Since this syndrome develops by excess free water intake in the setting of unsuppressable ADH release, fluid restriction which results in negative water balance (usually < 1 liter/day) will restore the osmolality toward normal.[1] When neurological irritability or seizures accompany the rapid development of acute hyponatremia, the osmolality should be restored toward normal more quickly than fluid restriction alone will allow. Hypertonic saline infusion results in a transient rise of serum Na concentration, but the concomitant volume expansion induces a prompt natriuresis and return of hypo-osmolality. One useful technique to avoid this volume expansion is to administer furosemide 40 mg orally then rigorously replace the urine volume by normal saline. Since furosemide causes a hypotonic diuresis, this maneuver results in constant body volume and increased osmolality. Great care, however, must be taken to replace the diuretic-induced urine volume with normal saline solution. If this is not performed rigorously, volume depletion with resultant thirst may induce water drinking and worsening of the hyponatremia. In addition, severe fluid restriction may not be wise in patients receiving chemotherapy, since a maximal urine volume is desirable to obviate the risk of uric acid and xanthine-induced nephrolithiasis, and cyclophosphamide-induced cystitis.[19] In such patients, pretreatment with intravenous fluids may reduce the morbidity.

When SIADH is a chronic or recurrent problem, treatment with demeclocycline (7-chloro-6-demethyltetracycline) can partially inhibit the action of ADH with few side effects.[21] A dose-related effect of this drug, when administered in doses of 0.6–1.2 g/day, induces a reversible partial or complete nephrogenic diabetes insipidus, and may be of substantial benefit for patients with tumor-induced SIADH.

Hyponatremia may also be seen in patients with salt-losing nephropathy. Such patients usually are volume depleted and have a diffuse interstitial nephritis. Acute myeloid leukemia and multiple myeloma may result in this type of renal salt wasting and hyponatremia.[14,22] Finally, patients with myelomatosis may have high serum concentrations of cationic paraproteins and resultant hyponatremia.[23]

Hypernatremia

Disruption of the hypothalamic thirst center may result in mild volume depletion and hypernatremia.[24,25] Lesions of the hypothalamus and supracellular region may cause decreased vasopressin release in addition to adypsia, and both abnormalities together cause hypernatremia. Furthermore, when patients are unable to obtain fluids despite intact thirst stimulation, hypernatremia may result. Thus patients with intracerebral tumors and altered levels of consciousness may become hyperosmolar.[26] Finally, patients with diabetes insipidus with inadequate fluid replacement may become hypernatremic. The therapy for hypovolemic hypernatremia is to replace the fluid volume deficit. While the serum Na concentration is initially high, total body Na may be normal or decreased, and care must be taken to replete both water and sodium. Patients with hypothalamic lesions may be unable to regulate ADH secretion normally, and rehydration with hypotonic fluids may cause hyponatremia.[25]

Diabetes Insipidus

Central diabetes insipidus (DI) may result from anatomic derangement of the supraoptic paraventricular nucleii or the posterior lobe of the hypophysis. Primary brain tumors, metastatic brain tumors, and lymphoma have been associated with this defect in ADH secretion.[27] In addition, DI is often seen following craniotomy for resection of tumors. Patients with myeloblastic and lymphocytic leukemia have been described with DI, and demonstrate either leukemic infiltrates or thrombosis in small vessels of the hypothalamic nucleii and posterior lobe of the hypophysis.[28] This is a rare disorder, found to occur in 1 out of 1864 patients with leukemia.[29]

In *nephrogenic diabetes insipidus* (NDI), ADH is secreted normally, but the kidney does not respond appropriately to this hormone. Normal concentrating ability is impaired and polyuria results. This syndrome can be seen with several metabolic abnormalities found in patients with neoplasms. Sustained hypokalemia can produce polyuria and impaired renal concentrating ability. Tumors such as villous adenoma of the colon, other colonic carcinomas, and non-insulin-secreting islet-cell adenomas of the pancreas can result in diarrhea, secondary hyperaldosteronism, and resultant hypokalemia. Hypercalcemia, a consequence of several neoplastic diseases including carcinoma of the lung, breast, stomach and pharynx, xanthogranuloma and multiple myeloma, or tumor metastasis[30] may result in reversible NDI. Radiation nephritis can also produce a defect in urine concentrating ability.[31]

These disorders are characterized by polyuria (volume as high as 15 liter/day) and a defect in concentrating ability. In complete central DI, urinary osmolality typically is between 50 and 200 mOsm/kg,[32] while in partial DI the urine is not concentrated maximally following dehydration, and usually is less than 450 mOsm/kg.[33] In both, a significant response to exogenous ADH is seen. The diagnosis can be made by a dehydration test closely monitored to avoid substantial volume depletion, and subsequent vasopressin administration. Treatment of short-term central DI with intermittent exogenous ADH (aqueous pitressin 2–6 units administered parenterally every 4–6 hours) has been suggested following hypophysectomy,[1] while pitressin tannate in oil 2.5 units administered parenterally every 48 hours, or lysine vasopressin nasal spray, can control chronic central DI. More recently a potent vasopressin analog (DDAVP) administered intranasally has been used successfully.[34] Nephrogenic DI may be separated from central DI by infusion of aqueous vasopressin. In NDI, there is no increase in urine osmolality following this infusion. Correction of the metabolic abnormality (hypokalemia or hypercalcemia) results in correction of the defect.

Disorders of Potassium Balance

Potassium homeostasis, like sodium balance, is characterized by the maintenance of total body stores within narrow limits by achieving a zero net balance between input and loss. When renal function is normal, 90 percent of ingested K is excreted in the urine daily, while approximately 10 percent is excreted in the feces. Disturbances in this overall balance can affect the extracellular K concentration: decreased renal excretion caused by renal failure or hypoaldosteronism can result in hyperkalemia, while increased renal excretion (mineralocorticoid excess, renal tubular acidosis, diuretic administration, magnesium deficiency) or increased gastrointestinal losses (diarrhea, villous adenoma) may induce hypokalemia.[35] On the basis of isotope dilution and total body counting of naturally occurring ^{40}K (Ref. 36) total body potassium content has been estimated at 31–57 mEq/kg body weight, or approximately 3,500 mEq. Since the concentration of potassium in extracellular fluid is approximately 4 mEq/liter, nearly 98 percent of total body potassium is located within cells. It is evident that relatively small shifts in the transmembrane distribution of potassium between the intra- and extracellular spaces can have dramatic effects on the serum K concentration. Thus, factors favoring K entry into cells (alkalosis, insulin, epinephrine, aldosterone) may result in hypokalemia, while conditions inducing cellular efflux of K (acidosis) lead to hyperkalemia.

Hypokalemia

This condition usually is defined as serum potassium less than 3.0 mEq/liter. The low level of potassium in extracellular fluid can result from a redistribution of potassium (favoring intracellular sites) or may represent a reduction in total body potassium from excessive losses (Table 3). The major cause of redistribution hypokalemia is alkalosis. Both respiratory and metabolic alkalosis produce a fall in serum potassium concentration. This may be particularly pertinent to patients with neoplastic diseases in two ways: (1) When anorexia and decreased fluid intake are coupled with vomiting, diarrhea, or "third-space" sequestration of fluid, volume contraction results. The obligatory diuresis of hypercalcemia may produce the same effect. Under these conditions, the kidneys generate more bicarbonate, and a "contraction alkalosis" develops.[37] Potassium then moves into cells, and hypokalemia may be seen. In addition, this

Table 3
Causes of Hypokalemia

---

1. Alkalosis—respiratory and metabolic
2. Excessive losses in the urine
    a) Diuretic drugs
    b) Syndromes of mineralocorticoid excess
        1. hyperaldosteronism
        2. Bartter's syndrome
        3. excessive renin production
        4. licorice ingestion
    c) Renal tubular acidosis
    d) Magnesium deficiency
3. Excessive loss from gastrointestinal tract
    a) Diarrhea
    b) Villous adenoma
4. Excessive losses from the integument
    a) Postburn hypokalemia

---

volume contraction induces secondary hyperaldosteronism, enhancing K transport into cells and increasing K secretion in the distal tubule and collecting duct of the kidney. This kaluresis results in negative K balance, a metabolic condition favoring maintenance of the metabolic alkalosis.[37] Treatment of this syndrome thus requires both volume replacement with saline and potassium repletion. (2) Patients with pulmonary lesions such as metastatic carcinoma,[38] or those with advanced disease who become critically ill, may have a primary respiratory alkalosis. The hypokalemia in these patients is of clinical importance, since the sensitivity of cardiac muscle to digitalis is increased, and skeletal muscle and nervous tissue irritability is reduced in the presence of hypokalemia.

Potassium deficiency may result from inadequate intake or from excessive losses in the urine or the gastrointestinal tract. A diet severely depleted of potassium can result in hypokalemia. Such severe dietary restriction, however, is seen only with starvation or intractable vomiting, conditions associated with volume contraction, metabolic alkalosis, and sometimes ketoacidosis. The serum K concentration in such patients reflects both total body depletion and transcellular redistribution caused by the acid-based abnormalities.

Excessive Losses in the Urine: Excess Mineralocorticoid Activity

Several neoplastic diseases are characterized by high mineralocorticoid production, kaluresis, and hypokalemia.

Primary hyperaldosteronism. First described by Conn in 1955,[39] *primary hyperaldosteronism* is produced by an adrenal adenoma. Patients with this syndrome demonstrate hypertension, hypokalemia, metabolic alkalosis, (sometimes) muscle weakness, nocturia-polyuria, headache, polydypsia, tetany, paresthesias, and paralysis. Localization of the tumor can be aided by arteriography, adrenal venography with selective blood sampling, and adrenal imaging with ^{131}I-19-iodocholesterol.[40] Clinical improvement can be expected in 95 percent of patients following removal of the adenoma.[41] While surgical treatment is preferred by most groups, the aldosterone blocking agent spironolactone may successfully control all manifestations of the disorder.

Cushing's syndrome. Usually produced by primary adrenal hyperplasia, Cushing's syndrome sometimes can be the result of malignant adrenal neoplasms or nonadrenal tumors.[42] In these cases, hypokalemia and alkalosis are more common than in adrenal hyperplasia.

Ectopic ACTH syndrome. ACTH produced by tumors of nonendocrine organs can result in elevation of plasma cortisol levels, Cushingoid appearance, hypertension, edema, and a hypokalemic alkalosis.[43] Ectopic tumor production of corticotrophin releasing factor[44] also can produce this syndrome. In a review of the literature, Azzopardi and Williams[45] found four general categories of such tumors: (1) oat-cell carcinoma of the bronchus; (2) endocrine tumors of foregut origin (bronchial carcinoids, islet-cell pancreatic carcinomas, epithelial thymomas, medullary carcinomas of the thyroid, and possibly parathyroid carcinomas); (3) pheochromocytomas and related tumors, and (4) certain ovarian tumors (e.g., arrhenoblastomas). The cause of hypokalemic alkalosis in the "ectopic" ACTH syndrome has not been established with certainty, but probably is related to high levels of DOC and corticosterone.[46] These tumors are usually autonomous and are rarely suppressed with dexamethasone.

Renin-secreting tumor. An intrarenal renin-secreting tumor producing hypertension, metabolic alkalosis, and hypokalemia has been described.[47] Adenomatous transformation of juxtaglomerular tissue is probably responsible for autonomous high levels of renin release and the consequent hyperaldosteronism. An ectopic renin-secreting carcinoma[48] also has been reported.

Acute myeloid leukemia. Hypokalemia, with serum potassium < 3.5, may be present in more than 60 percent of patients with acute myeloid leukemia and its variants.[49] Most patients excrete large quantities of potassium in their urine, and many have elevated levels of serum lysozyme.[50] While it has been postulated that lysozme interferes with renal tubular function and causes increased potassium secretion, a recent study of 12 patients with this disease showed no correlation between urine and serum lysozyme and a low serum potassium.[49] Two patients had hypokalemia but were not in negative potassium balance; a subsequent case report likewise showed hypokalemia without hyperkaluria.[51] Thus in some patients, the hypokalemia may be the result of potassium movement into cells. Long-term hypokalemia in this disease recently has been reported.[52]

Antibiotic therapy. Patients with leukemia or solid tumors are frequently treated with antibiotics for possible or demonstrable infection. Broad-spectrum therapy is often initiated, and hypokalemia may result. In one study of 23 febrile patients with leukemia and neutropenia treated with clindamycin, cephalothin, methacillin, carbenicillin, and gentamicin, 14 (62 percent) demonstrated serum potassium < 3.0 mEq/liter.[53] Penicillin or carbenicillin may act as nonreabsorbable anions, increasing distal tubular potassium secretion and producing hypokalemia.[54]

Excessive Losses from the Gastrointestinal Tract

Hormone producing tumors. Four hormone-producing tumors may result in diarrhea and hypokalemia.

1. Zollinger-Ellison syndrome: Gastrin-producing tumors of pancreatic non-beta islet cells can result in diarrhea[55] and increased intestinal secretion of potassium. The diarrhea is caused by the large volume of hydrochloric acid produced in the upper gastrointestinal tract and may be reduced or eliminated by aspiration of gastric juice with a nasogastric tube.[56]

2. Pancreatic cholera syndrome: Tumors of the pancreas elaborate vasoactive intestinal polypeptide (VIP), prostaglandins, or other hormones and produce watery diarrhea, hypokalemia, and achlorhydria (WDHA syndrome). One third of such tumors are non-insulin-secreting islet-cell adenomas. Severe hypokalemia from large diarrheal potassium loss is caused by large stool volume, often exceeding 6–8 liter/day. The absolute fecal losses of potassium may be 300 mEq/day.[57] Total pancreatectomy has been suggested to avert the complications of fluid and potassium loss. In one reported case[58] attempts to correct the dehydration by fluid and electrolyte infusion resulted in a massive increase in fecal water and electrolyte loss. Prednisone therapy dramatically stopped the diarrhea and was associated with a decrease in plasma VIP levels. Streptozotocin also has been used to treat this disorder.[59] A father and son were recently described with islet-cell adenomas producing severe watery diarrhea.[60] While tumor from both patients contained detectable gastrin and VIP, the father had Zollinger-Ellison syndrome and the son had WDHA. Thus, watery diarrhea may be mediated by different hormones in families having multiple endocrine neoplasia.

3. Medullary carcinoma of the thyroid: Watery diarrhea and potassium loss may be seen in about one third of patients with medullary carcinoma of the thyroid. It has been suggested that calcitonin may play a role in the pathogenesis of this diarrhea.[61]

4. Carcinoid tumors: These may cause intestinal hypermotility with diarrhea, vomiting, and resultant hypokalemia. Excess production of serotonin probably mediates these symptoms.[62]

Villous adenoma. Since the original description in 1954,[63] excessive potassium losses due to villous adenoma of colon and rectum have been widely confirmed. While less than 1 percent of patients with adenomas develop hypokalemia,[64] those who do generally have long-standing diarrhea. The potassium content of stool in these patients is not higher than the level found in other types of diarrhea. Since the stool volume, however, may achieve levels of 1,500–3,500 ml/day, absolute excretion rate of potassium has been estimated to equal approximately 50 mEq/day.

The source of stool potassium has not been established but may result from increased secretion of colonic mucosal cells owing to secondary hyperaldosteronism[65] from a secretagogue elaborated by the tumor,[66] or from excessive excretion of colonic mucus.[67]

Management of Hypokalemia

Sustained hypokalemia from any of these causes can produce widespread effects in the body,[68] and often must be managed as a medical emergency. Manifestations of this electrolyte disturbance may include paralysis, intestinal dilitation and necrosis, cardiac arrhythmias including premature atrial and ventricular beats, atrial tachycardia and flutter, altered sensitivity to digitalis, and necrosis of cardiac muscle. Hypokalemia can produce impairment of renal tubular function that usually returns to normal when potassium is repleted,[69] but may result in chronic interstitial nephritis.[70]

The clinical approach to the hypokalemic patient depends upon whether the serum abnormality is caused by a change in potassium distribution or by a total body deficit. In patients with total body volume depletion and metabolic alkalosis, therapy is directed toward correction of hypovolemia by infusion of normal saline. In those with increased total body volume, but decreased effective circulating volume, such as in hypoalbuminemia of nephrosis or hepatic failure and ascites, colloid infusion may be indicated. If sustained hypovolemia has resulted in secondary hyperaldosteronism, supplemental potassium will also be required.

When tumors are responsible for potassium loss, their removal restores the equilibrium. Nonetheless, immediate measures are required when patients are in negative potassium balance and potassium replacement is necessary. It has been estimated that a serum potassium of 3.0 represents a total body deficit of 100–200 mEq of potassium.[71] Further reduction of serum potassium reflect a deficit of 200–400 mEq per additional 1-mEq/liter fall in serum concentration. Mild potassium deficiency usually can be corrected by foods rich in potassium, or by supplemental KCl in liquid form or embedded in a waxy matrix ("slow potassium"). In potassium deficiency associated with complications KCl may be administered intravenously. Since cellular uptake of potassium may not be an immediate process, care must be exercised in arranging the rate of potassium administration to avoid hyperkalemia. As a general rule, the concentration of potassium should not exceed 60–80 mEq/liter of infusate, and the infusion rate should not exceed 30–40 mEq/hr. In severe, life-threatening hypokalemia, 20–30 mEq KCl may be added to 200 ml of intravenous solution, infused in 30–60 minutes through a central vein, and repeated as necessary. These highly concentrated solutions are traumatic to the veins and infusion may be very painful. Once the acute crisis is resolved, more conventional forms of potassium replacement should be used.

Hyperkalemia

Hyperkalemia, a serum potassium concentration greater than 5.5 mEq/liter, may result from redistribution between cellular and extracellular sites, or from total body excess (Table 4). In addition, the serum potassium concentration of a collected sample of blood may increase in vitro. Measurement of this falsely elevated potassium value could lead to erroneous conclusions regarding the in vivo potassium concentration.

Redistribution of Potassium: Metabolic Acidosis

Both respiratory and metabolic acidosis may be associated with increased levels of serum potassium.[72, 73] While this phenomenon was first thought to result from the loss of cellular potassium in exchange for hydrogen ion, it recently has been shown that plasma bicarbonate concentration may modulate the serum potassium level independent of both blood pH and renal potassium excretion.[74] Lactic acidosis may be seen in patients with acute leukemia, lymposarcoma, Hodgkin's disease, and Burkitt's lymphoma.[75–79] The observations that the acidosis improves during remissions[78] and that lactate concentration is higher in malignant pleural or ascitic fluid than in blood[79] suggest that malignant cells produce high concentrations of lactate, exceeding the ability of the liver and kidney to

Table 4
Causes of Hyperkalemia

---

1. Redistribution of potassium from the intracellular to the extracellular space
   a) Acidosis
   b) Hemolysis
   c) Tissue necrosis
2. Excessive potassium retention
   a) Renal failure
   b) Hyporeninemic hypoaldosteronism

---

metabolize and excrete this acid. Solid tumors also may result in lactic acidosis without evidence of tissue hypoxia. Two patients with oat-cell carcinoma and extensive metastatic replacement of liver tissue developed sudden lactic acidosis,[80] possibly because the liver could no longer metabolize lactic acid.

The serum bicarbonate and potassium concentrations of such patients should be carefully followed, since sudden acidosis or hypokalemia may be life-threatening. The treatment of chronic lactic acidosis may require oral bicarbonate therapy, while the emergent treatment of precipitous lactic acidosis and hyperkalemia may require large amounts of intravenous $NaHCO_3$ infusion. If measures cannot be taken to eliminate the source of the high lactate production the prognosis may be very poor.

Tissue Destruction

When a large mass of cells are destroyed rapidly, the high intracellular potassium content suddenly is infused into the extracellular space. Under normal conditions, the kidneys respond to such a potassium load by substantially increasing the rate of potassium secretion into tubular urine, preventing sustained hyperkalemia. Thus the hyperkalemia of tissue necrosis is usually transient, and is sustained only in patients with impaired renal function. Several published reports describe this combination of tissue necrosis and renal failure producing hyperkalemia. Five of 22 patients treated with chemotherapy for Burkitt's lymphoma developed hyperkalemia.[81] In this tumor, virtually all cells are in acute proliferation and are sensitive to chemotherapy. Thus a large tumor mass may be destroyed in a short period of time, and the serum potassium concentration rises dramatically. The hyperkalemia may be sustained by acute renal insufficiency, a condition caused by renal cortical infiltration with tumor cells, ureteral obstruction, or acute uric acid nephropathy, another common complication of chemotherapy. Likewise, a patient with lymphosarcoma who underwent rapid tumor lysis with vincristine, prednisone, and 6-mercaptopurine developed hyperkalemia and acute uric acid nephropathy despite pretreatment with allopurinol.[82] A patient with acute lymphatic leukemia developed life-threatening hyperkalemia with chemotherapy.[83] This phenomenon may have resulted from rapid lysis of leukemic white blood cells and solid leukemic tissue with concurrent acute renal failure. Finally, a patient with chronic lymphocytic leukemia developed severe hyperkalemia after splenic irradiation.[84] In all these cases, initial hyperkalemia was induced by a large amount of tumor tissue, a high sensitivity of the tumor to therapy, and a rapid destruction of cells after initiation of therapy. Sustained hyperkalemia was caused by renal insufficiency.

Pseudohyperkalemia

Elevation of the serum potassium concentration may result from the in vitro release of potassium from formed elements of blood. This may be seen when red blood cells hemolyse in vitro, or in patients with thrombocytosis where platelets release potassium during coagulation. A similar phenomenon has been described in patients with myeloproliferative disorders, where the increased numbers of white blood cells are the source of the high potassium concentration.[85,86] When the laboratory reports a high serum potassium concentration, it is important to distinguish between true hyperkalemia, a disorder requiring immediate therapy, and pseudohyperkalemia, a laboratory curiosity requiring no therapy at all. In addition to the history, platelet count, and white blood cell count, other tests to distinguish true and pseudohyperkalemia include measurement of the plasma potassium concentration in anticoagulated blood, and assessment of the electrocardiogram for evidence of true hyperkalemia.

Diagnosis and Management of Hyperkalemia

Hyperkalemia may be life-threatening, producing weakness, paralysis, quadraplegia,[87] ileus, depression of cardiac conduction, and ventricular fibrillation or asystole.[88] The electrocardiogram may serve as a sensitive indicator of potassium's effect on the heart. As the serum potassium level rises, the T waves become tall and peaked, the PR interval prolongs, and then P waves disappear with atrial standstill. As potassium levels rise higher, the QRS complexes widen and the R-R intervals become irregular. A conduction delay at the A-V junction causes the junctional pacemaker to accelerate, but conduction delay also can be measured in the His bundle, in the Purkinje network, and in the ventricular muscle. Finally, ventricular tachycardia that leads to ventricular fibrillation or to asystole is a terminal event.

Therapy for hyperkalemia is designed to (1) correct any existing acidosis, (2) acutely shift potassium into cells, (3) increase the overall excretion of this ion, and (4) eliminate the underlying cause of the disturbance. Furthermore, the action of high levels of extracellular potassium to depolarize cell membranes can be blocked by the administration of calcium and hypertonic NaCl. Both measures have been shown to cause an immediate improvement in hyperkalemia-induced conduction defects.[89]

The emergency treatment of severe hyperkalemia (serum potassium > 8.0 mEq/liter) therefore should include the following steps (Table 5): intravenous injection of 14 mEq $CaCl_2$, then injection of approximately 50 mEq $NaHCO_3$ or more if severe acidosis also is present. Hypertonic glucose 50 ml of 50-percent solution, then can be injected with 10 units of crystalline

Table 5
Emergency Treatment of Hyperkalemia

1. Infuse 14 mEq (1 ampule) CaCl₂ intravenously
2. Infuse 44 mEq (1 ampule) NaCHO₃ intravenously, and more if severe metabolic acidosis is present
3. Give 50 ml of 50 percent dextrose (1 ampule) intravenously with 10 units CZI insulin
4. Administer 25–50 grams Kay-Exalate by mouth with 50 ml 70-percent sorbitol, or 50 grams Kay-Exalate in a retention enema for at least 30 minutes
5. Repeat EKG, serum HCO₃, potassium, and consider repeat of 1, 2, and 4 above

zinc insulin. Total body potassium will be reduced by the kidneys thereafter if their function is intact, and may be aided by the oral or rectal instillation of the exchange resin sodium polystyrene sulfonate (Kayexalate). Approximately 1 mEq of potassium is bound in each gram of resin when the resin is in the gut long enough for maximal exchange. When Kayexalate is given by enema as a 50-gram bolus, at least 30 minutes of retention is necessary for adequate exchange. If administered orally, 25–50 grams of resin are ingested with 50 ml of 70-percent sorbitol solution to induce diarrhea. When renal function is impaired, hemo- or peritoneal dialysis may be necessary to assist in potassium elimination. It should be noted, however, that Kayexalate removes potassium more efficiently than does peritoneal dialysis, and is therefore the initial treatment of choice. When severe hyperkalemia produces rhythm disturbances, transvenous pacemaker insertion should be considered.

Abnormalities of Uric Acid Metabolism

Degradation of the purine nucleotides results in the formation of uric acid (2,6,8-trioxypurine), a substance only sparingly soluble in water and body fluids.[90] In most mammals uric acid is converted to the water-soluble allantoin by a hepatic uricase. Unfortunately, man lacks this enzyme and must contend with excretion of the less soluble uric acid. The mechanism of renal excretion involves filtration at the glomerulus, tubular reabsorption, and tubular secretion. When high serum uric acid and increased urinary excretion of uric acid are present, two types of abnormalities may occur. At pH 7.4, the hydrogen ion concentration of most body fluids, uric acid is almost exclusively in its salt form, sodium urate. Chronic hyperuricemia may result in deposition of urate crystals in the medulla and pyrimids of the kidneys, with consequent interstitial inflammation. In contrast, acidic urine (pH 5.5) contains approximately 50-percent sodium urate and 50-percent uric acid. When high concentrations of uric acid are excreted in relatively small volumes of urine, uric acid crystals deposit in the collecting ducts, pelvis, and ureters, and can result in renal stones and an obstructive uropathy.

Since uric acid is the product of purine catabolism, it is not surprising that diseases characterized by rapid cell turnover cause increased uric acid production and excretion. For example, Krakoff [91] found increased levels of serum and urine uric acid in patients with chronic granulocytic leukemia; both corrected toward normal following successful treatment. Likewise, patients with lymphomas [92] and many solid tumors[93] demonstrate hyperuricemia. While the elevated levels of uric acid rarely cause complications, treatment of such disorders with x-rays[94] or chemotherapy [95] can result in sudden severe hyperuricemia, acute renal failure, and death.

Acute Uric Acid Nephropathy*

Radiation or chemotherapy in patients with leukemia is frequently complicated by acute renal failure. The presence of elevated serum uric acid concentrations and thick precipitation of uric acid in the collecting tubules, ureters, and pelvis implicates acute uric acid obstruction in the pathogenesis of the azotemia.[96,97] Precipitation of calcium phosphate deposits also may play a role in renal insufficiency. Therapy for other tumors also may result in acute renal failure.[98,99] Since its recognition, this disorder has been treated by induction of copious urine flow with oral or intravenous fluids, alkalinization of the urine to increase the solubility of uric acid, and allopurinol, a competitive inhibitor of xanthine oxidase to reduce the serum concentration of uric acid. This therapy is given for days before the chemotherapy or radiation therapy, and has successfully decreased the incidence of acute renal failure.

Recent studies in a rat model of acute urate nephropathy[100] demonstrate that not only obstruction of the collecting ducts, but also obstruction of the distal renal vasculature may occur in this disease. Furthermore, clearance and micropuncture studies fail to demonstrate a major effect of urinary alkalinization in preventing this acute renal injury.[101] Thus, the advisability of alkali administration must be reconsidered, particularly in hypocalcemic patients. Raising the blood pH in such patients may reduce the plasma concentration of ionized calcium and induce tetany and seizures.

It is therefore recommended that before chemotherapy is initiated for leukemia, lymphoma, angioimmunoblastic lymphadenopathy, or solid

*See also p 252.

tumors with a large cell burden, allopurinol 300 mg/day be administered for several days. Liberal oral fluid ingestion also should be encouraged, and if the urine volume is less than approximately 3 liters/day, an intravenous fluid infusion of 2–3 liter/day should be performed immediately before and during chemotherapy. Serum uric acid, creatinine, potassium, calcium, and phosphorus levels should be carefully monitored, and urine volumes measured. If the serum uric acid level rises to >20 mg% and azotemia appears, consideration should be given to the institution of acute hemodialysis.

Hypouricemia

Hypouricemia has been reported in patients with Hodgkin's disease,[102] carcinoma of the lung,[103] and acute myeloid leukemia.[104] Each of these has been associated with an increased urinary excretion of uric acid, and in some cases other abnormalities of proximal renal tubular function including aminoaciduria and phosphaturia. In one study[104] pyrazinamide, a potent inhibitor of uric acid secretion, did not adequately suppress urate excretion, suggesting that these patients have a defect in proximal tubular reabsorption. Other neoplasms similarly have resulted in defective renal tubular function. The adult Fanconi syndrome has been found in patients with multiple myeloma and carcinomas of the pancreas and liver. In a recent report of patients with Hodgkin's disease and hypouricemia, the abnormally increased renal clearance of uric acid was correlated with the clinical activity of the lymphoma,[105] appearing only in patients with advanced disease.

No specific therapy is necessary for this disorder, but careful monitoring of the glomerular filtration rate and tubular function would seem prudent.

Disorders of Phosphate Metabolism

The normal 70-kg man contains approximately 700 grams of elemental phosphorus: 80 percent in bone, 9 percent in muscle, and the remaining 11 percent in other cells, where it serves as the major intracellular anion. Phosphate exists in organic and inorganic forms. The inorganic phosphate exists primarily as $H_2PO_4^-/HPO_4^{2-}$, but at high serum levels (8–10 mg/100 ml) a significant proportion is complexed with calcium in colloidal suspension. Phosphate is a key intermediary in cell metabolism as (1) a source of high-energy bonds (ATP); (2) a major component of the buffer system $H_2PO_4^-/HPO_4^{2-}$; (3) a controlling factor in red cell O_2 delivery through the modulation of 2,3-DPG levels; and (4) a key component of membrane phospholipids and nucleoproteins.

Phosphate balance is effected by the renal excretion of phosphate to equal the daily dietary load. The average oral intake is 1 g/day; 90 percent of this is absorbed in the gut and ultimately excreted by the kidneys. The serum phosphate concentration in the adult is maintained between 2.7 and 4.5 mg/100 ml. In the kidney non-protein-bound phosphate is filtered at the glomerulus, and 80–90 percent of the filtered load is reabsorbed, predominantly by the proximal tubule. Phosphate may also be secreted into the tubular lumen. Renal phosphate excretion is affected by the glomerular filtration rate, the concentration of serum phosphate, the volume status, and the phosphaturic effect of parathyroid hormone. The potential role of vitamin D or its active metabolites in phosphate homeostasis has been recently reviewed.[106]

Hypophosphatemia

Phosphate deficiency is commonly encountered in several clinical situations[107] (see Table 6). Of these, hyperalimentation-induced hypophosphatemia is a common syndrome in oncologic patients. While the nutritional recovery syndrome was first described in former prisoners of war, the metabolic consequences of refeeding a severely cachectic patient must be considered in cancer patients as well. The resumption of caloric intake, particularly carbohydrate, leads to accelerated cellular phosphate influx and systemic hypophosphatemia.

Severe hypophosphatemia, less than 1 mg/100 ml, results in dysfunction of several major organ systems. Hypophosphatemia may produce a decrease in red-blood-cell ATP content, with increased membrane fragility and hemolysis.[108] In the remaining red blood cells, decreased levels of 2,3-DPG shift the Bohr dissociation curve to the right, with consequent reduction of O_2 release at the tissue level.[109] Cardiac contractility is highly

Table 6
Causes of Phosphate Deficiency

1. Respiratory alkalosis
2. Diabetic ketoacidosis
3. Phosphate binders
4. Alcoholism
5. Hyperalimentation
6. Nutritional recovery syndrome

dependent upon availability of high-energy phosphate bonds. Severe reversible cardiomyopathy has been described in patients with hypophosphatemia.[110] Leukocyte functions, including chemotaxis, phagocytosis, and bactericidal activity are highly dependent on the availability of high-energy phosphate bonds. Hypophosphatemia reduces intracellular ATP and impairs its interaction with contractile proteins in the leukocyte cytoplasm.[111] When platelets are bathed in vitro in low-phosphate solutions, abnormalities of function have been shown. Clinical bleeding abnormalities, however, have not been reported in hypophosphatemia. Central nervous system functional integrity is dependent upon adequate O_2 delivery and intact cellular metabolism. A syndrome of metabolic encephalopathy characterized by seizures, coma, paresthesia, and weakness has been described in patients with reduced concentrations of serum phosphate.[112] Muscular weakness and acute rhabdomyolysis may occur in hypophosphatemic alcoholics.[107]

Therapy of hypophosphatemia consists of oral or parenteral administration of phosphate salts. Oral replacement is to be preferred, and phosphate-rich foods such as milk are particularly useful in patients with severe caloric deficits. More rapid oral replacement may be obtained with 15–30 ml of Na_2HPO_4 solution (Neutra-Phos) 3–4 times daily. Parenteral administration is reserved for severe hypophosphatemia. An initial dose of 2.5 mg/kg body weight of the commercially available potassium or sodium phosphate solutions (93 mg/ml) has been suggested. This may be administered over a 6-hour period with monitoring of serum phosphate levels and repeated as indicated by serum levels and clinical response.[113] Serious contraindications to the use of supplemental phosphate include hypercalcemia, acute or chronic renal failure (particularly with oliguria), and ongoing tissue injury and necrosis.

Hyperphosphatemia

The serum phosphate may rise when renal excretion is decreased, or when a sudden high phosphate burden exceeds the kidney's ability to excrete this anion. Such phosphate loads may come from oral intake, intravenous infusion, or tissue destruction and release of intracellular phosphate. Table 7 lists the common causes of hyperphosphatemia.

Sustained hyperphosphatemia may result in life-threatening metabolic abnormalities. When the serum concentration of phosphate exceeds 6–8 mg/100 ml colloidal complexes of calcium phosphate may be deposited in extraosseous locations,[114] and the serum level of ionized calcium may fall precipitously. This sudden hypocalcemia results in neuromuscular ir-

Table 7
Causes of Hyperphosphatemia

1. Decreased excretion
   a) renal failure
   b) hypoparathyroidism
2. Increased burden
   a) neoplastic diseases
   b) catabolic states, particularly lactic acidosis
   c) IV or oral PO_4 loading
   d) overdose of vitamin D or its metabolites

ritability, and patients may demonstrate positive Chvostek and Trousseau signs. Prolonged hypocalcemia may induce secondary hyperparathyroidism, and more severe hypocalcemia predisposes to tetany and grand mal seizures. The electrocardiogram is usually normal, but may show prolongation of the Q-T interval in some severe cases. Metastatic calcification may occur in any tissue, although the alkaline sides of acid-secreting epithelia (gastric mucosa, renal tubules, alveolar membranes) and vascular walls are usually the first to be affected. Extensive metastatic calcification may result in vascular occlusion and ischemia. Finally, vitamin D metabolism may be impaired in hyperphosphatemia.

The introduction of aggressive tumor chemotherapy has resulted in the evolution of a new treatment-related syndrome. Following the initiation of chemotherapy, patients may develop acute, severe hyperphosphatemia, hyperphosphaturia, and hypocalcemia. This clinical complex has been described following therapy for acute lymphocytic leukemia, Burkitt's lymphoma, Burkitt-cell leukemia, and ovarian dysgerminoma.[115-119] These tumors are all characterized by a high growth-rate with rapid cell turnover,[120] large tumor cell burden, and sensitivity to chemotherapeutic agents. Since lymphoblasts contain 4 times as much phosphate as do more mature cells, it is postulated that rapid lysis of numerous phorphorus-rich cells results in the release of large quantities of inorganic phosphate into the circulation. Calcium phosphate complexes may precipitate and severe hypocalcemia often results. Acute renal failure may occur simultaneously, possibly caused by deposition of calcium phosphate in the renal parenchyma or collecting system.[121] The resultant inability to excrete the phosphate load exacerbates the problem. The routine prophylactic use of urinary alkalinization combined with allopurinol for the prevention of uric acid nephropathy may predispose to more extensive renal deposition of calcium phosphate due to its decreased solubility in alkaline fluids. Hyperphosphatemia has also been reported to occur in catabolic states associated with lactic acidosis[122] and volume depletion.

The treatment of hyperphosphatemia includes reduction of any exogenous phosphate load, prevention of acute renal failure with maintenance of a normal glomerular filtration rate, oral phosphate binders, and supplemental calcium for symptomatic hypocalcemia. When chemotherapy is planned to treat tumors that have a known potential for rapid cell lysis, consideration should be given to more gradual chemotherapeutic regimens, or to debulking procedures to reduce the tumor mass prior to induction. Preexisting renal failure should be considered a relative contraindication to aggressive chemotherapeutic schedules. Prophylactic fluid administration and oral phosphate binders have been advocated prior to chemotherapy.[115]

Intravenous or oral phosphate preparations have been used to treat the sustained hypercalcemia seen in several oncologic diseases. Such therapy may result in extensive metastatic calcification and renal failure.[123] The use of more satisfactory agents for the treatment of hypercalcemia (e.g., mithramicin, calcitonin)should eliminate the need for phosphate loading.

Hypocalcemia and Malignancy

The normal physiology of calcium and states of hypercalcemia are extensively reviewed elsewhere in this symposium. The present discussion will be limited to the differential diagnosis of hypocalcemia associated with malignancy (Table 8)[124-128]. Radical neck surgery or extensive thyroidal surgery may result in inadvertent removal of the parathyroid glands and subsequent hypocalcemia. The diagnosis may be confirmed by measuring the level of parathyroid hormone. Hypocalcemia has been reported in some cases of medullary carcinoma of the thyroid, possibly due to the hypocalcemic effects of thyrocalcitonin.[125] Decreased serum calcium levels have also been described in the course of acute leukemia[126-128] and have usually been ascribed to a decreased serum albumin concentration or renal failure.

Several leukemic patients, however, have been reported with hypocalcemia, normal serum albumin concentrations, and no evidence of renal impairment.[126] Magnesium deficiency may lead to hypocalcemia, possibly by inducing a fall in parathyroid hormone release or by decreased end-organ response to the calcemic effects of parathyroid hormone.[129] Finally, hypocalcemia rarely has been described in patients with extensive osteo-

Table 8
Hypocalcemia Associated With Malignancy

1. Decreased serum albumin (nephrosis, cirrhosis, cachexia)
2. Parathyroid hormone deficiency
   a) surgical
   b) destruction by malignant disease
   c) congenital
   d) magnesium deficiency
3. Skeletal resistance to PTH
   a) uremia
   b) magnesium deficiency
   c) pseudohypoparathyroidism
   d) vitamin K deficiency
4. Hyperphosphatemia
5. Pancreatitis
6. Chemotherapeutic agents (mithramycin)
7. Extensive osteoblastic activity (carcinoma of breast, prostate)

blastic metastatic breast and prostatic cancer, presumably due to increased calcium utilization by the osteoblastic tissues.[130]

Disorders of Magnesium Homeostasis

Magnesium has received increased attention as an important intracellular cation. Abnormalities of magnesium metabolism may be seen in oncology patients, and may result in several clinical abnormalities.[131] Like potassium, most of the body's magnesium (2000 mEq) is contained in soft tissues and bone. Thus, the plasma magnesium concentration does not accurately reflect the status of body stores. Magnesium is absorbed via the GI tract and 20–30 percent is protein-bound in the plasma. The serum concentration is maintained between 1.8 and 3.0 mEq/liter. Magnesium excretion is dependent upon adequate renal function — it is filtered at the glomerulus and 90 percent is reabsorbed by the proximal tubule. Parathyroid hormone appears to increase magnesium reabsorption.[131]

Hypomagnesemia

The urinary excretion of magnesium is markedly increased by diuretics, hypercalcemia, certain drugs (gentamicin, cisplatin[132]), alcohol, and states of mineralocorticoid excess. Patients with excess GI fluid losses produced by vomiting, prolonged nasogastric suction, fistulae, or malabsorptive diseases may have increased magnesium losses. Hypomagnesemia is also found in patients with protein-calorie malnutrition and in patients with prolonged intravenous alimentation.

The symptoms of hypomagnesemia include neuromuscular irritability, cardiac arrythmias, and metabolic encephalopathy. Therapy of severe hypomagnesemia in the presence of normal renal function is best accomplished by parenteral administration of $MgSO_4$. This may be accomplished by infusing 2 mEq/kg body weight over 4 hours (1 gram $MgSO_4 \cdot 7H_2O$ is approximately equal to 8 mEq magnesium). Alternatively, 8–16 mEq may be given by intramuscular injection at 4–6-hour intervals during the first day of therapy. Frequent monitoring of serum levels in these patients is essential. Less severe deficiency states and conditions known to be associated with excessive losses may be treated with 0.25–0.5 mEq/kg of oral magnesium supplements per day. This can be in the form of magnesium hydroxide, or a 4-percent magnesium chloride–6-percent citrate solution which yields 0.8 mEq magnesium per ml.

Hypermagnesemia

Hypermagnesemia has been reported almost exclusively in patients with renal failure. It has also been described in patients with Addison's disease[131] and in patients receiving chemotherapy for malignant lymphomas.[133] Two patients developed elevated serum magnesium levels during chemotherapy, presumably due to the release of intracellular magnesium in tumor cells. When the serum magnesium concentration exceeds 5–6 mEq/liter, clinical signs of toxicity include weakness, hyporeflexia, bradycardia, and lethargy. Serum levels above 10 mEq/liter are associated with severe respiratory depression. Severe, life-threatening hypermagnesemia should be treated with the intravenous infusion of 5–10 mEq of calcium and acute hemodialysis.

References

1. Berl T, Anderson RJ, McDonald KM, et al: Clinical disorders of water metabolism. Kid International 10:117–131, 1976
2. Andersson B, McCann SM: The effect of hypothalamic lesions on the water intake of the dog. Acta Physiol Scand 35:312–320, 1955
3. Leaf A, Bartter FC, Santos RF, et al: Evidence in man that urinary

electrolyte loss induced by pitressin is a function of water retention. J Clin Invest 32:868–878, 1953

4. Alexander EA, Doner DW, Auld RB, et al: Tubular reabsorption of sodium during acute and chronic volume expansion in man. J Clin Invest 51:2370–2379, 1972

5. Schwartz WB, Bennett W, Curelop S: A syndrome of renal sodium loss and hyponatremia probably resulting from inappropriate secretion of antidiuretic hormone. Am J Med 23:529–542, 1957

6. Bartter FC, Schwartz WB: The syndrome of inappropriate secretion of antidiuretic hormone. Am J Med 42:790–806, 1967

7. Moses AM, Miller M, Streeten DHP: Pathophysiologic and pharmacologic alterations in the release and action of ADH. Metabolism 25:697–721, 1976

8. Sellwood RA, Spencer J, Azzopardi JG et al: Inappropriate secretion of antidiuretic hormone by carcinoma of the prostate. Br J Surg 56:933–935, 1969

9. Miller R, Ashkar FS, Rudzinski DJ: Inappropriate secretion of antidiuretic hormone in reticulum cell sarcoma. South Med J 64:763–764, 1971

10. Cassileth PA, Trotman BW: Inappropriate antidiuretic hormone in Hodgkin's disease. Am J Med Sci 265:233–235, 1973

11. Vorherr H, Massry SG, Utiger RD, et al: Antidiuretic principle in malignant tumor extracts from patients with inappropriate ADH syndrome. J Clin Endocrinol 28:162–168, 1968

12. Perks WH, Stanhope R, Green M: Hyponatremia and mesothelioma. Br J Dis Chest 73:89–91, 1979

13. Mir MA, Delamore IW: Hyponatraemia syndrome in acute myeloid leukemia. Br Med J 1:52–55, 1974

14. Mir MA, Delamore IW: The syndrome of inappropriate renal sodium wasting and hyponatraemia in acute myeloid leukaemia. Br J Hematol 28:149–150, 1974

15. McKee LC Jr: Hypocalcemia in leukemia. South Med J 68:828–832, 1975

16. Jaffe N, Kim BS, Vawter GF: Hypocalcemia—a complication of childhood leukemia. Cancer 29:392–398, 1972

17. Stuart MJ, Cuaso C, Miller C, et al: Syndrome of recurrent increased secretion of antidiuretic hormone following multiple doses of vincristine. Blood 45:315–320, 1975

18. Nicholson RG, Feldman W: Hyponatremia in association with vincristine therapy. Can Med Assoc J 106:356–357, 1972

19. DeFronzo RA, Calvin OM, Braine H, et al: Cyclophosphamide and the kidney. Cancer 33:483–491, 1974
20. Munro AH, Crompton GK: Inappropriate antidiuretic hormone secretion in oat cell carcinoma of bronchus. Aggravation of hyponatremia by intravenous cyclophosphamide. Thorax 27:640–642, 1972
21. Cherrill DA, State RM, Birge JR, et al: Demeclocycline treatment in the syndrome of inappropriate antidiuretic hormone secretion. Ann Intern Med 83:654–656, 1975
22. Kahn T, Levitt MF: Salt wasting in myeloma. Arch Intern Med 126:664–667, 1970
23. Bloth B, Christensson J, Mellstedt H: Extreme hyponatremia in patients with myelomatosis: an effect of cationic paraproteins. Acta Medica Scandia 203:273–275, 1978
24. Zazgornik J, Jellinger K, Waldausl W, et al: Excessive hypernatremia and hyperosmolality associated with germinoma in the hypothalmic and pituitary region. Europ Neurol 12:38–46, 1974
25. Lascelles PT, Lewis PD: Hypodipsia and hypernatremia associated with hypothalamic and suprasellar lesions. Brain 95:249–264, 1972
26. Schoolman HM, Dubin A, Hoffman WS: Clinical syndromes associated with hypernatremia. Arch Intern Med 95:15–23, 1955
27. Blotner H: Primary or idiopathic diabetes insipidus: A systemic disease. Metabolism 7:191–200, 1958
28. Miller VI, Campbell WG Jr: Diabetes insipidus as a complication of leukemia. Cancer 28:666–673, 1971
29. Williams HM. Diamond HD, Craver LF: The pathogenesis and management of neurological complications in patients with malignant lymphomas and leukemias. Cancer 11:76–82, 1958
30. Zeffrin JL, Heinemann HO: Reversible defect in renal concentrating mechanism in patients with hypercalcemia. Am J Med 33:54–63, 1962
31. Coburn JW, Kleeman CR, Rubini ME: Hyposthenuria in radiation nephritis in dogs: A specific tubular defect? Clin Res 12:249, 1964
32. Coggins CH, Leaf A: Diabetes insipidus. Am J Med 42:807–813, 1967
33. Miller M, Dalakos T, Moses AM, et al: Recognition of partial defects in antidiuretic hormone secretion. Ann Int Med 73:721–729, 1970
34. Edwards CRW, Kitau MJ, Chard T, et al: Vasopressin analogue DDAVP in diabetes insipidus: Clinical and laboratory studies. Br Med J 3:375–378, 1973
35. Kliger AS, Hayslett JP: Disorders of potassium balance, in Brenner

BM, Stein JH (eds): Acid-Base and Potassium Homeostasis. Church-hill Livingstone, 1978, pp 168–264

36. Anderson EC: Three component body composition analysis based on potassium and water determinations. Ann NY Acad Sci 110:189–212, 1963

37. Seldin DW, Rector FC Jr: The generation and maintenance of metabolic alkalosis. Kidney International 1:305–321, 1972

38. Emirgil C, Zsoldos S, Heinemann HO: Effect of metastatic carcinoma to the lung on pulmonary function in man. Am J Med 36:382–394, 1964

39. Conn JW: Part II — Primary aldosteronism: a new clinical syndrome. J Lab Clin Med 45:6–17, 1955

40. Brillon KE: An approach to early adrenal visualization in Conn's and Cushing's syndromes. J Endocrinology 68:40P, 1976

41. Conn JW, Knopf RF, Nesbit RM: Clinical characteristics of primary aldosteronism from an analysis of 145 cases. Am J Surg 107:159–172, 1964

42. Christy NP, Laragh JH: Pathogenesis of hypokalemic alkalosis in Cushing's syndrome. N Engl J Med 265:1083–1088, 1961

43. Rees LH: The biosynthesis of hormones by non-endocrine tumors — a review. J Endocrinology 67:143–175, 1975

44. Upton GV, Amatruda TT: Evidence for presence of tumor peptides with corticotropin releasing factor-like activity in the ectopic ACTH syndrome. N Engl J Med 285:419–424, 1971

45. Azzopardi JG, Williams ED: Pathology of non-endocrine tumors associated with Cushing's syndrome. Cancer 22:274, 1968

46. Schambelan M, Stockigt JR, Biglieri EG: Isolated hypoaldosteronism in adults. N Engl J Med 287:573–578, 1972

47. Conn JW, Cohen EL, Lucas CP, et al: Primary reninism. Arch Intern Med 130:682–696, 1972

48. Genest J, Rojo-Ortega JM, Kuchel O, et al: Malignant hypertension with hypokalemia in a patient with renin-producing pulmonary carcinoma. Trans Assoc Am Physicians 88:192–201, 1975

49. Mir MA, Brabin B, Tang OT, et al: Hypokalemia in acute myeloid leukaemia. Ann Intern Med 82:54–57, 1975

50. Pickering TG, Catovsky D: Hypokalemia and raised lysozyme levels in acute myeloid leukemia. Quart J Med 42:677–682, 1973

51. Kosmidis P, Jamse KM, Axelrod AR: Hypokalemia in leukemia. Ann Intern Med 82:854–855, 1975

52. Ledoux F, Bergerat JP, Vetter JM, et al: Long-term hypokalemia in acute myeloid leukemia. Arch Intern Med 138:1287–1290, 1978

53. Tattersall MHN, Battersby G, Spiers ASD: Antibiotics and hypokalaemia. Lancet 1:630–631, 1972
54. Klastersky J, Vanderkelen B, Daneau D, et al: Carbenicillin and hypokalemia. Ann Intern Med 78:774–775, 1973
55. Ellison EH, Wilson SD: The Zollinger-Ellison syndrome: Reappraisal and evaluation of 260 registered cases. Ann Surg 160:512–530, 1964
56. McGuigan JE: The Zollinger-Ellison syndrome and related diseases, in Sleisenger MH, Fordtran JS (eds): Gastrointestinal Disease. Philadelphia, W. B. Saunders, 1973, pp 743–750
57. Verner JV, Morrison AB: Endocrine pancreatic islet disease with diarrhea. Arch Intern Med 133:492–500, 1974
58. Barraclough MA, Bloom SR: Vipoma of the pancreas: Observations on the diarrhea and circulatory disturbances. Arch Intern Med 139:467–471, 1979
59. Kahn CR, Levy AG, Gardner JD, et al: Pancreatic cholera: beneficial effects of treatment with streptozotocin. N Engl J Med 292:941–945, 1975
60. Hutcheon DF, Bayless TM, Cameron JL, et al: Hormone-mediated watery diarrhea in a family with multiple endocrine neoplasms. Ann Intern Med 90:932–934, 1979
61. Gray TK, Bieberdorf FA, Fordtran JS: Thyrocalcitonin and the jejunal absorption of calcium, water, and electrolytes in normal subjects. J Clin Invest 52:3084–3088, 1975
62. Sjoerdsma A, Weissbach H, Terry LL, et al: Further observations on patients with malignant carcinoid. Am J Med 23:5–15, 1957
63. McKittrick LS, Wheelot EC Jr: Carcinoma of the Colon. Springfield, Ill., Thomas, 1954
64. Jahadi MR, Baldwin A: Villous adenomas of the colon and rectum. Am J Surg 130:729–732, 1975
65. Turnberg LA: Electrolyte absorption from the colon. Gut 11:1049–1054, 1970
66. Shields R: Absorption and secretion of electrolytes and water by the human colon with particular reference to benign adenoma and papilloma. Br J Surg 53:893–897, 1966
67. Duthie HL, Atwell TD: The absorption of water, sodium and potassium in the large intestine with particular reference to the effects of villous papillomas. Gut 4:373–377, 1963
68. Welt LG, Hollander W Jr, Blythe WB: The consequences of potassium depletion. J Chronic Dis 11:213–254, 1960

69. Relman AS, Schwartz WB: The nephropathy of potassium depletion: clinical and pathological entity. N Engl J Med 255:195–203, 1956

70. Cremer W, Bock KD: Symptoms and course of chronic hypokalemic nephropathy in man. Clin Nephrology 7:112–119, 1977

71. Schribner BH, Burnall JM: Interpretation of the serum potassium concentration. Metabol Clin Exp 5:468–479, 1956

72. Schribner BH, Fremont-Smith K, Burnell JM: The effect of acute respiratory acidosis on the internal equilibrium of potassium. J Clin Invest 34: 1276–1285, 1955

73. Swan RC, Pitts RF: Neutralization of infused acid by nephrectomized dogs. J Clin Invest 34:205–212, 1955

74. Fraley DS, Adler S: Isohydric regulation of the plasma potassium by bicarbonate in the rat. Kidney International 9:333–343, 1976

75. Roth GJ, Porte D Jr: Chronic lactic acidosis and acute leukemia. Arch Intern Med 125:317–321, 1970

76. Scheerer PP, Pierre PV, Schwartz DL, et al: Reed-Sternberg cell leukemia and lactic acidosis. N Engl J Med 270:274–278, 1964

77. Block JB: Lactic acidosis in malignancy and observations on its possible pathogenesis. Ann NY Acad Sci 230:94–102, 1974

78. Wainer RA, Wiernik PD, Thompson WL: Metabolic and therapeutic studies of a patient with acute leukemia and severe lactic acidosis of prolonged duration. Am J Med 55:255–260, 1973

79. Block JB, Bronson WR, Bell WR: Metabolic abnormalities of lactic acidosis in Burkitt-type lymphoma with malignant effusions. Ann Intern Med 65:101–108, 1966

80. Spechler SJ, Esposita AL, Koff RS et al: Lactic acidosis in oat cell carcinoma with extensive hepatic metastasis. Arch Intern Med 138:1663–1666, 1978

81. Arseneau JC, Canellos GP, Banks PM, et al: American Burkitt's lymphoma. A clinicopathologic study of 30 cases. Am J Med 58:314–321, 1975

82. Muggia FM: Hyperkalemia and chemotherapy. Lancet 1:602–603, 1973

83. Fennelly JJ, Smyth H, Muldowney FP: Extreme hyperkalaemia due to rapid lysis of leukaemic cells. Lancet 1:27, 1974

84. Kurlander R, Stein RS, Roth D: Hyperkalemia complicating splenic irradiation of chronic lymphocytic leukemia. Cancer 36:926–930, 1975

85. Bronson WR, DeVita VT, Carbone PP, et al: Pseudohyperkalemia

due to release of potassium from white blood cells during clotting. N Engl J Med 274:369–375, 1966

86. Ringelhann B, Laszlo E, Vajda L: Pseudohyperkalemia in acute myeloid leukaemia. Lancet 1:928, 1974
87. Bull GM, Carter AB, Lowe KG: Hyperpotassaemic paralysis. Lancet 2:60–63, 1953
88. Ettinger PO, Regan TJ, Oldewurtel HA: Hyperkalemia, cardiac conduction and the EKG: a review. Am Heart J 88:360–371, 1974
89. Chamberlain MJ: Emergency treatment of hyperkalaemia. Lancet 1:464–467, 1964
90. Gutman AB, Yu TF: Uric acid nephrolithiasis. Am J Med 45:756–779, 1968
91. Krakoff IH: Studies of uric acid biosynthesis in the chronic leukemias. Arthritis Rheum 8:772–779, 1965
92. Weisberger AS, Persky L: Renal calculi and uremia as complications of lymphoma. Am J Med Sci 225:669–676, 1953
93. Ultmann JE: Hyperuricemia in disseminated neoplastic disease other than lymphomas and leukemias. Cancer 15:122–129, 1962
94. Merrill D: Uremia following x-ray therapy in leukemia. N Engl J Med 222:94–97, 1940
95. Kjellstrand CM, Campbell DC II, VonHartizsch B: Hyperuricemic acute renal failure. Arch Intern Med 133:349–359, 1974
96. Kritzler RA: Anuria complicating the treatment of leukemia. Am J Med 25:532–538, 1958
97. Frei E III, Bentzel CJ, Rieselbach R, et al: Renal complications of neoplastic disease. J Chronic Dis 16:757–776, 1963
98. Muggia FM, Ball TJ Jr, Ultmann JE: Allopurinol in the treatment of neoplastic disease complicated by hyperuricemia. Arch Intern Med 120:12–18, 1967
99. Mazur EM, Lovett DH, Enriquez R, et al: Angioimmunoblastic lymphadenopathy, evolution to a Burkitt-like lymphoma. Am J Med 67:317–324, 1979
100. Conger JD, Falk SA, Guggenheim SJ, et al: A micropuncture study of the early phase of acute urate nephropathy. J Clin Invest 58:681–689, 1976
101. Conger JD, Falk SA: Intrarenal dynamics in the pathogenesis and prevention of acute urate nephropathy. J Clin Invest 59:786–793, 1977
102. Bennett JS, Bond J, Singer I, et al: Hypouricemia in Hodgkin's disease. Ann Intern Med 76:751–756, 1972

103. Weinstein B, Irreverre F, Watkin DM: Lung carcinoma, hypouricemia and aminoaciduria. Am J Med 39:520–526, 1965
104. Mir MA, Delamore IW: Hypouricaemia and proximal tubular dysfunction in acute myeloid leukaemia. Br Med J 3:775–777, 1974
105. Zamkoff K, Kaplan M, Gottlieb AJ: Hypouricemia in Hodgkin's disease. Relation to extent of disease. NY State J Med 78:1047–1049, 1978
106. Favus MJ: Vitamin D physiology and some clinical aspects of the vitamin D endocrine system. Med Clin North Am 62:1291–1317, 1978
107. Knochel JP: Pathophysiology and clinical characteristics of severe hypophosphatemia. Arch Int Med 137:203–220, 1977
108. Klock JC, Williams H, Mentzer WC: Hemolytic anemia and somatic cell dysfunction in severe hypophosphatemia. Arch Int Med 134:360–364, 1974
109. Alberti KGMM, Emerson PM, Darley JH, et al: 2,3-Diphosphoglycerate and tissue oxygenation in uncontrolled diabetes mellitus. Lancet 2:391–395, 1972
110. Darsee JR, Nutter DO: Reversible severe congestive cardiomyopathy in three cases of hypophosphatemia. Ann Intern Med 89:867–870, 1978
111. Craddock PR, Yawata Y, VanSanten L, et al: Acquired phagocyte dysfunction: a complication of the hypophosphatemia of parenteral hyperalimentation. N Engl J Med 290:1403–1407, 1974
112. Silvis SE, Paragas PD, Jr: Paresthesias, weakness, seizures, and hypophosphatemia in patients receiving hyperalimentation. Gastroenterology 62:513–520, 1972
113. Lentz RD, Brown DM, Kjellstrand CM: Treatment of severe hypophosphatemia. Ann Intern Med 89:941–944, 1978
114. Herbert LA, Lemann J, Peterson JR, et al: Studies of the mechanism by which phosphate infusion lowers serum calcium concentration. J Clin Invest 45:1886–1894, 1966
115. Zusman J, Brown DM, Nesbit ME: Hyperphosphatemia, hyperphosphaturia and hypocalcemia in acute lymphoblastic leukemia. N Engl J Med 289:1335–1340, 1973
116. Cadman EC, Lundberg WB, Bertino JR: Hyperphosphatemia and hypocalcemia accompanying rapid cell lysis in a patient with Burkitt's lymphoma and Burkitt cell leukemia. Am J Med 62:283–290, 1977

117. Armata J, Depowska T: Hyperphosphatemia and hypocalcemia in neoplastic disorders. N Engl J Med 290:858, 1974

118. Brereton HD, Johnson RE: Hyperphosphatemia and hypocalcemia in Burkitt lymphoma. Arch Intern Med 135:307–309, 1975

119. Lovett DH: Unpublished observations

120. Iversen U, Iverson OH, Bluming, AZ, et al: Cell kinetics of African cases of Burkitt lymphoma: a preliminary report. Europ J Cancer 8:305–308, 1972

121. Eltinger DS, Harker WG, Gerry HW, et al: Hyperphosphatemia, hypocalcemia, and transient renal failure. J Am Med Assoc 239:2472–2474, 1978

122. O'Connor LR, Klein KL, Bethune JE: Hyperphosphatemia in lactic acidosis. N Engl J Med 297:707–709, 1977

123. Ayala G, Chertow BS, Shah JH, et al: Acute hyperphosphatemia and acute persistent renal insufficiency induced by oral phosphate therapy. Ann Intern Med 83:520–521, 1975

124. Singer FR, Bethune JE, Massry SG: Hypercalcemia and hypocalcemia. Clin Nephrol 7:154–162, 1977

125. Melvin KEW, Tashjian AH, Jr: The syndrome of excessive thyrocalcitonin produced by medullary carcinoma of the thyroid. Proc National Acad Sci 59:1216–1222, 1968

126. McKee LC, Jr: Hypocalcemia in leukemia. Southern Med J 68:828–832, 1975

127. Jaffe N, Byung SK, Vawter GF: Hypocalcemia: a complication of childhood leukemia. Cancer 29:392–398, 1972

128. O'Reagon S, Carson S, Chesney RW, et al: Electrolyte and acid-base disturbances in the management of leukemia. Blood 49:345–353, 1977

129. Massry SG: Pharmacology of magnesium. Am Rev Pharmacol Toxicol 17:67–82, 1977

130. Raskin P, McClain C: Hypocalcemia associated with metastatic bone disease. Arch Intern Med 132:539–543, 1973

131. Massry SG, Seelig MS: Hypomagnesemia and hypermagnesemia. Clin Nephrol 7:147–153, 1977

132. Schilsky RL, Anderson T: Hypomagnesemia and renal magnesium wasting in patients receiving cisplatin. Ann Intern Med 90:929–931, 1979

133. Ilicin G: Serum copper and magnesium levels in leukemia and malignant lymphoma. Lancet 2:1036–1037, 1971

10

MANAGEMENT OF ACUTE RENAL
FAILURE ASSOCIATED WITH
NEOPLASTIC DISEASE

Marc B. Garnick
Robert J. Mayer

The term "acute renal failure" characterizes a rapid reduction in glomerular filtration rate and renal blood flow leading to the accumulation of nitrogen end-products (blood urea nitrogen and serum creatinine) with progression to the uremic syndrome.[1,2] Although acute renal failure occurs most commonly in the setting of oliguria (urine output of less than 400 ml/day) or anuria (urine output of less than 100 ml/day), the biochemical alterations associated with this medical emergency can develop without reduction in urinary output.[3]

This chapter will discuss the multiple etiologies of acute renal failure in the cancer patient (Table 1): (1) causes due to tumor invasion of the renal parenchyma, ureters, and bladder; (2) causes resulting from nephrotoxic products elaborated from the tumor itself or resulting from rapid tumor-cell destruction; (3) causes resulting from cytotoxic chemotherapy, radiotherapy, and antimicrobial therapy. Those aspects of chronic renal impairment, such as the nephrotic syndrome and electrolyte abnormalities that are associated with neoplastic disease and its treatment, will not be included.

Although not specifically caused by malignancy per se, acute renal failure in the cancer patient may have a pre-renal etiology. Such causes

Supported by NIH Grant CA17979-05.

Table 1
Causes of Acute Renal Failure
in Patients with Malignancy

---

1. Tumor Invasion
    (a) Replacement of the renal
         parenchyma
    (b) Obstructive uropathy
2. Tumor Metabolites
    (a) Paraproteins
    (b) Uric acid
    (c) Calcium
3. Complications of Therapy
    (a) Cytotoxic chemotherapy
        1. Methotrexate
        2. Streptozotocin
        3. Cis-platinum
    (b) Radiation nephritis
    (c) Antimicrobial agents

---

include intravascular fluid depletion resulting from gastrointestinal losses (vomiting and diarrhea), poor oral intake, hypoalbuminemia, hypotension, or hemorrhage.[4] Physiologically, the fluid loss diminishes both renal blood flow and the glomerular filtration rate, often resulting in oliguria. If appreciated at an early stage, this azotemic process is reversible by the replacement of intravascular volume with intravenous fluids or blood. Though not specific for patients with neoplastic disease, pre-renal azotemia as a cause of oliguria should be considered before invoking one of the more specific etiologies of renal failure that are discussed in this review.

Causes Due To Tumor Invasion of the Genitourinary Tract

Replacement of the Renal Parenchyma

Renal failure resulting from bilateral replacement of the kidneys by tumor has been reported in leukemia[5-8] and lymphoma.[9-21] While 30–50 percent of autopsied patients with leukemia may show infiltration of the kidneys by leukemic cells,[5,22] actual compromise of renal function is rare.[6] The leukemic infiltrate is usually diffuse, but may be nodular or focal[7,23] and may result in as much as a tenfold increase in kidney size.[5] Radiographically, renal enlargement and elongation of the calyces are common.[24] Among the leukemias, the form most commonly associated with acute renal failure is acute lymphocytic leukemia.[6-8] Radiation to the kidneys in doses of 600–1000 rads accompanied by cytotoxic chemotherapy is the treatment of choice for this condition.[6,8]

Renal parenchymal infiltration by Hodgkin and non-Hodgkin lymphomas has been reported in one third of autopsied cases.[18] Clinically, the diagnosis may be suggested by flank masses or enlarged renal outlines on radiograms, but uremia from lymphomatous renal infiltration can also occur in normal-sized kidneys.[13] Other clues include mild proteinuria without nephrotic syndrome[17] and hypertension, presumably due to distension of intrarenal arteries.[15] Pathologically, multiple discrete kidney nodules appear more frequently than diffuse enlargement.[17,18] Despite the high prevalence of lymphomatous renal infiltration, however, death directly attributable to acute renal failure secondary to such tumor invasion is uncommon. In a series of 696 cases of lymphoma, only 4 (0.5 percent) patients died from uremia.[18] In the absence of a previous diagnosis of lymphoma, acute renal failure of unknown etiology merits a kidney biopsy. In the setting of widespread lymphoma and enlarged kidneys, however, an invasive diagnostic procedure is usually not indicated. When lymphoma has been shown to be the cause of acute renal failure, radiotherapy[10,15] and chemotherapy[11,13,14,16] in conjunction with dialysis[12,16] have transiently improved renal function. Little has been reported concerning the treatment of such renal failure with the aggressive drug combinations that recently have proven so effective in disseminated non-Hodgkin lymphoma.[25-28] The use of such chemotherapeutic regimens with dose modifications for agents renally excreted (i.e. cyclophosphamide, bleomycin) offers intensive antitumor exposure to the kidneys and the remainder of the body as well and should be strongly considered in such situations.

Obstructive Uropathy

Uremia in the cancer patient otherwise unexplained by alternative causes (Table 1) should always suggest the possibility of ureteral or bladder-outlet obstruction. The onset of obstructive uropathy may be associated with pain in the abdomen or back. The development of asymptomatic anuria, seizures or obtundation, however, may often be the initial presenting feature of this syndrome.[29] Intravenous infusion pyelography may demonstrate enlarged kidneys and hydronephrosis.[29] Additional diagnostic information can be obtained by retrograde pyelography with ureteral catheterization[29] and abdominal ultrasonography[30] (Fig. 1).

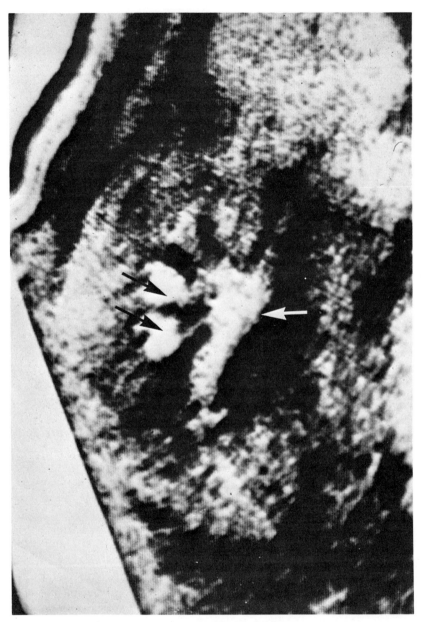

Fig. 1. *Ultrasonography depicts dilated calyces (dark arrows) and renal pelvis (white arrow) on longitudinal section of a hydronephrotic kidney in a patient with acute renal failure. (Courtesy of Edward H. Smith, M.D.)*

Bilateral ureteral obstruction may be caused by retroperitoneal or direct ureteral metastases from lymphomas or solid tumors. Kidney size may be normal, but bilateral hydronephrosis is present and retrograde pyelography usually demonstrates extrinsic ureteral obstruction. Lymphocytic lymphoma,[7,18,31-33] diffuse histiocytic lymphoma,[34,35] and Hodgkin's disease[33] have all been associated with this complication. Significant improvement in renal function has been reported following the use of radiotherapy[31] and chemotherapy.[31,33,35]

Bilateral ureteral obstruction caused by solid tumors resulting in acute renal failure have been reported in cervical,[36-39] gastric, [40,41] pancreatic,[42] colonic,[43] breast,[44,45] ovarian,[46] lung,[40] bladder,[47] and prostate[47] cancers. Uremia secondary to ureteral obstruction accounts for 60–80 percent of cervical carcinoma deaths.[37] Stomach[48] and colon[43] cancers metastatic to the bladder have also caused acute renal failure.

Diverting ureteral surgery followed by pelvic irradiation appears to be the treatment of choice.[38,48,49] Chemotherapy alone is inadequate in correcting the obstructive uropathy caused by nonlymphomatous solid tumors. The aggressiveness with which one approaches the treatment of urinary obstruction should be governed by the patient's general medical condition. In the face of widely disseminated incurable disease, the relatively pain-free demise from uremia may be more satisfactory than the protracted, often painful, and inevitable deterioration resulting from respiratory, cerebral, or other organ failure.

Causes Due to Tumor Metabolites

Paraproteinemic Nephropathy

Renal insufficiency occurs in 50–80 percent of patients with multiple myeloma.[50,51] Although deterioration of renal function is usually insidious, acute renal failure has been reported on numerous occasions.[52-55] Dehydration is undoubtedly the most important factor predisposing to acute oliguric renal failure in multiple myeloma patients.[51,56-58] Such dehydration may have contributed to the development of acute renal failure in previous patients with multiple myeloma following intravenous pyelography and venography. These case reports [59-63] formed the basis for the widespread acceptance that radiologic contrast studies in multiple myeloma patients were contraindicated.[61] Retrospective studies,[57,58] however, have suggested that such patients were usually dehydrated prior to the roentgenographic procedure and often had clinical evidence of preex-

isting renal insufficiency. Furthermore, some patients may have under-
gone abdominal compression during the radiologic examination, a procedure known to transiently further reduce renal function.[64] In recent
reviews summarizing 32 patients who developed radiocontrast-induced
acute renal failure, multiple myeloma was present in only one case, an
elderly female who had an elevated baseline serum creatinine.[65,66] Based
upon these studies, contrast procedures — pyelography, computerized
axial tomography, and angiography — may be performed in myeloma patients if adequate hydration is maintained throughout the procedure, and
hypotension and abdominal compression avoided.

The pathophysiology of renal insufficiency in multiple myeloma is
thought to result from both tubular precipitation of proteinaceous material
and glomerular damage from Bence-Jones proteins (light chain fragments)
causing tubular atrophy and glomerulitis.[50,51,67-70] The solubility of Bence-
Jones proteins decreases at an acid pH.[71] The tendency for patients with
oliguria to produce a more acid urine, thereby increasing the precipitation
of Bence-Jones proteins, emphasizes the need for adequate hydration.[51]
Once acute renal failure has developed in the myeloma patient, the potential for the return of normal renal function is poor, despite dialysis and
chemotherapy.[53,56,72] Hence, efforts in the myeloma patient should be directed towards the prevention of such a complication. The chronic use of
urinary alkalinizing agents and increased nocturnal fluid intake have
therefore been advocated, especially in patients excreting large quantities
of Bence-Jones proteins.[51]

Other hematologic malignancies associated with myeloma-type serum proteins have been incriminated in the development of acute renal
failure. Glomerular precipitation of PAS-positive macroglobulin in a patient with Waldenstrom's macroglobulinemia[73] and tubular precipitation
of monoclonal proteins in several patients with lymphoma[74] have been
reported.

Uric Acid

Acute renal failure resulting from uric acid nephropathy may occur
during the course and treatment of patients with leukemia and lymphoma.[75-77] This was clearly demonstrated when uric acid excretion was
measured in normal adults and untreated patients with leukemia.[78] The
former group excreted 6.5 mg of uric acid/kg day compared with 30.3 mg/
kg day in patients with acute lymphocytic leukemia, 13.0 mg/kg day in
patients with acute myelocytic leukemia and chronic myelocytic leukemia,
and 5.2 mg/kg day in patients with chronic lymphocytic leukemia. Uric

acid excretion seemed to correlate better with the type of underlying leukemia than with the absolute peripheral white blood cell count. Patients with "aleukemic" disease had elevated excretion values, while a normal excretion pattern was observed in patients with chronic lymphocytic leukemia having markedly elevated peripheral white blood cell counts.[78] Clinically, however, uric acid nephropathy is now most commonly seen immediately following the initial administration of chemotherapy or radiotherapy to patients with leukemia and lymphoma.[5,77,79] Prior to the introduction of allopurinol, serum uric acid values of 70 mg/dl were not uncommon in such settings[5] and levels as high as 87 mg/dl[80] have been reported.

Pathophysiologically, the renal medulla, distal tubule, and collecting duct appear to be the predominant sites of uric acid precipitation and subsequent damage.[81,82] This is logical since these anatomical regions of the nephron represent the areas where maximal urinary concentration[83] and acidification[84] occur. Furthermore, uric acid deposition has been shown to cause inflammatory vascular changes distinct from the tubular obstruction, resulting in nephrosclerosis and pyelonephritis.[82,85]

The prevention and treatment of uric acid nephropathy resulting from antitumor therapy is founded on three physical–chemical principles: (1) hydration, allowing adequate tubular fluid flow; (2) urinary alkalinization, increasing the solubility of uric acid; and (3) allopurinol administration, decreasing the formation of uric acid. Vigorous hydration increases uric acid clearance by preventing the urinary supersaturation of uric acid and the resulting formation of tubular crystals.[77,86] Uric acid solubility is further increased by urinary alkalinization. At a pH of 7.4, greater than 95 percent of urinary uric acid is dissociated into its more soluble ionized form.[5,75] Allopurinol and its metabolite, oxypurinol, are potent inhibitors of xanthine oxidase, the enzyme which converts hypoxanthine and xanthine to uric acid.[87] Additionally, allopurinol may reduce de novo purine synthesis by lowering levels of 5-phosphoribosylpyrophosphate through the inhibition of phosphoribosylpyrophosphate amidotransferase.[87] Based upon these principles, uric acid nephropathy should be preventable. In a patient potentially at risk, cytotoxic therapy should be withheld for at least 12 hours if possible, during which time a saline diuresis should be instituted, the urinary pH maintained at 7.0 with sodium bicarbonate, and allopurinol administered. Urinary alkalinization in excess of pH 7.5 does not further increase uric acid solubility but may lead to an unnecessary metabolic alkalosis.[75]

Although uncommon, the use of allopurinol may in itself lead to renal complications. The inhibition of xanthine oxidase may lead to the formation of xanthine stones with resulting nephropathy and renal failure.[88,89] As with uric acid, xanthine solubility is greater at a urinary pH of 7.0, thus further emphasizing the necessity for concomitant urinary hydration and alkalinization along with the use of allopurinol.[90] A hypersensitivity syndrome characterized by fever, eosinophilia, diffuse rash, and interstitial nephritis has been reported following allopurinol administration.[91] Renal function may diminish but returns to normal after discontinuation of the drug. These toxic effects associated with allopurinol underscore the importance of discontinuing this agent once a clinical remission has been achieved.

Hemodialysis with a hollow-fiber kidney appears to be the treatment of choice for oliguria secondary to uric acid nephropathy.[92] This technique of dialysis results in more effective uric acid clearance than peritoneal dialysis or coil hemodialysis.[92] Since uric acid nephropathy is usually an acute complication of antitumor therapy, aggressive management with such hemodialysis is indicated.

Hypercalcemia

Hypercalcemia may occur in patients with solid tumors such as breast, lung, and kidney carcinomas,[93] as well as such hematologic malignancies as multiple myeloma,[94] acute,[95,96] and chronic[97,98] leukemias and lymphoma.[99–101] Multiple pathogenetic mechanisms have been described to explain the hypercalcemia. These include bony destruction by metastatic tumor with subsequent calcium release into the blood, often exacerbated in the bedridden, dehydrated patient; the elaboration of tumor products containing parathyroid hormone-like activity; and the increase in plasma calcium caused by hormonal therapy, especially in patients with breast cancer.[102,103] Possible additional mechanisms include an osteoclastic-like property recently recovered from malignant plasma cells in patients with multiple myeloma[104] and the elaboration of prostaglandins in patients with a variety of solid tumors.[105]

The presence of chronic hypercalcemia alters both kidney structure and function. Degeneration and necrosis of tubular epithelium followed by intraluminal deposition of such necrotic debris and cast formation subsequently lead to atrophy and dilatation of the tubules and interstitial nephritis.[106,107] Functional impairments found in the early stages of hypercalcemia include hyposthenuria and insensitivity to antidiuretic hormone with associated polyuria, nocturia, and polydipsia.[94] The acute onset of severe hypercalcemia or chronic exposure of the renal tubules to elevated calcium levels may lead to a reduction in the glomerular filtration rate and in renal blood flow, resulting in acute renal failure.[107]

The therapeutic modalities employed in the treatment of hypercalcemia are numerous, but should always be used in conjunction with therapy of the underlying malignant disease. Such therapeutic modalities have been the subject of recent reviews.[102,108]

Causes due to Therapy

Cytotoxic Chemotherapy

Methotrexate

Methotrexate is excreted by the kidneys.[109] If renal function is compromised, methotrexate serum levels remain elevated and marrow suppression, mucositis, and dermatitis ensue.[110] Nephrotoxicity may occur rarely, however, following the use of conventional doses of methotrexate in patients with previously normal renal function.[111] In a series of 13 patients with advanced carcinomas, methotrexate in doses of 0.5 mg/kg to 3 mg/kg resulted in elevation in blood urea nitrogen and creatinine in 5 patients. Three of these patients had persistent azotemia at the time of their deaths. Autopsy examination of the kidneys demonstrated extensive necrosis of the tubular epithelial cells.[111]

In the past several years, the use of far higher doses of methotrexate accompanied with citrovorum factor rescue has assumed an increasingly important role in cancer chemotherapy.[112] At such high doses, a 50-percent elevation from the baseline serum creatinine has been reported in 60 percent of patients 24 hours after receiving methotrexate.[113] Three of the 33 patients included in the latter study died with acute renal failure. Postmortem examination of the kidneys demonstrated bilateral renal enlargement, amorphous yellow tubular precipitates shown immunologically to be methotrexate (Fig. 2), and high levels of methotrexate throughout the renal parenchyma.[113]

Vigorous hydration and urinary alkalinization have substantially reduced the incidence of acute renal failure secondary to the administration of high-dose methotrexate.[114] Prior to the initiation of such therapy, patients should have a normal intravenous pyelogram and a creatinine clearance of at least 60 ml/min/1.73 M². Methotrexate, like uric acid, is more soluble at an alkaline urinary pH. The use of hydration and sodium bicar-

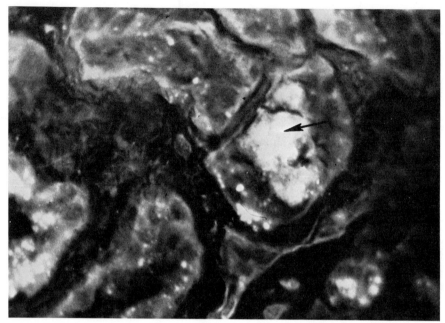

Fig. 2. *Kidney biopsy from a patient treated with 3 g/M² of methotrexate who became dehydrated and developed acute renal failure despite citrovorum factor rescue. The renal tissue was stained with fluoresceinated rabbit antimethotrexate antibody and demonstrates methotrexate precipitation (arrow) in a renal tubule. (Courtesy of Susan W. Pitman, M.D.)*

bonate alkalinization has markedly reduced the incidence of methotrexate-induced nephrotoxicity.[114] Whether this reduction is secondary to an augmentation in the glomerular filtration rate brought about by the increased fluid intake or urinary alkalinization, or even a combination of both, has not yet been adequately investigated.

If methotrexate nephrotoxicity develops, plasma clearance of the drug is prolonged.[115] Efforts should be directed to the prevention of such toxicities as myelosuppression and mucositis since hemodialysis,[116] peritoneal dialysis,[116] and hemoperfusion[117] have proven ineffective in augmenting methotrexate clearance. Such prevention, in our experience, may be achieved through the continued use of intravenous citrovorum factor (100 mg/M² every 3 hours)[118] and concomitant intravenous thymidine (8 g/M² daily via continuous infusion)[119] until renal function recovers and serum methotrexate levels are undetectable.

Streptozotocin

Streptozotocin is a nitrosourea which has been used successfully in the treatment of pancreatic islet-cell tumors.[120,121] Renal toxicity is the major dose-limiting side effect. In a group of 52 patients treated for islet-cell tumors, 65 percent developed nephrotoxicity and 5 patients died of acute renal failure.[120] Toxicity appears to be dose-related as renal impairment has been reported rarely at doses below 1.5 g/M² week or 500 mg/M² day × 5. The earliest manifestation of renal toxicity is mild proteinuria,[122] but with continued treatment, proximal renal tubular damage may ensue.[123] Hypophosphatemia, and subsequently a florid Fanconi syndrome, as well as azotemia have all been reported following streptozotocin administration.[123] The mechanism of drug-induced renal injury is related to the normal excretion of 10–20 percent of unaltered drug into the renal tubule, where it is concentrated and may spontaneously release an active methylating agent.[124] The appearance of proteinuria in patients receiving streptozotocin should cause temporary discontinuation of this drug until urinary findings return to normal.

Cis-Dichlorodiammineplatinum (II)

Cis-platinum has recently assumed an important role in the treatment of genitourinary carcinomas, cancer of the ovary, and squamous-cell carcinoma of the head and neck.[125,126] Nephrotoxicity was documented in both preclinical animal[127] and human toxicologic studies.[128,129] Renal biopsies[130] and postmortem examinations of the kidneys[128,129] have demonstrated nonspecific hyaline droplet degeneration involving the proximal tubular epithelium, thickening of the tubular basement membranes, and renal tubular necrosis. The glomeruli in these studies were normal. Despite the restriction of structural abnormalities to the tubules, functional abnormalities related to cis-platinum reflect altered glomerular filtration rate.[128,129] Such a diminution in the creatinine clearance appears to be dose-related and becomes clinically apparent 7–14 days after drug administration.[128,129] Early human studies with cis-platinum showed that the decrease in glomerular function was irreversible once it had occurred[130] and that changes in renal function proved to be the dose-limiting toxicity necessitating drug discontinuation.[131] Preliminary evidence has suggested that patients receiving potentially nephrotoxic antibiotics[129,132] or having such conditions damaging to the kidney as preexisting nephrosclerosis[133] or concomitant hyperuricemia[134] are at increased risk for the development of renal damage from cis-platinum exposure. Pretreatment hydration with intravenous saline[135] and mannitol[136,137] appears to diminish the degree of renal functional impairment induced by this heavy metal.

Antitumor Agents Requiring Dose Modifications in Renal Failure

Little is known concerning dose modifications of renally excreted cytotoxic agents in patients with renal failure. Table 2 summarizes the information that is available. Those drugs, which are both excreted by and toxic to the kidney (methotrexate, streptozotocin, cis-platinum), are contraindicated in patients with impaired renal function. Data are presently inadequate regarding the potential for dialysis of streptozotocin and cis-platinum. As mentioned previously, methotrexate is not significantly dialyzed in humans.[116,117] Cyclophosphamide is an alkylating agent whose metabolites are predominantly excreted in the urine[138] and are toxic[139] and carcinogenic[140] to the bladder mucosa. Animal studies suggest that cyclophosphamide may be dialyzable,[141] but no experience in humans has been reported. It would seem advisable to reduce the dose of cyclophosphamide in patients with renal failure who are not undergoing dialysis, but it may well be that higher doses can be given to those individuals who are receiving regular dialysis. Cytotoxic agents such as bleomycin,[142,143] melphalan,[144] and purine antagonists (6-mercaptopurine and azathioprine)[145] are partially excreted through the kidney. In the case of bleomycin, pharmacologic studies have demonstrated decreased drug excretion in the setting of renal failure.[142,143] None of these agents is known to be nephrotoxic. Patients with impaired renal function who are receiving these drugs on an intermittent schedule most likely require no dose modification. However, when these agents are administered to patients with renal failure on a daily or continuous infusion regimen, consideration might be given to a slight dose reduction.

Table 2
Renally Excreted Cytotoxic Agents Requiring Dose Alterations in Patients with Kidney Failure

Contraindicated	Moderate Dose Reduction	Slight Dose Reduction
Methotrexate	Cyclophosphamide	Bleomycin
Streptozotocin		Melphalan
Cis-platinum		6-Mercaptopurine
		Azathioprine

Other Agents Possibly Causing Renal Failure

Abnormalities in renal function have been reported in a small group of patients treated with high doses of mitomycin-C.[146] Three of 42 patients who had received cumulative doses of greater than 1.5 mg/kg during a 6-month period developed increases in serum creatinine. Renal function should be monitored in patients receiving mitomycin-C.

The nitrosoureas, methyl CCNU[147,148] and CCNU,[149] have been associated with chronic renal failure characterized by a progressive elevation in the serum creatinine. Such impaired renal function with methyl CCNU appears related to the cumulative dose administered, and has rarely been observed unless greater than 1500 mg/M² has been given.

Adriamycin has recently been implicated in a single case report to be a potential nephrotoxic chemotherapeutic agent.[150] The pathologic lesions demonstrated by renal biopsy in this patient resemble those experimentally induced in rats treated with the related anthracycline, daunorubicin.[151] The absence of other reports linking anthracyclines with renal failure suggest that this phenomenon is extremely rare.

The use of nonspecific immunostimulants (e.g. *Corynebacterium parvum*) may lead to nephrotoxicity.[152] The mechanism for this uncommon finding appears to be a proliferative glomerulonephritis, presumably caused by the deposition of antigen-antibody complexes on the glomerular basement membrane, leading to a nephrotic syndrome and an elevation of the serum creatinine. This condition appears to resolve spontaneously when the immunotherapy is withdrawn.

Radiation Nephritis

The delivery of greater than 2300 rads of radiotherapy to the whole of both kidneys during a 4–5-week period may lead to a clinical syndrome known as radiation nephritis.[153–155] This syndrome may be acute or chronic. Acute radiation nephritis usually appears 6–13 months following the completion of abdominal radiotherapy.[154] Patients may complain of headache and shortness of breath which may herald the onset of malignant hypertension and acute renal failure. Microscopic hematuria, albuminuria, and hyaline and granular casts are the usual urinary findings. The prognosis of acute radiation nephritis is directly related to the presence or absence of hypertension.[155] The development of malignant hypertension leads to death in 50 percent of patients, while in those recovering, gradual diminution in renal function over a 10-year period may lead to eventual chronic renal failure.[155,156] Radiation damage to one kidney has also been associated with the development of severe hypertension.[157] The recognition of such a complication is crucial since clinical improvement has resulted from the surgical removal of the damaged kidney.

The recognition of radiation nephritis as a clinical entity and the introduction of megavoltage technology has led to the development of improved techniques of renal shielding. Furthermore, the administration of intra-arterial epinephrine into the renal artery during abdominal radiotherapy allows blood vessels in normal renal tissue to constrict, creating a relatively hypoxic environment, thereby permitting a total radiation dose of greater than 2300 rads to be delivered.[158] These data are preliminary and the long-term effects of such high-dose irradiation are unknown.

Antimicrobial Agents

The nephrotoxicity of antimicrobial agents has been reviewed recently.[159] Particularly pertinent to the treatment of the patient with cancer have been several reports linking the commonly used broad-spectrum antibiotic combination, gentamicin and cephalothin, with acute renal failure.[160-164] In the largest of these series, [164] 119 severely ill individuals with known malignancy were given this two-drug antibiotic combination. Fifty patients survived and 69 died. Of the 69 who expired, 33 (48 percent) demonstrated evidence of tubular injury and 14 of these 33 developed renal failure. This nephrotoxicity is not dose-dependent, but susceptibility to tubular damage appears greater if hypotension from hemorrhage, sepsis, or dehydration occurs. Furthermore, as previously discussed, the renal failure associated with gentamicin and cephalothin seems to be augmented by the concomitant administration of cis-platinum.[129,132] The risk of renal failure is apparently less, however, if gentamicin is given together with a penicillin derivative.[165] Based on these data, the choice of an aminoglycoside and a cephalosporin antibiotic in combination should be made with caution.

Conclusion

This review has described the diverse settings in which acute renal failure may develop in patients with neoplastic disease. As improved results of cancer therapy have prolonged survival in many malignancies, the prevention, early recognition, and treatment of renal failure has gained increasing importance. Attention to the medical circumstances that may contribute to renal insufficiency during times of diagnosis and treatment of neoplastic disease can decrease the risk of this complication. Renal failure due to direct infiltration of the kidneys by potentially treatable tumors, however, should not be a contraindication to the administration of maximal therapy.

References

1. Levinsky NG, Alexander EA: Acute renal failure, in Brenner BM, Rector FC (eds): The Kidney. Philadelphia, W.B. Saunders, 1976, Chap 21, pp 806–837
2. Luke RG: Acute renal failure. Hosp Med 6:62–75, 1970
3. Levinsky NG: Management of emergencies: V. Acute renal failure. N Engl J Med 274:1016–1018, 1966
4. Fichman M, Bethune J: Effects of neoplasms on renal electrolyte function. Ann NY Acad Sci 230:448–472, 1974
5. Frei E, Bentzel CJ, Rieselbach R, et al: Renal complications of neoplastic disease. J Chronic Dis 16:757–776, 1963
6. Lundberg WB, Codman ED, Finch SC, et al: Renal failure secondary to leukemic infiltration of the kidneys. Am J Med 62:636–642, 1977
7. Merrill D, Jackson H: The renal complications of leukemia. N Engl J Med 228:271–276, 1943
8. Stoffel TJ, Nesbit ME, Levitt SH: The role of radiotherapy in renal involvement in acute childhood leukemia. Radiology 117:687–694, 1975
9. Aledort LM, Hodges M, Brown JA: Irreversible renal failure due to malignant lymphoma. Ann Int Med 65:117–121, 1966
10. Armstrong D, Myers WPL: Renal failure incident to reticulum cell sarcoma of the kidneys: Response to radiotherapy. Ann Intern Med 65:109–117, 1966
11. Champion AE, Coup AJ, Hancock BW: Hodgkin's disease and chronic renal failure. Cancer 38:1867–1868, 1976
12. Duncan H, Elliot W, Hall M, et al: Acute renal failure complicating a reticulosis: Remission following haemodialysis. Br Med J 1:1130–1132, 1963
13. Ellman L, Davis J, Lichtenstein NS: Uremia due to occult lymphomatous infiltration of the kidneys. Cancer 33:203–205, 1974
14. Jones WG: Reversible lymphomatous non-obstructive uropathy. Br J Urol 47:524, 1975

15. Kanfer A, Vandewalle A, Morel-Marager L, et al: Acute renal insufficiency due to lymphomatous infiltration of the kidneys. Cancer 38:2588–2592, 1976

16. Lizzi F, Tartaglia A, Propp S: Reversible uremia secondary to renal replacement by lymphoma. NY State J Med 71:360–363, 1971

17. Martinez-Maldonado M, Ramirez de Arellano GH: Renal involvement in malignant lymphomas: A survey of 49 cases. J Urol 95:485–488, 1966

18. Richmond J, Sherman RS, Diamond HD, et al: Renal lesions associated with malignant lymphomas. Am J Med 32:184–207, 1962

19. Wallach JB, Sharfman WB, Angrist AA: Uremia due to replacement of renal parenchyma by tumor. J Urol 67:623–628, 1952

20. Watson EM, Sauer HR, Sadugor MG: Manifestations of lymphoblastomas in the genito-urinary tract. J Urol 61:626–642, 1949

21. Wolfsohn AW: Uremia due to renal lymphomatosis. Ann Int Med 53:197–203, 1960

22. Sternby NH: Studies in enlargement of leukaemic kidneys. Acta Haemat 14:354–362, 1955

23. Meyer LM: Pathology of the genitourinary tract in leukemia. Urol Cut Rev 45:693–695, 1941

24. Gowdy JF, Neuhauser EBD: The roentgen diagnosis of diffuse leukemic infiltration of the kidneys in children. Am J Roentgen 60:13–21, 1948

25. DeVita VT, Canellos GP, Chabner B, et al: Advanced diffuse histiocytic lymphoma, a potentially curable disease: Results with combination chemotherapy. Lancet 1:248–250, 1975

26. Rodriguez V, Cabanillas F, Burgess MA, et al: Combination chemotherapy ("CHOP-Bleo") in advanced (non-Hodgkin) malignant lymphoma. Blood 49:325–333, 1977

27. Schein PS, DeVita VT, Hubbard S, et al: Bleomycin, adriamycin, cyclophosphamide, vincristine and prednisone (BACOP) combination chemotherapy in the treatment of advanced diffuse histiocytic lymphoma. Ann Intern Med 85:417–422, 1976

28. Skarin AT, Rosenthal DS, Moloney WC, et al: Combination chemotherapy of advanced non-Hodgkin lymphoma with bleomycin, adriamycin, cyclophosphamide, vincristine and prednisone (BACOP). Blood 49:759–770, 1977

29. Pillay VKG, Dunea G: Clinical aspects of obstructive uropathy. Med Clin North Am 55:1417–1427, 1971

30. Smith EH, Bartrum RJ: Ultrasound and renal failure, in Griffiths HJ

(ed): Radiology of Renal Failure. Philadelphia, W.B. Saunders, 1976, Chap 10, pp 227–238

31. Abeloff MD, Lenhard RE: Clinical management of ureteral obstruction secondary to malignant lymphoma. Johns Hopkins Med J 134:34–42, 1974

32. Shivers CH de T, Axelrod HD: Lymphoblastomatous nephropathy. J Urol 65:380–385, 1951

33. Williams G, Peet TND: Bilateral ureteral obstruction due to malignant lymphoma. Urology 7:649–651, 1976

34. Brewer WR, Wei Lan C, Bunts RC: Complete bilateral ureteral obstruction from leukemia and lymphoma. J Urol 98:186–190, 1967

35. Koziol I: Reticulum cell sarcoma: Unusual cause of ureteral obstruction. Urology 4:456–458, 1974

36. Aldridge CW, Mason JT: Ureteral obstruction in carcinoma of the cervix. Am J Obstet Gynecol 60:1272–1280, 1950

37. Beach EW: Urologic complications of cancer of the uterine cervix. J Urol 68:178–189, 1952

38. Chua DT, Iliya FA, O'Leary JA, et al: Palliative urinary diversion in patients with advanced carcinoma of the cervix. Cancer 20:93–95, 1967

39. Van Dyke AH, van Nagell JR: The prognostic significance of ureteral obstruction in patients with recurrent carcinoma of the cervix uteri. Surg Gyn Obstet 141:371–373, 1975

40. Presman D, Ehrlich L: Metastatic tumors of the ureter. J Urol 59:312–325, 1948

41. Tock EPC, Wee AST: Bilateral ureteric metastases causing complete anuria. Br J Urol 40:421–424, 1968

42. Schmidt JD: Bilateral ureteral obstruction due to cancer of the pancreas. J Urol 106:652–654, 1971

43. Mayer RJ, Garnick MB: Unpublished data

44. Geller SA, Lin CS: Ureteral obstruction from metastatic breast carcinoma. Arch Pathol 99:476–478, 1975

45. Grabstald H, Kaufman R: Hydronephrosis secondary to ureteral obstruction by metastatic breast cancer. J Urol 102:569–576, 1969

46. Alexander S, Kim K, Pinck BD, et al: Metastatic ureteral tumors. J Urol 110:288–293, 1973

47. Chisholm GD, Shackman R: Malignant obstructive uremia. Br J Urol 6:720–726, 1968

48. Goldstein AG: Metastatic carcinoma of the bladder. J Urol 98:209–215, 1967

49. Washington JA, Holland JM, Ketchum AS: Return of renal function following diversion of the obstructed ureter. Cancer 18:1457–1461, 1965

50. Martinez-Maldonado M, Yium J, Suki WN, et al: Renal complications in multiple myeloma: Pathophysiology and some aspects of clinical management. J Chronic Dis 24:221–237, 1971

51. Rees ED, Waugh WH: Factors in the renal failure of multiple myeloma. Arch Int Med 116:400–405, 1965

52. Booth, LJ, Minielly JA, Smith EKM: Acute renal failure in multiple myeloma. Can Med Assoc J 111:334–335, 1974

53. Bryan CW, Healy JK: Acute renal failure in multiple myeloma. Am J Med 44:128–133, 1968

54. Healy JK: Acute oliguric renal failure associated with multiple myeloma: Report of three cases. Br Med J 1:1126–1130, 1963

55. Holman RL: Complete anuria due to blockage of renal tubules by protein casts in a case of multiple myeloma. Arch Pathol 27:748–752, 1939

56. Cohen HJ, Rundles, RW: Managing the complications of plasma cell myeloma. Arch Intern Med 135:177–184, 1975

57. Myers GH Jr, Witten DM: Acute renal failure after excretory urography in multiple myeloma. Am J Roentgen 113:583–588, 1971

58. Morgan C Jr, Hammack WJ: Intravenous urography in multiple myeloma. N Engl J Med 275:77–79, 1966

59. Bartels ED, Brun GC, Gammeltoft A, et al: Acute anuria following intravenous pyelography in a patient with myelomatosis. Acta Medica Scandia 150:297–302, 1954

60. Killman S, Gjorup S, Thaysen JH: Fatal acute renal failure following intravenous pyelography in a patient with multiple myeloma. Acta Medica Scandia 158:43–46, 1957

61. Leucutia T: Multiple myeloma and intravenous pyelography. Am J Roentgen 85:187–189, 1961

62. Myhre JR, Brodwall EK, Knutsen SB: Acute renal failure following intravenous pyelography in cases of myelomatosis. Acta Medica Scandia 156:263–266, 1956

63. Perille PE, Conn HO: Acute renal failure after intravenous pyelography in plasma cell myeloma. JAMA 167:2186–2189, 1958

64. Bradley SE, Bradley GP: The effect of increased intra-abdominal pressure on renal function in man. J Clin Invest 26:1010–1022, 1947

65. Byrd L, Sherman RL: Radiocontrast-induced acute renal failure: A clinical and pathophysiologic review. Medicine 58:270–279, 1979

66. Cohen M, Meyers AM, Milne FJ, et al: Acute renal failure after use of radiographic contrast media. South Afr Med J 54:662–664, 1978

67. Blackman SS Jr, Barker WH, Buell MV, et al: On the pathogenisis of renal failure associated with multiple myeloma. Electrophoretic and chemical analysis of protein in urine and blood serum. J Clin Invest 23:163–166, 1944

68. DeFronzo RA, Humphrey RL, Wright JR, et al: Acute renal failure in multiple myeloma. Medicine 54:209–223, 1975

69. Zlotnick A, Rosenmann E: Renal pathologic findings associated with monoclonal gammopathies. Arch Intern Med 135:40–45, 1975

70. DeFronzo RA, Cooke CR, Wright JR, et al: Renal function in patients with multiple myeloma. Medicine 57:151–166, 1978

71. Putnam FW, Easley CW, Lynn LT, et al: Heat precipitation of Bence-Jones proteins. I. Optimum conditions. Arch Biochem Biophys 83:115–130, 1959

72. Richards AI, Hines JD: Recovery from acute renal failure in plasma cell leukemia. Am J Med Sci 266:293–297, 1973

73. Argani I, Kipkie GF: Macroglobulinemic nephropathy: Acute renal failure in macroglobulinemia or waldenstrom. Am J Med 36:151–157, 1964

74. Burke JF, Flis R, Lasker N, et al: Malignant lymphoma with "myeloma kidney" acute renal failure. Am J Med 60:1055–1060, 1976

75. Gutman AB, Yu TF: Uric acid nephrolithiasis. Am J Med 45:756–779, 1968

76. Kjellstrand CM, Campbell DC II, Von Hartitzsch B, et al: Hyperuricemic acute renal failure. Arch. Intern Med 133:349–359, 1974

77. Rieselbach RE, Bentzel CJ, Cotlove E, et al: Uric acid excretion and renal function in the acute hyperuricemia of leukemia: Pathogenesis and therapy of uric acid nephropathy. Am J Med 37:872–884, 1964

78. Sandberg AA, Cartwright GE, Wintrobe MM: Studies on leukemia. I. Uric acid excretion. Blood 11:154–166, 1956

79. Kiely JM, Wagoner RD, Holley KE: Renal complications of lymphoma. Ann Intern Med 71:1159–1173, 1969

80. Alsarraf D, Reese L: Management of acute renal failure due to marked hyperuricemia. Can Med Assoc J 106:352–354, 1972

81. Epstein FH, Pigeon G: Experimental urate nephropathy: Studies of the distribution of Urate in renal tissue. Nephron 1:144–157, 1964

82. Kanwar YS, Manaligod JD: Leukemic urate nephropathy. Arch Pathol 99:467–472, 1975

83. Jamison RL: Urinary concentration and dilution, in Brenner M, Rector FC (eds): The Kidney. Philadelphia, W.B. Saunders, 1976, Chap 11, pp 391–440

84. Rector FC: Renal acidification and ammonia production; chemistry of weak acids and bases; buffer mechanisms, in Brenner M, Rector FC (eds): The Kidney. Philadelphia, W.B. Saunders, 1976, Chap 9, pp 318–342

85. Klineberg JR, Bluestone R, Schlosstein L, et al: Urate deposition disease — how is it regulated and how can it be modified? Ann Intern Med 78:99–111, 1973

86. Conger JD, Falk SA: Intrarenal dynamics in the pathogenesis and prevention of acute urate nephropathy. J Clin Invest 59:786–793, 1977

87. Rastegar A, Thier SO: The physiologic approach to hyperuricemia. New Engl J Med 286:470–476, 1972

88. Ablin A, Stephens BG, Hirata T, et al: Nephropathy, xanthinuria and orotic aciduria complicating Burkitt's lymphoma treated with chemotherapy and allopurinol. Metabolism 21:771–778, 1972

89. Bano P: Xanthine nephropathy in a patient with lymphosarcoma treated with allopurinol. N Engl J Med 283:354–357, 1970

90. Seegmiller JE: Xanthine stone formation. Am J Med 45:780–783, 1968

91. Gelbart DR, Weinstein AB, Fajordo LF: Allopurinol-induced interstitial nephritis. Ann Int Med 86:196–198, 1977

92. Steinberg SM, Galen MA, Lazarus JM, et al: Hemodialysis for acute anuric uric acid nephropathy. Am J Dis Childh 129:956–958, 1975

93. Myers WPL: Hypercalcemia in neoplastic disease. Cancer 9:1135–1140, 1956

94. Muggia FM, Heinemann HO: Hypercalcemia associated with neoplastic disease. Ann Intern Med 73:281–290, 1970

95. Benvenisti DS, Sherwood LM, Heinemann HO: Hypercalcemic crisis in acute leukemia. Am J Med 46:976–984, 1969

96. Zidar BL, Shadduck RK, Winkelstein A, et al: Acute myeloblastic leukemia and hypercalcemia: A case of probable ectopic parathyroid hormone production. N Engl J Med 295:692–694, 1976

97. Ballard HS, Marcus AJ: Hypercalcemia in chronic myelogenous leukemia. N Engl J Med 282:663–665, 1970

98. Haskell CM, DeVita VT, Canellos GP: Hypercalcemia in chronic granulocytic leukemia. Cancer 27:872–880, 1971

99. Kabakow B, Mines MF, King FH: Hypercalcemia in Hodgkin's disease. N Engl J Med 256:59–62, 1957

100. Moses AM, Spencer H: Hypercalcemia in patients with malignant lymphoma. Ann Intern Med 59:531–536, 1963

101. O'Regan S, Carson S, Chesney RW, et al: Electrolyte and acid–base disturbances in the management of leukemia. Blood 49:345–353, 1977

102. Deftos LF, Neer R: Medical management of the hypercalcemia of malignancy. Ann Rev Med 25:323–331, 1974

103. Besarab A, Caro JF: Mechanisms of hypercalcemia in malignancy. Cancer 41:2276–2285, 1978

104. Mundy GR, Raisz LG, Cooper RA, et al: Evidence for the secretion of an osteoclast stimulating factor in myeloma. N Engl J Med 291: 1041–1046, 1974

105. Demers LM, Allegra JC, Harvey HA, et al: Plasma prostaglandins in hypercalcemic patients with neoplastic disease. Cancer 39:1159–1162, 1977

106. Epstein F: Calcium nephropathy, in Strauss MB, Welt LG (eds): Diseases of the Kidney. Boston, Little, Brown & Company, 1971, Chap 24, pp 903–931

107. Suki WN, Eknoyan G: Tubulo-interstitial disease, in Brenner BM, Rector FC (eds): The Kidney. Philadelphia, W.B. Saunders, 1976, Chap 25, pp 1113–1144

108. Mazzaferri EL, O'Dorisio TM, LaBuglio A: Treatment of hypercalcemia associated with malignancy. Sem Oncol 5:141–153, 1978

109. Chabner BA, Myers CE, Coleman CN, et al: The clinical pharmacology of antineoplastic agents. N Engl J Med 292:1107–1113, 1159–1168, 1975

110. Ojima O, Anderson LL, Collins GJ, et al: Pharmacologic studies of methotrexate in cancer patients with uropathy. Arch Surg 100:173–177, 1970

111. Condit PT, Changes RE, Joel W: Renal toxicity of methotrexate. Cancer 23:126–131, 1969

112. Frei E III, Jaffe N, Tattersall MHN, et al: New approaches to cancer chemotherapy with methotrexate. N Engl J Med 292:846–851, 1975

113. Pitman SW, Parker LM, Tattersall MHN, et al: Clinical trial of high-dose methotrexate (NSC-740) with citrovorum factor (NSC-3590) — Toxicologic and therapeutic observations. Cancer Chemotherapy Rep (Part 3) 6:43–49, 1975

114. Pitman SW, Frei E III: Weekly methotrexate–calcium leukovorin rescue: Effect of alkalinization on nephrotoxicity; pharmacokinetics in the CNS; and use in CNS non-Hodgkin's lymphoma. Cancer Treat Rep 61:695–701, 1977

115. Stoller RG, Hande KR, Jacobs SA, et al: Use of plasma pharmaco-kinetics to predict and prevent methotrexate toxicity. N Engl J Med 297:630–634, 1977
116. Hande KR, Balow JE, Drake JC, et al: Methotrexate and hemodialysis (Letter). Ann Intern Med 87:495–496, 1977
117. Gibson TP, Reich SD, Krumlovsky FA, et al: Hemoperfusion for methotrexate removal. Clin Pharmacol Ther 23:351–355, 1978
118. Frei E III, Blum RH, Pitman SW, et al: High-dose methotrexate with citrovorum factor rescue: Rationale and spectrum of antitumor activity. Am J Med 68:370–376, 1980
119. Ensminger WD, Frei E III: The prevention of methotrexate toxicity by thymidine infusions in humans. Cancer Res 37:1857–1863, 1977
120. Broder LE, Carter SK: Pancreatic islet cell cancer. II. Results of therapy in 52 patients. Ann Intern Med 79:108–118, 1973
121. Schein PS, DeLellis RA, Kahn CR, et al: Islet cell tumors: Current concepts and management. Ann Intern Med 79:239–257, 1973
122. Schein P, Kahn R, Gorden P, et al: Streptozotocin for malignant insulinomas and carcinoid tumor. Report of eight cases and review of literature. Arch Intern Med 132:555–561, 1973
123. Sadoff L: Nephrotoxicity of streptozotocin (NSC-85998). Cancer Chemother Rep (Part 1) 54:457–459, 1970
124. Myerowitz RL, Sartiano GP, Cavallo T: Nephrotoxic and cytoproliferative effects of streptozotocin: Report of a patient with multiple hormone-secreting islet cell carcinoma. Cancer 38:1550–1555, 1976
125. Rozencweig M, Von Hoff DD, Slavik M, et al: Cis-Diamminedichloroplatinum II: A new anticancer drug. Ann Intern Med 86:803–812, 1977
126. Einhorn LH, Williams SD: The role of cis-platinum in solid-tumor therapy. N Engl J Med 300:289–291, 1979
127. Leonard BJ, Eccleston E, Jones D, et al: Antileukaemic and nephrotoxic properties of platinum compounds. Nature 234:43–45, 1971
128. Higby DJ, Wallace HJ, Holland JF: Cis-diamminedichloroplatinum (NSC-119875): A Phase I study. Cancer Chemother Rep (Part 1) 54:459–463, 1973
129. Talley RW, O'Bryan RM, Gutterman JU, et al: Clinical evaluation of toxic effects of cis-diamminedichloroplatinum (NSC-119875)—Phase I clinical study. Cancer Chemother Rep (Part 1) 57:465–471, 1973
130. Dentino M, Luft FC, Yum MN, et al: Long-term effect of cis-diamminedichloride platinum (CDDP) on renal function and structure in man. Cancer 41:1274–1281, 1978

131. Gottlieb JA, Drewinko B: Review of current clinical status of platinum coordination complexes in cancer chemotherapy. Cancer Chemother Rep 59:621–628, 1975

132. Gonzalez-Vitale JC, Hayes DM, Cvitkovic E, et al: Acute renal failure after cis-dichlorodiammineplatinum (II) and gentamicin–Cephalothin therapies. Cancer Treat Rep 62:693–698, 1978

133. Hardaker WT, Stone RA, McCoy R: Platinum nephrotoxicity. Cancer 34:1030–1032, 1974

134. Rossof AH, Slayton RE, Perlia CP: Preliminary clinical experience with cis-diamminedichloroplatinum (II) (NSC-119875, CACP). Cancer 30:1451–1456, 1972

135. Stark, JJ, Howell SB, Carmody J: Prevention of cis-platinum nephrotoxicity. Clin Res 25:412A, 1977

136. Gonzalez-Vitale JC, Hayes DM, Cvitkovic E, et al: The renal pathology in clinical trials of cis-platinum (II) diamminedichloride. Cancer 39:1362–1371, 1977

137. Hayes DM, Cvitkovic E, Goldbey RB, et al: High-dose cis-platinum diammine dichloride: Amelioration of renal toxicity by mannitol diuresis. Cancer 39:1372–1381, 1977

138. Bagley CM, Bostick FW, DeVita VT: Clinical pharmacology of cyclophosphamide. Cancer Res 33:226–233, 1973

139. Johnson WW, Meadows DC: Urinary-bladder fibrosis and telangiectasia associated with long-term cyclophosphamide therapy. N Engl J Med 284:290–294, 1971

140. Wall RL, Clausen KP: Carcinoma of the urinary bladder in patients receiving cyclophosphamide. N Engl J Med 293:271–273, 1975

141. Galletti PM, Pasqualino A, Geering RG: Hemodialysis in cancer chemotherapy. Trans Am Soc Art Int Org 12:20–24, 1966

142. Crooke ST, Luft F, Broughton A, et al: Bleomycin serum pharmacokinetics as determined by a radioimmunoassay and a microbiologic assay in a patient with compromised renal function. Cancer 39:1430–1434, 1977

143. Crooke ST, Presayko AW: Bleomycin pharmacokinetics in patients with varying renal function. Proc Am Soc Clin Oncol 18:C–79a, 1977

144. Speed DE, Galton DAG, Swan A: Melphalan in the treatment of myelomatosis. Br Med J 1:1664–1669, 1964

145. Anderson RJ, Gambertoglio JG, Schrier RW: Immunosuppressive and antineoplastic agents, in Clinical Use of Drugs in Renal Failure. Springfield, Ill., Charles C. Thomas, 1976, Chap 9, pp 173–184

146. Liu K, Mittleman A, Sproul EE, et al: Renal toxicity in man treated with mitomycin C. Cancer 28:1314–1320, 1971

147. Harmon WE, Cohen HJ, Schneeberger EE, et al: Chronic renal fail-
      ure in children treated with methyl CCNU. N Engl J Med 300:1200–
      1203, 1979
148. Nichols WC, Moertel CG: Personal communication
149. Morton DL: CCNU nephrotoxicity following sustained remission in
      oat cell carcinoma. Cancer Treat Rep 63:226–227, 1979
150. Burke JF, Laucius JF, Brodovsky HS, et al: Doxorubicin hydrochlo-
      ride-associated renal failure. Arch Intern Med 137:385–388, 1977
151. Buss H, Lamberts B: The kidney glomerulus of the rat during exper-
      imental daunomycin-nephrosis. A comparative transmission and
      scanning electron microscopic study. Beitr Pathol Bd 148:360–387,
      1973
152. Dosik GM, Gutterman JU, Hersh EM, et al: Nephrotoxicity from
      cancer immunotherapy. Ann Intern Med 89:41–46, 1978
153. Kunkler PB, Farr RF, Luxtom RW: The limit of renal tolerance to
      x-rays: An investigation into renal damage occurring following the
      treatment of the testes by abdominal baths. Br J Radiol 25:190–201,
      1952
154. Luxton RW: Radiation nephritis. Quart J Med 22:215–242, 1953
155. Luxton RW: Radiation nephritis: A long-term study of 54 patients.
      Lancet 2:1221–1224, 1961
156. Rubenstone AI, Fitch LB: Radiation nephritis. A clinicopathologic
      study. Am J Med 33:545–554, 1962
157. Levitt WM: Radiation nephritis. Br J Urol 29:381–382, 1957
158. Steckel RJ, Tobin PL, Stein JJ, et al: Intra-arterial epinephrine protec-
      tion against radiation nephritis. A progress report. Radiology
      92:1341–1345, 1969
159. Appel GB, Neu HC: The nephtotoxicity of antimicrobial agents. N
      Engl J Med 296:663–670, 722–728, 784–787, 1977
160. Bobrow SN, Jaffe E, Young RC: Anuria and acute tubular necrosis
      associated with gentamicin and cephalothin. JAMA 222:1546–1547,
      1972
161. Cabanillas F, Burgos RC, Rodriguez RC, et al: Nephrotoxicity of
      combined cephalothin-gentamicin regimen. Arch Intern Med
      135:850–852, 1975
162. Fillastre JP, Laumonier R, Humbert G, et al: Acute renal failure as-
      sociated with combined gentamicin and cephalothin therapy. Br
      Med J 2:396–397, 1973
163. Kleinknect D, Ganeval D, Droz D: Acute renal failure after high
      doses of gentamicin and cephalothin. Lancet 1:1129, 1973

164. Plager JE: Association of renal injury with combined cephalothin-gentamicin therapy among patients severely ill with malignant disease. Cancer 37:1937–1943, 1976
165. Wade JC, Petty BG, Conrad G, et al: Cephalothin plus an aminoglycoside is more nephrotoxic than methicillin plus an aminoglycoside. Lancet 2:604–606, 1978

11

ACUTE INFECTION IN PATIENTS WITH MALIGNANT DISEASE

Victorio Rodriguez
Steven J. Ketchel

During this decade, the useful lives of many cancer patients have been prolonged through the application of various therapeutic advances in chemotherapy, surgery, radiation therapy, and immunotherapy. Concomitantly, progress made in the management of complications in these patients has become an integral part of the successful treatment of the cancer patient.[1] In spite of this progress, infection remains the most frequent serious complication in cancer patients during therapy and is the most frequent cause of death in such patients.[2-4]

There are several reasons for the high incidence of infection in cancer patients, and although most are due to the effects of the underlying malignancy, they are also in part related to the combined effects of the tumor and its treatment. Thus surgery, chemotherapy, and radiotherapy contribute to the alteration of the normal anatomical barriers which render the host susceptible to invasion by environmental pathogens or by organisms from the patients' own flora. In addition, chemotherapy and radiotherapy decrease the inflammatory and immune responses of the host. Perhaps the single most important factor which predisposes cancer patients to infection is neutropenia. Neutropenia can result from the underlying disease (in hematologic malignancies) or the treatment (in most cancer patients receiving intensive radiotherapy or chemotherapy). Studies in patients with acute leukemia have demonstrated that the frequency of infection is inversely related to the number of circulating granulocytes. Bodey et al.[5]

demonstrated that in those patients with acute leukemia who had less than 100 neutrophils/mm^3 in the peripheral blood, there were 43 episodes of infection per 1,000 days; this incidence of infection decreased to 19 episodes per 1,000 days when the polymorphonuclear count was between 100 and 500/mm^3, and fell even lower when the count was between 500 and 1,000/mm^3. Furthermore, recovery from severe infection in most neutropenic patients depends upon their ability to respond to the infectious process with an increased production of granulocytes.[1] Thus, the response of granulocytopenic patients with infections to some of the available antibiotics is suboptimal.[6] Since neutropenia is common during cancer treatment, there is a continual risk of infection in cancer patients. It is therefore important that medical oncologists become aware of these complications and their management.

In this paper, we attempt to update our previous review on the most frequent types of acute infections, their clinical manifestations, and available antimicrobial therapies.[7]

Most Frequent Infections in Patients with Malignant Diseases

Cancer patients are most frequently affected by bacterial infections. This has been well demonstrated in studies on the causes of death, which indicate that the majority of patients with acute leukemia, solid tumors, and lymphomas die of bacterial infection.[2-4] Seventy-six percent of infections causing death in patients with acute leukemia, 87 percent in lymphoma patients, and 93 percent in patients with solid tumors are due to bacterial organisms (Table 1). The majority of these bacterial infections are caused by gram-negative bacilli, with *Escherichia coli*, Klebsiella-Entero-

Table 1
Infection as Cause of Death in Cancer Patients

	Acute Leukemia	Lymphoma	Solid Tumors
Number of patients studied at autopsy	315	206	816
Number dying of infection (%)	234 (74)	104 (51)	380 (47)
Percent due to bacterial infections	76	87	93
Percent due to gram-negative bacilli	78	60	68

Table 2
Infections During Chemotherapy
of Cancer Patients

Type	Percent
Disseminated	35
Pneumonia	34
Cellulitis	12
Urinary tract	7
Gastrointestinal	4
Upper respiratory	3
Anorectal	3
Miscellaneous	2

bacter organisms, and *Pseudomonas* spp. the most common pathogens causing death in these patients.[2-4]

Infection is not only a major problem as the cause of death in cancer patients, but is also a major complication during remission-induction therapy. In a recent study of the causes of fever in 494 adults with acute leukemia during a 6-year period, infection occurred in 64 percent of 1,894 episodes.[8] Similar findings also have been observed in patients with lymphoma and solid tumors during intensive remission-induction therapy.[9,10] The most frequent types of infection seen in these patients are shown in Table 2. Disseminated infection, pneumonia, and cellulitis occur more frequently. Urinary-tract, gastrointestinal, and upper-respiratory-tract infections occur less frequently. Anorectal infections, although of low frequency, are especially important because they may originate disseminated infection. Pelvic inflammatory disease, peritonitis, meningitis, and other miscellanous infections are less common.

The organisms that most frequently cause infections in patients with acute leukemia are listed in Table 3. They are representative of the most likely organisms to infect the compromised host during intensive remission-induction therapy. *Pseudomonas aeruginosa* used to be the most frequent pathogen until 1970. Since the introduction of carbenicillin the mortality rate, and subsequently the proportion of infections caused by *Pseudomonas*, have substantially decreased.[4,11] However, the incidence of infections caused by pathogens of the Enterobacteriaceae group has increased to the point that today *E. coli*, *Klebsiella*, and *Enterobacter* spp. are the most common causes of gram-negative bacillary infections during induction therapy and are the causes of most deaths due to infection in patients with advanced malignancies.[4,8] Salmonella infections may rarely be

Table 3
Organisms Causing Infection During
Chemotherapy of Cancer Patients

Type	Percent
Gram-negative bacilli	51
Gram-positive organisms	4
Anaerobes	2
Fungal	6
Multiple	9
Viral	0.7
Pneumocystis and toxoplasma	0.5
Unidentified	27

seen in patients with solid tumors. Infections caused by *Legionella pneumophila* have been found with increasing frequency in recent years.[12]

With less frequency, acute infections may also be produced by other bacterial and nonbacterial pathogens listed in Table 3. Infections caused by gram-positive organisms were very frequent before the availability of effective penicillins. Since the introduction of methicillin those infections caused by *Staphylococcus aureus* and Streptococci have substantially decreased. Resurgent staphylococcal infections, however, have been found in hospital populations of cancer patients, and thus today the incidence may be slightly higher than it was a few years ago. Although much rarer, infections caused by *Listeria monocytogenes* may occur, particularly in patients with lymphoma or leukemia.

Anaerobic infections occur with low incidence; they account for less than 5 percent of the infections developing during induction chemotherapy in the leukemic population.[8] Of these, infections caused by *Clostridium* and *Bacteroides* spp. have been most frequently seen; however, other less recognized anaerobic pathogens, such as *Corynebacterium* spp., *Propionibacterium acnes*, and *Bacillus* spp. are being seen more often as pathogens in these patients. Recently, mycobacterial disease has been described as an emergent problem in patients with malignant disease and should be considered a definite risk, especially in individuals with hairy-cell leukemia, lymphomas, and carcinomas of the lung.[13]

Fungal infections in patients with cancer have been appearing with increasing frequency during recent years. In a study of fungal infections found at autopsy in 161 leukemic patients, the yearly frequency of fungal infections increased from 10 percent to greater than 30 percent during a 10-year period. *Candida* sp. accounted for the majority of these infections.[14] In large cancer institutes, the incidence of serious *Candida* infections is approximately 10–25 percent; however, less than 10 percent are recognized early and most are identified postmortem. In patients with acute leukemia, the overall incidence of *Candida* septicemia has increased from 2 to 6 percent during the last 5 years. Unfortunately, the majority of serious fungal infections are seldom diagnosed antemortem due to the lack of specific signs and symptoms and the lack of reliable diagnostic laboratory tests. Isolation of *Candida* spp. from clinical specimens is seldom helpful in establishing the diagnosis because the organism is ubiquitous. The organism is cultured from blood specimens of only 25 percent of patients with disseminated candidiasis. Serological tests are often not helpful in the patient whose antibody titer fails to rise because of impaired immunological mechanisms. Recently, characteristic skin lesions have been identified that may aid in the diagnosis of systemic candidiasis.[15] Aspergillosis and phycomycosis have become progressively more frequent in recent years and are rarely diagnosed antemortem because the organisms are cultured infrequently from these patients. Cryptococcosis is an infection likely to develop in a high proportion of patients with lymphomas. The cryptococcal antigen test has proven to be very useful in diagnosing cryptococcosis in these patients.

Viral infections are also of concern among the patient undergoing cancer chemotherapy. Although their incidence ranks low in the spectrum of infections, they may become overwhelming and rapidly disseminated. *Herpes simplex* and *herpes zoster* infections are most frequent. *Herpes zoster* occurs commonly in patients with malignant lymphomas and in children with acute leukemia. It has been recognized that the more intense the therapeutic regimen the greater the susceptibility to viral infections, especially *herpes zoster*. Studies of patients who have received combination therapy with irradiation and chemotherapy indicate that the incidence of *herpes zoster*, with its potential of dissemination, is higher than in those receiving chemotherapy or radiotherapy alone.[16] Other viral infections such as cytomegalic inclusion disease are being recognized more frequently, particularly in patients undergoing bone marrow transplantation.

Parasitic infections, specifically those produced by *Pneumocystis carinii* and *Toxoplasma gondii*, appear to be increasing in frequency among patients receiving cancer chemotherapy and chronic immunosuppression. *Pneumocystis carinii* infections occur mainly in children undergoing continuous myelosuppressive therapy. The syndrome this infection commonly presents is an acute interstitial pneumonitis and it is being detected more frequently in cancer patients in intensive and prolonged chemotherapy or extensive radiation programs.[17] *Toxoplasma gondii* is a parasite which can be pathogenic to debilitated hosts and appears as disseminated infection in many myelosuppressed patients.[18] This organism can be transmitted by blood products transfused to the patient; thus it has the potential of becoming an acute problem.

Diagnosis of Infection in Cancer Patients

The diagnosis of bacterial infections in cancer patients is often difficult. Most of the patients have impaired host defenses and frequently are severely neutropenic. Consequently, the mechanisms of inflammatory response of the host are decreased or suppressed. The classical clinical manifestations of infection therefore may be absent or atypical in many patients. The diagnosis of bacterial infections relies upon the diagnostic tools available in clinical medicine. If a cancer patient develops fever during neutropenia, infections should be strongly suspected. A complete physical examination with special attention to the lungs, the postauricular, perianal, inguinal, and axillary areas should be performed since these are often sites of infection which can be missed in an incomplete physical examination. Prior to initiating therapy, cultures of blood, urine, throat, and any obvious site of infection should be obtained for aerobic and anaerobic organisms and atypical pathogens. Cultures should be repeated daily while fever persists. Roentgenologic examination of chest and sinuses as clinically indicated are helpful. Biopsy of skin lesions for histologic and microbiologic studies may lead to the identification of the pathogenic organisms.

Fever is a valuable diagnostic sign in the cancer patient. In our experience, fever greater than 101°F not related to transfusion of blood products is a sign which heralds severe infection in about 80 percent of patients with advanced malignancies and neutropenia. Furthermore, as can be seen in Figure 1, the fatality rate of cancer patients with severe infection is very high within the initial 48 hours after development of infection if no prompt, adequate therapy is initiated.[19-21] Consequently, fever is a sign that should not be masked with nonspecific therapy, but rather should impel the physician to a thorough diagnostic workup and immediate, if not simultaneous, initiation of antibiotic therapy.

Studies on the causes of fever in patients with acute leukemia demonstrate that fever is usually due to infection. During hospitalization for remission-induction therapy, the patients spend a third of their days in the hospital with fever, and over 60 percent of the febrile episodes are due to

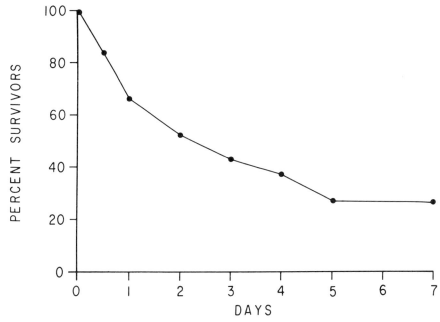

Fig. 1. *Depicts the survival curve of cancer patients with gram-negative bacteremia prior to effective antibacterial therapy. Mortality can be as high as 50 percent during the initial 48 hours if prompt therapy is not initiated.* [19-21]

infection.[8] In 35 percent of the episodes the origin of the fever cannot be determined, but fever occurs most often when the patients have severe neutropenia.

Studies similar to those performed on patients with acute leukemia have also been conducted in patients with lymphoma and metastatic carcinoma, and indicate that during myelosuppressive therapy most febrile episodes are due to infection.[9,10] In a substantial number of cancer patients, no etiologic factor can be recognized as producing fever and they are listed as being of unknown origin (FUO).[22,23] Since patients with impaired host defenses often fail to develop other clinical signs of infection, it is likely that a substantial proportion of such FUO episodes are actually due to infection. We therefore recommend instituting broad-spectrum antibiotic therapy in these patients since it is often difficult to differentiate infectious and noninfectious fevers in the neutropenic patient. About two thirds of patients with FUO become afebrile after initial adequate antimicrobial therapy is commenced.[22] This suggests that an unidentified infection may be present and responding; one which, if not treated sufficiently, may lead to an unnecessarily high mortality rate. Because the diagnostic signs of infection may be scanty in the neutropenic cancer patient, the physician must develop high degrees of suspicion to identify infection in these patients. Skin lesions such as ecthyma gangrenosum in *Pseudomonas* infections,[19] or the lesions of disseminated *Candida* infections,[15] may assist in the early diagnosis of severe infection. Systemic candidiasis may also be diagnosed by characteristic focal, white, occular lesions on the surface of the retina. The bone marrow examination used in searching for granulomas may be of aid in diagnosing fungal or mycobacterial disease; bone marrow cultures may be positive in systemic infections.

It has been our practice to do a "prednisone test" in febrile patients not responding to antibacterial therapy after 7 days of unidentified infection. The test consists of oral administration of 10–15 mg of prednisone 4 times a day for 2 days. If the patient becomes rapidly afebrile and the fever reappears after the prednisone is discontinued, it is likely that the patient has a fungal infection.[24] This test is not specific but is suggestive of fungal infection in the febrile patient with compromised host defenses who has failed to respond to antibiotics and it may suggest the necessity for antifungal therapy. A typical response to the prednisone test in a patient who was proven to have a fatal fungal infection is shown in Figure 2.

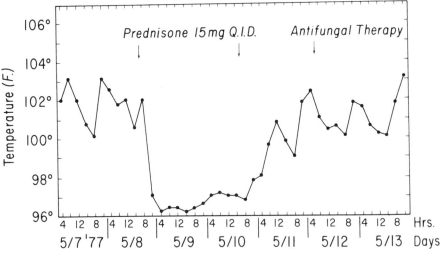

Fig. 2. *The prednisone test (10–15 mg 4 times a day during 48 hr) in a patient with a proven fatal* Candida *infection.*

Management of the Febrile Cancer Patient

Hospitalized cancer patients who are neutropenic should have their temperatures taken frequently. Similarly, patients in remission who continue to receive maintenance chemotherapy during which periods of neutropenia might occur should be instructed to take their temperatures frequently and report to the physician if fever of 101°F or greater occurs. Studies of various gram-negative bacillary septicemia in patients with malignancies indicate that fever of 101°F or greater is the commonest sign of infection in these patients.[19-21] Furthermore, progression of infection in these patients is so overwhelming and rapid that if no attention is paid to the earliest signs of infection, the physician can expect a high fatality rate which varies from 18 percent to greater than 40 percent during the first 48 hours. Hence, after appropriate cultures have been obtained antibiotic therapy should be instituted promptly. In febrile patients with adequate neutrophil counts, antibiotic therapy may be delayed while under careful observation if no other signs of infection are present. However, patients with gastrointestinal or genitourinary tumors are susceptible to gram-negative bacillary septicemia after diagnostic or surgical procedures, and delaying antibiotic therapy may be detrimental. Whenever the presence of infection is strongly suspected, it is advisable to institute antibiotics promptly after obtaining appropriate diagnostic studies.

Currently, the best choice for neutropenic patients is carbenicillin or ticarcillin plus a cephalosporin and/or an aminoglycoside. The doses recommended for cancer patients are listed in Table 4. Patients with adequate neutrophils may be given an aminoglycoside with or without carbenicillin, a cephalosporin, or an antistaphylococcal penicillin. Patients with tumors of the gastrointestinal or genitourinary tract should initially receive clindamycin or chloramphenicol for possible anaerobic infections. Appropriate adjustments of antibiotic therapy should be made after the results of cultures and in vitro sensitivity tests become available.

In the neutropenic patient, once antibiotic therapy has been initiated a decision must be made concerning the duration of therapy. If the patient has an identified infection or FUO which responds to antibiotic therapy, this therapy should be continued for about 1 week, or 3 days after becoming afebrile, whichever is longer. Those antibiotics which are not appropriate based upon culture results, however, should be deleted. Although most patients who become afebrile shortly after antibiotic therapy is initiated, and have no apparent site of infection, might not be infected, about 20 percent of them are eventually proven to have infection and some patients die if antibiotic therapy is discontinued prematurely.[22,23] Antibiotic

Table 4
Antimicrobial Agents for Treatment of Infection in the Compromised Host

	Indications	Dose
Penicillins		
Penicillin G	Gram(+) cocci, Clostridium infections	600,000 units q4h
Methicillin	Penicillin G-resistant S. aureus	1 g q4-6h
Ampicillin	H. influenza, E. coli, P. mirabilis, Gram(−) cocci	1 g q4h
Carbenicillin	Ps. aeruginosa, Proteus sp.	5 g q4h
Ticarcillin	Ps. aeruginosa, Proteus sp.	3.5 g q4h
Cephalosporins		
Cephalothin	E. coli, P. mirabilis, Klebsiella sp., Gram(+) cocci	2 g q6h
Cefazolin	E. coli, P. mirabilis, Klebsiella sp., Gram(+) cocci	1 g q6h
Cefamandole	Like cephalothin or slightly more active	1–2 g q6h
*Aminoglycosides**		
Kanamycin	Gram(−) bacilli except Ps. aeruginosa & many S. marcescens	150 mg/M^2 q6h*
Gentamicin	Gram(−) bacilli & methicillin-resistant Staph. aureus	50 mg/M^2 q6h*
Tobramycin	Gram(−) bacilli & methicillin-resistant Staph. aureus	50 mg/M^2 q6h*
Amikacin	Gram(−) bacilli including Ps. aeruginosa & some gentamicin-resistant organisms	150 mg/M^2 q6h*
Sisomicin	Similar to gentamicin	40 mg/M^2 q6h*
Polypeptides		
Polymyxin B	Gram(−) bacilli except Proteus sp. & many S. marcescens	25 mg/M^2 q6h
Colistin	Gram(−) bacilli except Proteus sp. & many S. marcescens	50 mg/M^2 q6h
Miscellaneous		
Chloramphenicol	Salmonella	500 mg/M^2 q6h
Clindamycin	Anaerobes, mainly Bacteroides	600 mg/M^2 q6h
Trimethoprim & Sulfamethoxazole	Gram(−) except Pseudomonas, P. carinii	20 mg tid / 100 mg/kg tid
Antifungal		
Amphotericin B	Systemic fungal infection	20–40 mg/M^2/day
5-Fluorocytosine	Candidiasis, cryptococcosis	1 g/M^2 q6h
Miconazole	Systemic infections, mainly Candidiasis	600 mg–1 gram

therapy should therefore be continued in such patients for a minimum of 1 week, or until the patient's neutropenia recovers. A substantial number of neutropenic patients with identified infections who fail to respond to appropriate antibiotic therapy will respond to the addition of white blood cell transfusions. Therefore, if feasible, the administration of white blood cell transfusions to neutropenic patients who have failed to respond to 2 or 3 days of antibiotic therapy is recommended. Obviously, if the causative organism is found to be resistant to the original antibiotic regimen, appropriate antibiotics should be administered. Those patients failing to respond to antibiotics and white blood cell transfusions should be placed on other appropriate antibiotic regimens. The neutropenic patient with persistent fever despite antibiotic therapy and no identified infection offers a therapeutic dilemma. We also administer white blood cell transfusions to these patients. If they fail to respond, they become candidates for a therapeutic trial of amphotericin B, since they have a high probability of fungal infection. All antimicrobial agents are discontinued in those patients who fail to respond to amphotericin B and they are reevaluated for evidence of infection.

Management of Identified Bacterial Infection in the Cancer Patient

Broad-spectrum antibiotic therapy should be instituted promptly when the neutropenic patient develops fever because infection is likely to disseminate widely and rapidly. The currently available antimicrobial agents are listed in Table 4, but only the most recently available will be described.

Single Antibiotics

The aminoglycoside antibiotics have gained wide acceptance because of their broad spectrum of activity. Gentamicin sulfate is active against most gram-negative bacilli, including *Pseudomonas aeruginosa*, and has been used extensively in cancer patients. Using an intermittent dosage schedule of 30 mg/M^2 (0.75 mg/kg) intravenously every 6 hours, the response rate of gentamicin therapy was 51 percent in gram-negative bacilli infections in cancer patients.[25] The results of gentamicin treatment of gram-negative bacilli infections in cancer patients are listed in Table 5. Although gentamicin is very effective against infections in patients with adequate neutrophils, it is suboptimal in patients who are neutropenic at the initiation of infection or in those patients whose neutrophil count falls

Table 5
Single Antibiotic Therapy Against Most Common Gram-Negative
Bacillary Infections in Cancer Patients

Antibiotic	Escherichia coli		Klebsiella Enterobacter-Serratta		Pseudomonas	
	Number	% Cure	Number	% Cure	Number	% Cure
Gentamicin	8	75	22	52	22	45
Tobramycin	11	36	20	60	10	40
Amikacin*	9	78	14	88	3	100
Sisomicin*	3	67	19	73	8	25
Carbenicillin	8	50	14	7	59	75
Ticarcillin	11	9	10	0	20	80
Cephalosporins	21	62	40	15	—	—

*Amikacin and sisomicin were given by continuous infusion to some of these patients.

Table 6
Effect of Neutrophil Count on Response to Antibiotic Therapy

Antibiotic	Neutrophil Count/mm³					
	<100		101–1000		>1000	
	# Pts	% Cure	# Pts	% Cure	# Pts	% Cure
Gentamycin	23	22	17	53	24	79
Tobramycin	21	24	10	70	28	79
Amikacin*	25	64	24	63	10	80
Sisomicin*	20	50	14	71	4	75
Carbenicillin	16	75	26	88	9	50
Ticarcillin	12	92	4	75	4	100
Cephalosporin	33	24	33	67	14	50

Pts = Patients.
*Amikacin and sisomicin were given to some of these patients by continuous infusion.

during their infection (Table 6). The failure of gentamicin in neutropenic patients does not appear to be due to inadequate serum concentrations or to the emergence of resistant organisms. The current recommended dose should be at least 40–50 mg/M² every 6 hours. Nephrotoxicity is a special concern in cancer patients because they often receive multiple courses of gentamicin therapy and because the frequency of nephrotoxicity increases after multiple courses. Occasionally patients develop acute renal failure after only a few days of therapy.

Tobramycin is also an aminoglycoside antibiotic with a spectrum of activity similar to gentamicin but with more activity in vitro against *P. aeruginosa;* most organisms resistant to gentamicin are also resistant to tobramycin. Tobramycin used in an intermittent dosage schedule of 50 mg/M² (1.25 mg/kg) intravenously every 6 hours during 82 infections in cancer patients produced an overall response rate of 54 percent.[26] The majority of infections were caused by *E. coli, P. aeruginosa,* and *Klebsiella pneumoniae* (Table 5). Like gentamicin, tobramycin is quite effective in patients with adequate circulating neutrophils but is only minimally effective in patients with neutropenia (Table 6). Failure of the neutropenic patient is not related to emergence of resistant organisms or to inadequate serum concentrations, nor is it related to inadequate serum inhibitory activity. The major toxicity of tobramycin is renal, but it appears to be somewhat less nephrotoxic than gentamicin.

Amikacin is an aminoglycoside antibiotic chemically related to kanamycin which has a broad spectrum of in vitro activity against most gram-negative bacilli. It is resistant to some inactivating enzymes for other aminoglycosides, and therefore is active against strains of gram-negative bacilli which are resistant to other aminoglycoside antibiotics. Amikacin has been extensively evaluated for treatment of infections in patients with cancer.[27] Patients with adequate neutrophil counts received amikacin alone, employing an intermittent infusion schedule. Neutropenic patients received amikacin alone or in combination with carbenicillin. Amikacin was administered to these patients by a continuous infusion schedule. Of 99 infections occurring in neutropenic patients, amikacin cured 66 percent of 59 infections treated with amikacin alone and 73 percent of 40 infections treated with the addition of carbenicillin. Amikacin cured 60 percent of 156 infections in patients with adequate neutrophil counts. The majority of infections were pneumonias and septicemias. The most commonly identified pathogens were *E. coli*, organisms of the *Klebsiella-Enterobacter-Serratia* group and *P. aeruginosa*. Seventy-five percent of infections produced by these organisms were cured with amikacin (Table 5). An additional 24 infections produced by strains of gram-negative bacilli resistant in vitro and clinically to other aminoglycoside antibiotics were treated with amikacin.[27] Thirteen (54 percent) infections were cured. Comparative studies of amikacin with other aminoglycosides have demonstrated similar clinical activity and toxicity. The major advantage of amikacin is its activity against infections produced by strains of gram-negative bacilli resistant to other aminoglycoside antibiotics; therefore it is a valuable antimicrobial agent for such life-threatening occasions.

Sisomicin is a new aminoglycoside antibiotic produced by *Micromonospora inyoensis*. Its spectrum of activity in vitro is similar to gentamicin but it is more active against some strains of gram-negative bacilli. Studies of sisomicin alone and in combination with carbenicillin or clindamycin have been conducted for the treatment of infections in cancer patients.[28] Sisomicin alone was administered to patients failing to respond to other antibiotic therapy, and cured 53 percent of 73 infectious episodes. Sisomicin plus carbenicillin was used as initial therapy and this combination cured 71 percent of 133 episodes of infection. Patients with adequate neutrophils were treated with sisomicin alone or in combination with clindamycin during 31 infectious episodes and 77 percent were cured. Neutropenic patients who received sisomicin alone were randomly allocated to receive the antibiotic by intermittent or continuous infusion. The response rates were 46 percent and 61 percent, respectively. Response to sisomicin alone is also related to the patients' neutrophil count. Nephrotoxicity occurred during 11 percent of febrile episodes in patients who initially had normal renal function. Ototoxicity occurred infrequently.

The penicillins are bactericidal antibiotics and are the most effective group of antibiotics for use in patients with impaired host defenses. Even in neutropenic patients, these antibiotics cure the majority of infections caused by sensitive organisms.[1] Before the availability of methicillin *Staphylococcus aureus* was the leading cause of fatal infections in cancer patients, whereas at present few patients die of these infections if treated promptly with one of the antistaphylococcal penicillins.

The penicillin which has been studied most extensively in cancer patients is carbenicillin because of its activity against *P. aeruginosa*.[11] It is also active against both indole-positive and indole-negative *Proteus* spp., and some *Enterobacter* spp. and *E. coli*. In the treatment of systemic infections, the total daily dose of carbenicillin should be at least 30 grams (5 grams every 4 hours). The overall response rate in a large series of *Pseudomonas* infections in cancer patients was 75 percent. Carbenicillin is effective even in patients with severe neutropenia (Table 6).

Ticarcillin is another semisynthetic penicillin which has a spectrum of activity similar to carbenicillin but is somewhat more active against *P. aeruginosa* in vitro. Ticarcillin at a dose of 3.5 grams every 4 hours administered to cancer patients with *Pseudomonas* infections cured about 80 percent of their infections.[29] Like carbenicillin, ticarcillin is effective regardless of the patient's neutrophil count. Unfortunately, organisms resistant to carbenicillin are also resistant to ticarcillin.

Toxicity with these semisynthetic penicillins is related to their sodium content, since they are disodium salts. Electrolyte imbalance (hypokalemia, hypernatremia) and fluid overload occur due to the excessive amount of sodium which is administered with therapeutic doses of carbenicillin and ticarcillin.

Combination of Antibiotics

No single antibiotic has a sufficiently broad spectrum of activity to be used alone as initial therapy for presumptive infection in cancer patients since they are susceptible to such a wide variety of organisms. Regimens which have become especially popular as initial therapy for presumed infection are carbenicillin plus an aminoglycoside and carbenicillin plus a cephalosporin.[30-35] It is not clear what is the most optimum regimen, but carbenicillin or ticarcillin should be included in the initial therapy chosen, especially in neutropenic patients.

The combination of carbenicillin plus an aminoglycoside has become popular as initial therapy for presumed infection in cancer patients because of its broad spectrum of activity and the in vitro synergism of these two classes of antibiotics against some strains of *P. aeruginosa*. The overall

Table 7
Initial Therapy of Infections with Antibiotic
Combinations in Cancer Patients

Combination	Number of Infections	Percent Cure
Carbenicillin + Gentamicin	114	58
Carbenicillin + Gentamicin*	115	67
Carbenicillin + Amikacin*	102	68
Carbenicillin + Sisomicin*	93	67
Ticarcillin + Tobramycin	40	92
Amikacin + Cephalothin	30	83
Carbenicillin + Cephalosporin	208	53
Carbenicillin + Kanamycin	48	58
Gentamicin + Cephalothin	33	79
Gentamicin + Chloramphenicol	31	68

*Aminoglycoside antibiotic administered by continuous infusion.[33]

response rate in a collated series of 114 infections in which the patients received carbenicillin plus gentamicin was 58 percent (Table 7). The response rate was better for Pseudomonas infections than for infections caused by other susceptible gram-negative bacilli. Several other antibiotic combinations have produced equally good results, although only a few comparative trials have been conducted.

The combination of carbenicillin and amikacin has been studied as initial therapy of presumed infection in a randomized study also comparing carbenicillin plus gentamicin and carbenicillin plus sisomicin. The aminoglycosides were administered by continuous infusion.[33] The overall cure rate for each antibiotic combination was similar, being 67 percent for carbenicillin plus gentamicin, 68 percent for carbenicillin plus amikacin, and 67 percent for carbenicillin plus sisomicin. Gram-negative bacilli were the most frequent pathogens isolated and responded equally well to the three antibiotic combinations (67, 64, and 74 percent). Also, the cure rate among infections produced by multiple organisms which are notoriously difficult to treat was excellent (60, 100, and 88 percent).

In a comparative study of ticarcillin plus tobramycin versus carbenicillin plus gentamicin in 82 compromised hosts, the former combination was more efficacious (92 percent) than the latter (71 percent); most infections were caused by Pseudomonas organisms. The majority of patients, however, had cystic fibrosis and only 10 cancer patients were entered in the study.[34]

Amikacin plus cephalothin as an empiric regimen for granulocytopenic cancer patients has been reported as producing an overall response rate of 83 percent. However, the response rate was only 53 percent in microbiologically documented bacterial infections, but increased to 76 percent when patients received granulocyte transfusions.[35]

The combination of carbenicillin plus cephalothin has been compared with the combination of carbenicillin and kanamycin in a randomized study of 98 infections in neutropenic cancer patients.[36] The majority of infections were pneumonias, septicemias, and cellulitis caused by *P. aeruginosa, K. pneumoniae,* and *Enterobacter* spp. The overall response rates for the two regimens were similar (60 versus 58 percent). The response rate for *Pseudomonas* infections was nearly 90 percent for both regimens.

The combination of gentamicin and cephalothin has been compared to the combination of gentamicin and chloramphenicol in a randomized study of 86 infections in neutropenic patients.[37] The combination of gentamicin and cephalothin was superior (79 versus 68 percent). The superiority of this combination was most apparent in patients with septicemia (89 versus 56 percent). Even among those infections caused by organisms which were resistant to cephalothin, but sensitive to chloramphenicol in vitro, the response rate was higher for gentamicin plus cephalothin (93 versus 57 percent).

The combination of sulfamethoxazole and trimethoprim (Bactrim) has been given orally to 35 cancer patients with infections.[38] Thirty-two patients did not respond to an initial antibiotic regimen that consisted primarily of carbenicillin and an aminoglycoside. The overall cure rate was 54 percent. The most common infecting organism was *K. pneumoniae* and 45 percent responded. Overall, 47 percent of the patients whose neutrophil count remained unchanged or decreased responded, while 61 percent of those whose neutrophil count increased responded. Thus, it appears that the sulfamethoxazole–trimethoprim combination is useful in the treatment of serious infections in cancer patients who do not respond to initial antibiotic therapy.

Management of Nonbacterial Infections

Nonbacterial infections are less common in cancer patients than those produced by gram-negative bacteria, but usually are as severe and often are life-threatening. These infections are usually caused by fungal, viral, or protozoal organisms, many of which are pathogens able to survive within macrophages. Resistance to pathogens able to survive intracellularly is largely dependent upon cellular immunity, which is often compromised in cancer patients; hence their susceptibility to such infections and the high morbidity and mortality rates that ensue if they are not treated properly.

Disseminated candidiasis is most difficult to diagnose early and treat adequately. In cancer patients the diagnosis should be entertained, particularly in those febrile patients not responding to adequate antibacterial therapy for unidentified infection. Systemic candidiasis needs to be treated with amphotericin B in daily doses ranging from 0.5 to 1.0 mg/kg. However, the response rate in these patients is only about 20 percent. Although therapy with amphotericin B has traditionally been initiated in doses of less than 5 mg (in patients with chronic fungal disease) with gradual dose escalation, this method of administration is suboptimal in neutropenic cancer patients with systemic candidiasis since the infection might rapidly become overwhelming and fatal. Thus, we recommend initiation of therapy with a starting dose of 0.3 mg/kg and rapid escalation to full daily doses. The dose of amphotericin B should be dissolved in 500 ml of 5 percent dextrose and infused in about 4 hours to minimize the chills and fever which occur during administration. Local phlebitis at the site of administration may occur and the addition of 100 units of heparin to the intravenous solution may decrease this complication. Amphotericin B produces severe nephrotoxicity with prolonged administration and because of this complication therapy often needs to be modified before complete clinical improvement has occurred. 5-Fluorocytosine in oral doses of 3 grams every 6 hours also has been used in our patients, and in approximately a third of the cases improvement of the infection can be achieved. *Candida* organisms, however, rapidly become resistant to 5-fluorocytosine; consequently, it is not a very reliable drug for the therapy of severe fungal infections. In addition, since it needs to be administered orally, absorption might not be reliable in these severely ill patients. Toxicity effects of 5-fluorocytosine are mainly leukopenia, rash, and elevation of the serum glutamic oxaloacetic transaminases.

Aspergillosis is also a common fungal infection in cancer patients; it is found at autopsy in over 10 percent of patients with acute leukemia. It therefore should be suspected most frequently among the acute opportunistic infections, particularly in far-advanced patients. The response to amphotericin B is poor in advanced infection, but with early use of aggressive invasive diagnostic techniques prompt diagnosis of aspergillus infection is possible and successful amphotericin therapy has been accomplished.[39] *Torulopsis glabrata* also has been recognized as an important pathogen in cancer patients. The organism is sensitive to amphotericin B and 5-fluorocytosine, and therapy with either of these agents should be initiated if the diagnosis is made.

In cryptococcosis, which frequently causes infections in patients with lymphoma, amphotericin B and 5-fluorocytosine have been used successfully for therapy.[40] When cryptococcosis is found in the central nervous system, the intrathecal administration of amphotericin B is usually necessary. Doses of 0.25–0.5 mg can be administered intrathecally every other day. Therapy with 5-fluorocytosine is not very reliable because of the rapid development of resistance.

New antifungal agents like clotrimazole and miconazole, which are imidazole derivatives, have been introduced recently. Both are effective in vitro against a variety of fungi. Clotrimazole is used orally but is poorly absorbed and produces suboptimal results. Miconazole has shown clinical success in initial trials in cancer patients, used in doses of 600–1200 mg 3 times daily, particularly in *Candida* infections.[41]

Most patients who develop serious viral infections are usually receiving antitumor agents and adrenal corticosteroids. Most serious viral infections in cancer patients are caused by DNA viruses such as cytomegalic virus, *herpes simplex,* and *herpes zoster.* Recently, adenine arabinoside (Ara-A) has given promising results in *herpes simplex* infections.[42] In our experience, Ara-C (Cytarabine) in small doses (30–50 mg/M^2 day × 5 days) also may be therapeutically efficacious in desperately ill patients with *herpes zoster* infection. Recently, the use of transfer factor has yielded initial promising results in seriously ill cancer patients.[43] Since the therapy of viral infections is still suboptimal, prevention is extremely important. Patients with disseminated *herpes simplex* or *zoster* should be isolated to avoid spread to other patients. Cancer patients should also avoid smallpox vaccination.

Among the protozoal infections, *Pneumocytitis carinii* and *T. gondii* are the most common in cancer patients. Therapy of pneumocytosis with pentamidine isothianate at a dose of 4 mg/kg day is effective in 50 percent of the patients. Unfortunately, this drug produces renal dysfunction in a few patients. The use of trimethoprim and sulfamethoxazole recently has been found helpful in patients with *P. carinii* and offers an excellent alternative to pentamidine. It is also very effective prophylactically in patients susceptible to develop *P. carinii* infection during immunosuppression.[44] Treatment of toxoplasmosis can be successful with pyrimethamine and triple sulfa. Dosages should be high initially (75–200 mg of Daraprim on the first day) and then reduced to 25 mg daily for 4 weeks; sulfa (4 g/day) is given concomitantly.

Management of Gram-Negative Shock

Gram-negative bacillary septicemia may be associated with endo-toxin shock and catastrophic effects in patients. Vasoconstriction and ve-nous pooling with hypotension and narrow pulse pressure, accompanied by disseminated intravascular coagulation, the development of shock lung, and poor tissue perfusion are seen in gram-negative shock. Respira-tory failure is a very common fatal sequela of endotoxin shock. Severe metabolic acidosis is the consequence of tissue anoxia. Hepatic ischemia leads to jaundice, and decreased renal blood flow leads to oliguria.

The treatment of infections with antibiotics has substantially im-proved but the early recognition, understanding, and treatment of endo-toxin shock, especially that of the early, impending forms, has not ad-vanced sufficiently. This is unfortunate because endotoxin shock is the cause of death for most patients with septicemia from gram-negative ba-cilli. The patient with chills and fever (or hypothermia), prostration, tachycardia and tachypnea, hypotension, peripheral cyanosis, cold and clammy extremities, oliguria, and mental obtundation should be attended to immediately. One should gather clues of the cause of infection such as leukopenia and immunosuppression, indwelling catheters, perforated ul-cerated viscera, or instrumentation of the genitourinary tract. Appropriate cultures of blood and other sites should be collected and a combination of appropriate antibiotics should be administered as already discussed. The central venous pressure, urine output, vital signs, and estimates of pe-ripheral resistance and stroke volume should be obtained. After the ad-ministration of an empirically chosen antibiotic combination (as de-scribed above) the following additional measures are essential in the management of endotoxin shock:

1. Opening of airway (if obstructed), administration of O_2 (if pO_2 de-creased) or supported respiration by volume-cycled respirator.
2. Fluid repletion as guided by central venous pressure. For this pur-pose, dextran or albumin, electrolyte or bicarbonate solutions, or plasma may be used. At 12–14 cm of central venous water pressure, furosemide may be given to avoid overloading of circulation.
3. Vasoactive drugs should be employed with extreme care if augmenta-tion of intravascular volume does not reverse the signs of peripheral vasoconstriction. Either the alpha, beta-adrenergic agonist dopamine hydrochloride or beta-adrenergic isoproterenol are recommended. Dopamine is administered in doses of 2–5 mg/kg min but this may be

increased to 20 mg/kg min. Isoproterenol should be used (only after the plasma volume has been fully repleted) in doses ranging from 0.5 to 5.0 mg/min.

4. Digitalization with cedilanid or digoxin for increased central venous pressure or increased pulmonary artery wedge pressure should be considered.

5. Corticosteroids in large doses (15–30 mg methylprednisolone sodium succinate per kg; 3 mg dexamethasone phosphate per kg) to decrease peripheral resistance, and suppress systemic reactions to endotoxins, are frequently given.

Disseminated intravascular coagulation is a potentially fatal complication of endotoxin shock. The underlying condition should be treated first and most vigorously. Should, however, the extent of disseminated intravascular coagulation increase and the underlying condition progress, attempts to inhibit circulating thrombin with the administration of heparin are fully justified. Treatment of this condition is extremely complex; it requires a constant level of heparin and an adequate level of endogenous alpha 2-antithrombin. Treatment failures should be recognized early and further attempts at treatment with heparinized whole blood or plasma should be made promptly. However, replacement of clotting factors before the cessation of intravascular clotting could aggravate the consumption coagulopathy. When consumption coagulopathy is brought under control, the endogenous replacement of clotting factors is usually rapid and fibrinolysis ceases.

Protected Environment Programs for Cancer Patients

As infection is a common complication in patients with cancer receiving intensive therapy, and since most of the affecting pathogens are from the endogenous microbial flora, attempts to decrease the patient's flora and prevent acquisition of infection have been made. In the 1960s, studies of the use of protected environment with prophylactic antibiotics (PEPA programs) were initiated.

Initial studies used the "Life Island,"[45] an air-tight bubble enclosing a bed. Subsequently, laminar-air-flow (LAF) rooms have been introduced allowing greater patient mobility, increased number of air exchanges (380/ hr versus 13/hr) and decreased air turbulence when compared to the Life Island units.[46] Oral nonabsorbable antibiotics are administered to suppress bowel flora. With these regimens, the majority of initial bacterial strains are suppressed with a low acquisition rate for new organisms.[47] Greater than 90 percent of bacterial strains are eliminated from stool cultures with only 15 percent new strains appearing and only 16 percent of patients still having a positive stool culture for pathogens. More difficulty is noted with fungi: 44 percent eliminated, 20 percent new strains, and 66 percent pathogenic fungi in stools. Elimination of organisms from other sites is less satisfactory, and while many strains isolated are nonpathogenic, improved techniques of decontamination are required. *Candida* spp. and *P. aeruginosa* are the most commonly persisting pathogens.

The first major study of the usefulness of protected environments (PE) in acute leukemia was undertaken at the M. D. Anderson Hospital.[48] Thirty-three patients with acute leukemia treated in a PEPA program were retrospectively matched for all known pretreatment prognostic variables with patients treated out of a PE. Patients treated in a PE experienced fewer infectious episodes at all granulocyte levels. More patients in the PE group received an adequate trial of therapy. The remission rate in the PE group, although higher, was not significantly better than the control groups. However, an impressive prolongation of remission duration and duration of survival was noted in the PE group, the difference being attributed to the higher doses of chemotherapy that could be given to the patients treated in the PE because of the decreased incidence of infection.

In a recent study 145 leukemic patients were randomized to (1) PE plus oral nonabsorbable and absorbable antibiotics; (2) PE plus systemic antibiotics; or (3) systemic antibiotics alone in a general ward. All patients received intensive chemotherapy with adriamycin, cytosine arabinoside, vincristine, and prednisone, and immunotherapy with BCG.[49] Seventy-three of the 145 patients developed 102 infections. Thirty-one of these infections were fatal. The 145 patients spent a total hospitalization period of 8,540 days and during 5,073 days, they had a neutrophil count of less than 500/mm³; during 3,674 days (65 percent of the time) they had severe neutropenia (a neutrophil count of less than 100/mm³). Comparing the 63 patients treated in a PE unit with the 82 patients treated out of a PE unit (Table 8), the proportion of patients who developed major infections, the rate of fatal infections, and the proportion of infections at all levels of neutropenia were lower inside a PE than outside. The proportion of patients who survived long enough to receive an adequate trial was higher in the PE (97 percent) than out of the units (82 percent). The complete remission (CR) rate was 71 percent in and 43 percent out of a PE unit, a statistically significant difference (P greater than 0.01). The median survival time was 72 weeks for patients in a PE, compared with 42 weeks for patients outside

Table 8
Infections During Remission-Induction Chemotherapy in Protected
Environments (PEs)

	Acute Leukemia		Lymphomas	
	In PE	No PE	In PE	No PE
Number of patients	63	82	30	28
Percent of patients with infection	41	57	7	29
Percent of patients with fatal infection	13	28	0	4
Percent of days with severe neutropenia and infection	18	28	3	27

a PE, and the difference of survival curves was highly statistically significant (P less than 0.01).[49]

Similar experiences have been obtained in patients with malignant lymphoma treated with intensive combination chemotherapy.[50] Fifty-eight patients were randomly allocated to receive three courses of chemotherapy to induce remission with CHOP-Bleo on the protected-environment–prophylactic-antibiotic (PEPA) program (30 patients) or as controls (28 patients). The frequency of infection was significantly lower among the patients on the PEPA program, and dosage escalation of the chemotherapeutic agents was accomplished more often among these patients. Dosage escalation did not increase the complete remission rate, but did reduce the relapse rate and significantly reduced the fatality rate. The duration of remission and survival was significantly longer for those patients who received dosage escalation.

This modality of supportive care (PEPA program) has also been employed in recent years to intensify remission-induction therapy of patients with sarcomas[51] and breast cancer,[52] with encouraging preliminary results in relation to the reduction of risk of infection and increased response to intensive chemotherapy.

Recent reports suggest that without protected environment units, effective prophylaxis ("gut sterilization") may be obtained with the combination of Trimethoprim and sulfamethoxazole (TS).[44,53] In a study designed to prevent P. carinii in leukemic children, all other bacterial infections were also reduced in the group of patients receiving prophylaxis with TS.[44] In a randomized study of prophylaxis with TS in granulocytopenic patients the percentage of febrile granulocytopenic days was significantly less in patients receiving TS than in controls, and bacteremias were eliminated in the patients receiving TS.[53]

Summary

Infection is a major cause of morbidity and mortality in cancer patients. This chapter reviews most common types of infection and their current therapies. When the patient with cancer has fever or other signs and symptoms suggesting infection, it should be considered an oncologic emergency, especially in the neutropenic patient. Efforts should be made to identify the etiologic organism so that the correct antibiotic regimen can be instituted. Early initiation of treatment, however, is imperative to prevent death from gram-negative septicemia. Therefore, therapy is often started on a presumptive basis with a combination of broad-spectrum antibiotics. Patients whose fever and signs of infection persist in spite of adequate antibiotic therapy and in whom no bacterial organism has been clearly identified as the source of infection should be considered to have a fungal infection an be given a trial of antifungal therapy. The appropriate guidelines for the management of acute opportunistic infection are stressed. The rationale and results of pilot studies in suppression of endogenous flora to minimize risk of infections during chemotherapy are discussed.

References

1. Bodey GP: Infectious complications in the cancer patient. Current Prob Cancer 1(12):1–63, 1977
2. Inagaki J, Rodriguez V, Bodey GP: Causes of death in cancer patients. Cancer 33:568–573, 1974
3. Feld R, Bodey GP, Rodriguez V, et al: Causes of death in patients with malignant lymphoma. Am J Med Sci 268:97–106, 1974
4. Chang HY, Rodriguez V, Narboni G, et al: Causes of death in adults with acute leukemia. Medicine 55:259–268, 1976
5. Bodey GP, Buckley M, Sathe YS, et al: Quantitative relationships between circulating leukocytes and infection in patients with acute leukemia. Ann Intern Med 64:328–340, 1966
6. Rodriguez V, Bodey GP: Antibacterial therapy—special considerations in neutropenic patients. Clin Haematol 5:347–360, 1976
7. Ketchel SJ, Rodriguez V: Acute infections in cancer patients. Sem Oncol 5:167–179, 1978
8. Bodey GP, Rodriguez V, Chang HY, et al: Fever and infection in leukemic patients. A study of 494 consecutive patients. Cancer 41:1610, 1978

9. Feld R, Bodey GP: Infections in patients with malignant lymphoma treated with combination chemotherapy. Cancer 39:1018–1025, 1977

10. Livingston RB, Einhorn LH, Bodey GP, et al: COMB (cyclophosphamide, oncovin, methyl-CCNU and bleomycin): A four-drug combination in solid tumors. Cancer 36:327–332, 1975

11. Bodey GP, Whitecar JP Jr, Middleman E, et al: Carbenicillin therapy of pseudomonas infections. JAMA 218:62–66, 1971

12. Swartz M: Clinical aspects of Legionnaire's disease. Ann Intern Med 90:492–495, 1979

13. Feld R, Bodey GP, Groschel D: Mycobacteriosis in patients with malignant disease. Arch Intern Med 136:67–70, 1976

14. Bodey GP: Fungal infections complicating acute leukemia. J Chronic Dis 19:667–687, 1966

15. Bodey GP, Luna M: Skin lesions associated with disseminated candidiasis. JAMA 229:1466–1468, 1974

16. Ruckdeschel JC, Schimpff SC, Smyth AC, et al: Herpes zoster and impaired cell-associated immunity to the varicella-zoster virus in patients with Hodgkin's disease. Am J Med 62:77–85, 1977

17. Hughes WT: Protozoal infections in haematological diseases. Clin Haematol 5:329–345, 1976

18. Kirck T, Remington TS: Toxoplasmosis in the adult. An overview. N Engl J Med 298:550–553, 1978

19. Whitecar JP Jr, Bodey GP, Luna M: Pseudomonas bacteremia in cancer patients. Am J Med Sci 260:216–223, 1970

20. Umsawasdi T, Middleman EA, Luna M, et al: Klebsiella bacteremia in cancer patients. Am J Med Sci 265:473–482, 1973

21. Grose WE, Rodriguez V, Norek G, et al: Escherichia coli bacteremia in patients with malignant diseases. Arch Intern Med 138:1230–1233, 1978

22. Rodriguez V, Burgess MA, Bodey GP: Management of fever of unknown origin in cancer patients with neoplasma and neutropenia. Cancer 32:1007–1012, 1973

23. Pizzo PA, Robichaud KT, Gill FA, et al: Duration of empiric antibiotic therapy in granulocytopenic patients with cancer. Am J Med 67:194–200, 1979

24. Bodey GP, Groschel DH, Lichtiger B, et al: Supportive care in the management of cancer patients, in Clark RL, Howe CD (eds): Cancer Patient Care at M. D. Anderson Hospital and Tumor Institute. Yearbook Medical Publishers, Inc., Chicago, 1976, pp 571–605

25. Bodey GP, Middleman E, Umsawasdi T, et al: Infections in cancer

patients. results with gentamicin sulfate therapy. Cancer 29:1697–1701, 1972

26. Valdivieso M, Horikoshi N, Rodriguez V, et al: Therapeutic trials with tobramycin. Am J Med Sci 268:149–156, 1974

27. Valdivieso M, Keating MJ, Feld R, et al: Review of experience with amikacin and other aminoglycoside antibiotics in the treatment of infectious complications in patients with cancer. Am J Med (US Amikacin Symposium):204–211, 1977

28. Bodey GP, Cabanillas F, Feld R, et al: Sisomicin alone and in combination for therapy of infections in cancer patients in, Proceedings of the European Sisomicin Symposium, May 6–7, 1977. Princeton, NJ, Excerpta Medica, 1977

29. Rodriguez V, Bodey GP, Horikoshi N, et al: Ticarcillin therapy of infections. Antimicrob Ags Chemother 4:427–431, 1973

30. Rodriguez V, Whitecar JP Jr, Bodey GP: Therapy of infections with the combination of carbenicillin and gentamicin. Antimicrob Ags Chemother 386–390, 1969

31. Schimpff S, Satterlee W, Young VM, et al: Empiric therapy with carbenicillin and gentamicin for febrile patients with cancer and granulocytopenia. N Eng J Med 284:1061–1065, 1971

32. Bodey GP, Valdivieso M, Feld R, et al: Carbenicillin plus cephalothin or cefazolin as therapy for infections in neutropenic patients. Am J Med Sci 273:309–318, 1977

33. Keating MJ, Bodey GP, Rodriguez V: A randomized comparative trial of three aminoglycosides — comparison of continuous infusion of gentamicin, amikacin and sisomicin combined with carbenicillin in the management of infections in neutropenic patients with malignancies. Medicine 58:159–170, 1979

34. Pardy MF, Neu HC: A comparative study of ticarcillin plus tobramycin versus carbenicillin plus gentamicin for the treatment of serious infections due to gram-negative bacilli. Am J Med 64:961–966, 1978

35. Hahn DM, Schimpff SC, Young DM, et al: Amikacin and cephalothin: Empiric regimen for granulocytopenic cancer patients. Antimicrob Ags Chemother 12:618–624, 1977

36. Middleman EA, Watanabe A, Kaizer H, et al: Antibiotic combinations for infections in neutropenic patients. Evaluations of carbenicillin plus either cephalothin or kanamycin. Cancer 30:573–579, 1972

37. Valdivieso M, Bodey GP, Burgess MA, et al: Therapy of infections in neutropenic patients. Results with gentamicin in combination with cephalothin or chloramphenicol. Med Pediat Oncol 2:99–108, 1976

38. Grose EW, Bodey GP, Rodriguez V: Sulfamethoxazole–trimethoprim for infections of cancer patients. JAMA 237:352–354, 1977

39. Pennington JE: Aspergillus pneumonia in hematologic malignancies: Improvement in diagnosis and therapy. Arch Intern Med 137:769–771, 1977

40. Utz JP, Garriques IL, Sande MA, et al: Therapy of cryptococcosis with a combination of fluocytosine and amphotericin B. J Infect Dis 132:368–373, 1975

41. Rodriguez V: Miconazole therapy of fungal infections in cancer patients, in Proceedings of the 17th Interscience Conference on Antimicrobial Agents and Chemotherapy, New York, October 12–14, 1977. American Society Microbiology, 1977, Abstract 407

42. Whitley RJ, Soong SJ, Dolin R, et al: The collaborative study group: Adenine arabinoside therapy of biopsy-proved herpes simplex encephalitis. National Institute of Allergy and Infectious Diseases collaborative antiviral study. N Engl J Med 297:289–294, 1977

43. Ketchel SJ, Rodriguez V, Gutterman JU, et al: A study of transfer factor for opportunistic infections in cancer patients. Med Pediat Oncol 6(4):295–301, 1979

44. Hughes WH, Kuhn S, Chandhary S, et al: Successful chemoprophylaxis for pneumocystic carinii pneumonitis. N Engl J Med 279:1419–1422, 1977

45. Schwartz SS, Perry S: Patient protection in cancer chemotherapy. JAMA 197:623, 1966

46. Bodey GP, Freireich EJ, Frei E III: Studies of patients in a laminar air flow unit. Cancer 24:972, 1969

47. Bodey GP, Rosenbaum B: Effect of prophylactic measures on the microbial flora of patients in protected environment units. Medicine (Baltimore) 53:209, 1974

48. Bodey GP, Gehan EA, Freireich EJ, et al: Protected environment–prophylactic antibiotic program in the chemotherapy of acute leukemia. Am J Med Sci 262:138, 1971

49. Rodriguez V, Bodey GP, Freireich EJ, et al: Randomized trial of protected environment–prophylactic antibiotics in 145 adults with acute leukemia. Medicine 57:253–263, 1978

50. Bodey GP, Rodriguez V, Cabanillas F, et al: Protected environment–prophylactic antibiotic program for malignant lymphoma. Randomized trial during chemotherapy to induce remission. Am J Med 66:74–81, 1979

51. Rodriguez V, Bodey GP: Effect of protected environments plus oral

prophylactic antibiotics (PEPA) on the incidence of infections in cancer patients (PTS) during intensive chemotherapy, in Proceedings of the 16th Interscience Conference on Antimicrobial Agents and Chemotherapy, Chicago, October 1976. American Society Microbiology, 1976, Abstract 331

52. Bodey GP, Legha SS, Blumenschein GR, et al: Randomized trial of protected environment–Prophylactic antibiotic program (PEPA) in breast cancer, in Proceedings of the 70th Annual Meeting of American Association of Cancer Research. New York, American Association for Cancer Research, 1979, Abstract 671

53. Gurwith MJ, Brunton JL, Lank BA, et al: Prospective controlled investigation of prophylactic trimethoprim–sulfamethoxazole in hospitalized granulocytopenic patients. Am J Med 66:248–256, 1979

12

PULMONARY EMERGENCIES IN NEOPLASTIC DISEASE

George P. Canellos
Gary Cohen
Marshall Posner

Dyspnea is one of the most distressing and morbid complications that neoplastic disease or its treatment can impart to man. As opposed to dyspnea due to cardiogenic causes, in the cancer patient it usually follows an unrelenting and fatal course. There are instances, however, where embolic, infectious, or inflammatory complications can be reversed by appropriate treatment and supportive care. Further, where cytotoxic chemotherapy is effective symptomatic lung infiltration by tumor can be controlled and in some instances cured.

In most patients, pulmonary treatment and related symptoms are usually insidious in onset and represent a subacute or chronic management problem. Acute pulmonary decompensation related to a tumor itself is rare and more likely related to cancer treatment and compromise of host defenses. Usually the physician is faced with a history of cough and dyspnea which has evolved over days to weeks. In most instances there will be abnormalities in the chest x-ray; the lung is accessible by a variety of techniques to assist in the diagnosis. The pathogenesis and differential diagnosis of acute pulmonary failure in neoplastic disease is the subject of this chapter.

Dyspnea Indirectly Related to Neoplasia

Infection

Pulmonary infections are the direct cause of death in 15–25 percent of patients dying with cancer. While most of these infections are due to gram-negative bacteria, there are a significant number due to fungi, viruses, parasites, and mycobacteria.[1-5]

At some time during the course of the illness the patient with neoplasia is a compromised host. The immune system may be severely impaired by the tumor itself, as in multiple myeloma, Hodgkin's disease, and chronic lymphocytic leukemia, or as a result of tumor mass causing partial obstruction of bronchi, as in carcinoma of the lung predisposing to pulmonary infection. Leukopenia or immunosuppressive therapy can limit the patient's defenses.[6] Often minor infections progress rapidly, necessitating emergent measures. Physical examination may not be helpful in patients with leukopenia as they may not have evidence of consolidation or rales.

The predominant symptoms in patients with pulmonary infection are fever, cough, dyspnea, and chest pain, although in a number of series a small percentage of symptomatic pulmonary infections presented without fever.[7-9] In the evaluation of the cancer patient presenting with acute respiratory insufficiency and hypoxemia, a complicating infection should be considered. Initial laboratory evaluation should include multiple cultures of blood, and gram stain and culture of sputum. A chest x-ray may not distinguish between bacterial pneumonia and other causes. In one series, localized consolidation on chest x-ray was associated with bacterial infection in only 40 percent of cases[9]; conversely, in a series of gram-negative bacterial pneumonias, localized consolidation was seen in only 40 percent of patients.[7] The presence of a cavitary lesion may suggest fungal or mycobacterial infection, but can be associated with bacterial infection as well.[6,7] Thus, sputum examination for fungi and mycobacteria, particularly in endemic areas, is essential. Pneumonia in the patients with a solid tumor is largely secondary to gram-negative bacteria. The predominant gram-negative organisms are *Klebsiella*, *Pseudomonas*, and *Escherichia coli*.[1-3]

Following the clinical and bacteriologic evaluation of the patient, supportive respiratory measures should be instituted. Pneumonia in leukopenic patients is an emergency and should be treated with broad-spectrum antibiotics. A semisynthetic penicillin with activity against *Pseudomonas* as well as an aminoglycoside should be used. At least 50 percent of deaths from sepsis are secondary to pneumonia. This is particularly true of patients with leukopenia or hematologic malignancies with compromised immunity such as those with chronic lymphocytic leukemia.[1-3,10] Patients with normal leukocyte counts who are clinically stable may not require hospitalization. Unsuspected septicemia may evolve from a pulmonary focus and close communciation should be maintained in the event of rapid clinical deterioration.

Pulmonary Hemorrhage

Pulmonary hemorrhage in the cancer patient may be the result of at least three separate processes. It may accompany the acute respiratory distress syndrome with disseminated intravascular coagulation (DIC). This is more frequently seen in acute promyelocytic leukemia, but has also been noted in prostatic cancer, other types of leukemia, and multiple myeloma.[11,12] This form of pulmonary hemorrhage is associated with marked abnormalities in coagulation tests such as partial thromboplastin time and platelet count (see Chapter 7).

Pulmonary hemorrhage rarely may also be the result of severe thrombocytopenia secondary to chemotherapy.[13] This complication has been less frequent since the advent of platelet support. Finally, pulmonary hemorrhage may be secondary to tumor necrosis or erosion of a blood vessel. This form may present as minimal hemoptysis or fever or as a life-threatening hemorrhage into the lung.[14] Radiographically a diffuse pattern similar to pulmonary edema may be seen, although consolidation of a single lobe, nodular densities, and unilateral pulmonary infiltrates have also been reported.[15] If DIC is suspected, treatment with heparin, fresh-frozen plasma, and platelets may be life-saving.[11,12] Treatment of the underlying disease is essential to reverse the precipitating pathophysiologic mechanisms, including an attempt at remission induction of the leukemia.

Management of hemoptysis and hemorrhage associated with tumor necrosis and erosion of blood vessels depends upon the quantity of expectorated blood. Massive life-threatening hemoptysis is defined as the expectoration of >200 ml in 24 hours, or as a single expectoration of that amount.[16] A chest x-ray may show a major tumor mass, but is usually not helpful as any site within the lung may be responsible for the hemoptysis. Patients with extensive hemoptysis should have 4–6 units of blood available for transfusion. A thoracic surgeon should evaluate the patient and a bronchoscopy should be considered within the first 24 hours to identify the site of hemorrhage. Coagulation abnormalities, if present, should be corrected before invasive procedures.

Massive hemorrhage may require intubation, either with a Carlens tube by an experienced anesthesiologist or, in an emergency situation, with a regular large endotracheal tube. Intubation of the bronchus contralateral to the bleeding site and placement of the patient with the bleeding site down will protect the unaffected lung. Surgery for the removal of the bleeding segment or ligation of a vessel are the procedures of choice. Rebleeding is likely if surgery is not undertaken.[16,17] If the patient is inoperable or a poor candidate for surgery, arterial embolization of the bleeding bronchial artery may be considered.[18,19] Rarely, chronic intermittent pulmonary bleeding can result in pulmonary hemosiderosis.

Pulmonary Embolus

Pulmonary embolus is the cause of death in approximately 5 percent of patients with cancer.[1,2,20,21] Mucinous tumors such as pancreatic and gastric carcinomas may be associated with an increased incidence of pulmonary emboli or Trousseau's syndrome of migratory thrombophlebitis.[22-24] Pulmonary embolus is otherwise extremely rare among hematologic malignancies, especially among the acute leukemias.[25] Patients with cancer may have other predisposing factors to the development of thrombophlebitis and pulmonary embolus including a hyperfibrinogenemia, debility, obesity, and immobilization.[21,26,27] The presentation is that of sudden onset of chest pain, dyspnea, fever, or hemoptysis. The presentation of this symptom complex in patients with a hematologic malignancy in the absence of obvious phlebitis should suggest infection. In a series of cancer patients with a deep-vein thrombophlebitis 10 of 32 patients presented with pulmonary embolus; 6 of 32 subsequently experienced pulmonary embolus in which 4 were fatal.[28]

Physical examination may demonstrate a pleural effusion or a pleural friction rub in an acutely dyspneic patient. The patient should be examined for phlebitis. Once the initial diagnostic studies have been performed, evaluation should include a prompt lung scan or ventilation perfusion scan and arteriography if necessary.[27] Treatment should be initiated with heparin prior to diagnosis in cases where a strong suspicion of pulmonary embolus exists and contraindications such as thrombocytopenia or bleeding are absent. Treatment is usually initiated with a bolus injection of 4,000 units of heparin intravenously, followed by continuous infusion of between 800 and 1000 units of heparin per hour adjusted to maintain the partial thromboplastin time between 1½ and 2½ times normal.

Dyspnea Related to Tumor Progression

Airway Obstruction

Patients with solid tumors may develop stenosis of the airway, either from direct tumor growth into the lumen or from compression by external masses. Primary carcinomas of the trachea are extremely rare but secondary tracheal involvement can be seen with carcinomas of the thyroid, lung, or esophagus. The evaluation and therapy of these lesions has been discussed in an earlier chapter and will not be reviewed here.

A mediastinal mass can occasionally cause significant tracheal stenosis even in the absence of symptoms. The caliber of the airway should be closely examined on plain film of the chest, especially with rapidly growing tumors such as the lymphomas, since this finding constitutes a medical emergency which must be treated with radiotherapy.

Obstruction of airways in the lower respiratory tract is not limited to bronchogenic carcinoma since peribronchial metastases can occur with several different tumors. The initial symptoms of such obstruction may be localized pneumonia which is either recurrent or does not resolve appropriately with adequate therapy. Bronchoscopy or bronchography should always be performed in this situation.

Tumor Infiltration

Solid tumors and malignant lymphoma can occasionally cause diffuse reticulonodular infiltrates, usually with hilar lymph node involvement. This may be confused with other disorders as discussed in a later section, but due to the diffuse involvement of bronchial mucosa and peribronchial lymphatics with tumor, the diagnosis can be made with transbronchial biopsy. The presence of lymphangitic tumor is a very grave prognostic sign since this represents an advanced stage of the disease. In the absence of a response to systemic therapy, the survival after diagnosis is approximately 8 weeks. There are anecdotal reports, however, that symptoms of dyspnea can be ameliorated by steroids. In contrast, chemotherapy usually has a significant impact on survival when lymphangitic disease results from breast cancer, lymphoma, or other treatable tumors. Patients with marked leukocytosis (white counts >100,000) are at risk to develop respiratory symptoms on the basis of a generalized thrombosis of arterioles and capillaries by leukemic blasts.[29] The lungs may also show septal and alveolar edema, but there are no perivascular or parenchymal infiltrates. Dyspnea in these patients usually has a sudden onset and emergency measures should be aimed at prompt reduction of the peripheral white count via hydroxyurea (50 mg/kg/day PO), or centrifugation leukapheresis.[29,30] The syndrome occurs most often in patients with myeloblastic leukemias and only rarely in the lymphocytic types. This may be due to the decreased deformability of large myeloblasts leading to stasis and thrombosis in arterioles and capillaries. Hyperviscosity is not usually found in these patients since anemia compensates for the increased white cell volume. However, when patients with acute leukemia are transfused an acute leukostasis syndrome can develop.[31] Red cell transfusions, therefore, should be avoided until the white count is below 100,000/mm^3.

Pleural Effusions

Pleural effusion is a frequent cause of respiratory distress in the cancer patient.[32] Although the diagnosis and therapy of effusions in the general population is a source of much debate, the emergency management of the cancer patient with respiratory embarrassment is obvious—therapeutic thoracentesis. Nevertheless, total management of the effusion must be appropriately initiated by the emergency physician to prevent increased morbidity and the loss of important diagnostic information.

The symptoms of pleural effusion are dyspnea, cough, or pain, and any of these may bring the patient to the emergency ward. Although pain and cough can occasionally be ameliorated by the evacuation of an effusion, there is only rarely a need for relief of those symptoms as an emergency in the patient with known cancer. However, the patient with undiagnosed cancer who presents with one of the above symptoms may have an effusion on the roentgenogram.[33] Such a patient may benefit from an early well-planned diagnostic thoracentesis. The dyspnea of effusion can be chronic and stable, slowly progressive, or rapidly progressive. The latter may even mimic acute pulmonary embolism, and is the most important indication for emergency therapeutic thoracentesis.

The presence of pleural effusion alone can rarely cause paradoxical pulse and decreased voltage on the cardiogram, suggesting a pericardial effusion. On the other hand, mild-to-moderate subjective dyspnea may occasionally be related to fluid accumulation of less than 300 ml despite a normal arterial pO$_2$. These symptoms are often relieved by thoracentesis and may be related to a neurogenic reflex from receptors in the pleura.[34] Thus pleural effusion should always be considered in the differential diagnosis of the dyspneic patient with cancer.

Radiographic Studies

A pleural effusion is easily recognized on the chest film and may inadvertently direct attention away from other important findings in the patient with respiratory distress. As discussed in this and other chapters, some causes are easily treatable. For example, pneumothorax, pericardial effusion, cardiomegaly, and some pneumonias may be obscured if a large left-sided effusion is present. A mediastinal mass is occasionally present in association with effusion in the patient with lymphoma. In these cases, the effusion may completely resolve with therapy.

When effusion is suspected, a postero-anterior and lateral view is usually sufficient to detect as little as 50–100 ml of fluid. A comparison with old films is essential since the x-ray picture of an effusion can be mimicked by chronic radiation fibrosis, previous infection or surgery, previous effusion, healing tumor, etc. If the effusion is present to the same extent as in the past, it is unlikely to explain an acute exacerbation of dyspnea; when flattening of the costo-phrenic angle is noted for the first time, decubitus films should be obtained to rule out loculation of the effusion which might suggest a more chronic process. Although the presence of loculation may not alter the need for diagnostic or therapeutic thoracentesis, it increases the risk of complication from the procedure and may mitigate in favor of an ultrasound-directed tap or direct insertion of a chest tube.[35,36]

Therapeutic Thoracentesis

When clinical and radiographic signs suggest unilateral effusion a therapeutic thoracentesis should be performed. This can usually be done safely as an outpatient procedure. Hypoxia may actually be increased from 2 to 24 hours after removal of large amounts of fluid from the pleural space, although the etiology of this phenomenon is uncertain. A routine post-thoracentesis film must be obtained to rule out pneumothorax.

Diagnostic Thoracentesis

There are numerous studies in the medical literature which suggest that the specific etiology of an effusion can be determined from laboratory analyses of the fluid. Previous studies have evaluated protein content and characterization, enzymes, trace minerals, pH, special tumor markers, cytogenetics, cytology, and other characteristics with varying degrees of success.[37-44] A Mayo Clinic study doubted the cost-effectiveness of analyses of the standard practice of bacteriologic studies except in highly suspicious cases (e.g., purulent fluid).[45] They suggested the determination of protein and cytology only. Our experience has shown the biochemical separation of transudates and exudates to be the most useful. The now-standard method of Lyte et al. utilizes only the value for LDH (lactic acid dehydrogenase) and protein taken simultaneously from the fluid and the serum.[37] An exudate is defined by any one of the following: (1) an LDH in fluid greater than 200; (2) a ratio of the LDH in the fluid divided by the LDH in the serum greater than 0.6; (3) a ratio of fluid protein divided by serum protein greater than 0.5. Etiologic consideration should also be given to congestive heart failure, hypoproteinemia, and nephrotic states.

Other diagnostic studies may be obtained on the basis of the appearance of the effusion. A milky fluid might be chylous and suggest thoracic duct obstruction. Purulent effusions must be evaluated for an infectious etiology, although malignant exudates in the lymphoproliferative disorders may mimic this appearance. In that particular instance, cytology may be very helpful. The presence of blood is, of course, consistent with malignancy, but may also suggest pulmonary embolus and tuberculosis.[46]

Therapy

Some authors have suggested that treatment be tailored according to the cellularity of the effusion.[47,48] A cellular effusion would be expected to respond to intracavitary therapy, and an effusion with less than 1,000 cells/mm^3 would require a sclerosing agent. A highly malignant effusion would indicate the need for isotope or intracavitary chemotherapeutic agents. This plan links treatment to the probable pathogenesis but it has been propagated in the literature with no scientific basis. Despite a multitude of studies with intracavitary agents including tetracycline, quinacrine,[26] mustard, bleomycin, and others, no study divided their results according to cellularity, nor were the treatment failures analyzed.[49-52] We have reviewed over 100 effusions in patients with proven malignancy at the SFCI and have found that only 40 percent had malignant cells in the fluid. Nevertheless, there has been no difference in response to treatment in those with and without cellular effusions. Ten percent of patients had effusions which were transudative and usually were attributable to causes other than pulmonary involvement by tumor. Some of these responded to diuretics alone.

Results of treatment are extremely difficult to compare in the literature because of nonuniformity of patients, procedures, therapeutic agents, doses, and definitions of response. It is clear, however, that chest tube drainage alone affords a finite success rate in controlling pleural effusion, and most intracavitary agents, whether chemotherapeutic, purely sclerosing, or isotopic, provide a small increase in effectiveness.[51] The common denominator is the complete evacuation of pleural fluid and a sufficient dose of the intracavitary agent. Effective pleural drainage for purposes of subsequent sclerosis is usually not obtained by thoracentesis alone.

Pleurodesis with intracavitary agents is only indicated in cases where previous therapeutic thoracentesis has been successful in ameliorating symptoms, but was followed by reaccumulation of fluid. Occasionally a patient receiving chemotherapy such as high-dose methotrexate may require pleurodesis to avoid accumulation of drug which could result in alteration of the half-life and increased toxicity.[32] Other options for long-term treatment of effusions include radiation to the mediastinum[6] or hemithorax, open thoracotomy with talc or pleurectomy, and systemic therapy.[52,53] We favor the latter where effective therapy exists. If pleurodesis is required, we routinely use 1 gram of tetracycline in 100 ml of normal saline after 24–48 hours of chest tube drainage. We feel that intrapleural tetracycline is as effective as any agent currently in use and the complication rate is less.

Acute Pulmonary Complications of Tumor Therapy

Bronchospasm and Anaphylaxis

Acute bronchospasm and anaphylaxis may occur following administration of certain chemotherapeutic agents. The sudden onset of wheezing, respiratory distress, or cardiovascular collapse in a patient who has just received, or is in the process of receiving, chemotherapy should suggest the diagnosis of anaphylactic reaction.[54–56] Rapid treatment is essential following immediate termination of the infusion. Wheezing and mild dyspnea may be treated with benadryl 50 mg and hydrocortisone 100 mg intravenously. In patients with acute cardiovascular collapse or severe dyspnea, epinephrine 0.4 mg (1:1000 dilution) intravenously or subcutaneously may be life-saving. Vasopressors may be required to maintain blood pressure, as well as intubation for ventilatory support in severely hypoxemic patients. While this is a rare complication, it is treatable, and the physician should be aware of the potential of these agents for causing acute anaphylactic reactions. It is most commonly seen following bleomycin and L-asparaginase infusions but has also been noted following intravenous treatment with alkylating agents, especially intravenous melphalan and cis-dichlorodiammineplatinum.[54-59]

Radiation Pneumonitis

Radiation therapy to the thoracic cage can result in injury to the lung. The majority of patients can develop, in time, asymptomatic abnormalities. The incidence of clinically significant radiation pneumonitis is difficult to determine but does appear to be less than 5 percent of patients. The risk is higher in patients with bronchogenic carcinoma or Hodgkin's disease where radiation therapy is a major therapeutic modality. Radiographic evidence of radiation fibrosis has been noted in 65 percent of a group of 20 patients with Hodgkin's disease who received mediastinal radiation.[60] The Stanford series showed a 6.4-percent incidence of pneumonitis in patients receiving mediastinal radiation.[61] The incidence of pneumonitis and/or radiation fibrosis is considerably higher (33 percent) when lung is also irradiated. The incidence would be expected to decrease with the use of improved techniques of dose monitoring and shielding, and improved megavoltage equipment.

The factors contributing to development of radiation injury to lungs include dose, volume of lung irradiated, and dose rate. The risk of developing pneumonitis following whole-lung irradiation falls on an extremely steep dose curve of Rets delivered versus probability of disease.[62] Between 500 and 800 Ret, the probability varies from 5 percent to almost 100 percent.[63] In addition to the dose rate and volume, factors such as previous irradiation and chemotherapy may also contribute to the radiation damage. Chronic lung disease per se does not increase the risk.

Certain antineoplastic agents are known to enhance the radiation effect. These include actinomycin D and adriamycin. The role of actinomycin D is supported by experimental data showing a synergistic action when the drug preceded radiation.[64]

A number of drugs associated independently with pulmonary reactions may also enhance the toxicity of radiation. In addition, the concomitant administration of radiation and bleomycin may be associated with a higher risk of pulmonary disease.[65,66]

In patients with Hodgkin's disease receiving combined modality treatment, there is a risk of precipitating radiation pneumonitis following the abrupt cessation of the prednisone dose as is called for in the second and fourth cycles of the MOPP program. The 14 days of prednisone are sufficient to reactivate latent lung damage by radiation administered 6 months to 9 years prior to MOPP chemotherapy.[67] The risk appears to be low, occurring in 7 out of 150 cases, but of sufficient gravity to warrant omission of prednisone in those previously irradiated who are to be treated with MOPP at Stanford.

The clinical characteristics of radiation damage to the lungs can be divided into two phases: acute radiation pneumonitis and chronic pulmonary fibrosis. Pulmonary emergencies are rare in the latter circumstance except when complicated by secondary infection and/or progression of lymphangitic metastases.

Acute radiation pneumonitis in most instances is asymptomatic but unless extensive lung volume is treated it is rarely fatal. The onset is usually insidious, occurring 2–6 months after radiation therapy. The earlier onset generally predicts a more serious disorder. The most significant symptom is dyspnea, although a nonproductive cough and fever may be seen. In its most severe form, these symptoms precede a picture of respiratory failure, cyanosis, and tachypnea. Radiographic abnormalities are always present in symptomatic cases and can appear worse than the clinical condition. This is in contradistinction to lymphangitic metastases, which do not often reflect the severity of dyspnea in the chest film. The abnormalities, which can vary from blurring of pulmonary markings to dense opacification, will have anatomic borders which correspond to the margins of the treatment port. Reactions following mediastinal radiation can obscure cardiac borders and give the appearance of mediastinal widening. Pleural effusions, hemoptysis, and cavitation are distinctly rare.

The histopathologic changes associated with acute radiation injury include blood vessel abnormalities with engorgement and/or thrombosis; edema; desquamation of hyperplastic but atypical aveolar lining cells; deposition of fibrin and/or hyaline membranes within alveolar spaces; and thickening of septal walls.[68]

The acute effects of radiation on tumor can result in massive necrosis, resulting in complications such as hemorrhage. Acute obstruction of the major airways rarely can result from the swelling of an endobronchial tumor following radiation. It can be prevented by administering steroids 1 day prior to and for several days after the initiation of therapy.[63] The management of acute radiation pneumonitis depends upon its severity, but in circumstances where the patient is symptomatic, corticosteroids should be given immediately. Prednisone in a dose range of 60–100 mg will promptly control symptoms. Delay in steroid administration may decrease their effectiveness.[69] Prophylactic steroids are to be discouraged except in the unusual circumstances mentioned above.

Transfusion Reactions

The limiting toxicity of many treatment protocols is bone marrow depression. Consequently, attempts have been made to ameliorate this toxicity via blood product support. Therapy with packed red blood cells is commonly used for symptoms of dyspnea and fatigue or prophylactically in the patients with an hematocrit < 30 percent. Similarly, platelets are routinely used therapeutically in the patient with consumption coagulopathy and prophylactically for drug-induced nadirs < 20–30,000/mm³. White-cell transfusions are not yet standard practice, but can be important adjunctive therapy in the patient with documented sepsis with leukopenia. Despite the obvious benefits of blood component therapy, an increase in respiratory distress has occasionally resulted; it is usually easily treatable by the alert clinician.

The transfusion of red blood cells is now highly quality controlled, and significant respiratory distress is rare. However, reactions can still occur from improperly labeled or unmatched blood or from reactions to minor antigens in the patient with multiple transfusions. The symptoms of fever and urticaria are most common and are easily treated by antihistamines and discontinuation of transfusion. The main differential in the patient who develops respiratory distress during supportive therapy is the distinction between circulatory overload and acute bronchospasm.

More recently, a new symptom complex has been described in the transfused patient consisting of fever, nonproductive cough, diffuse pulmonary infiltration lasting up to 3 days, and eosinophilia.[70-72] Leukoagglutinins are the presumed etiology of this syndrome of "noncardiac" pulmonary edema which has been reproduced by as little as 50 ml of blood containing a high titer of such antibodies. The pathophysiology has not been well worked out but may include granulocyte microemboli or venoconstriction as a result of factors released in the complement cascade.[73] A recent study has identified C5a as a cause of granulocyte aggregation in patients undergoing filtration leukapheresis.[74] Transfusion of these granulocytes results in a higher proportion of allergic manifestations than from granulocytes obtained by centrifugation. The dyspnea of leukoagglutinin reactions is usually self-limited and routine respiratory support is indicated.[70]

Circulatory Overload

There are three main reasons for iatrogenic volume overload in the cancer patient: (1) red-cell transfusions in a compensated patient, (2) overzealous hydration or intravenous administration with therapeutic intent, and (3) excessive hydration in conjunction with chemotherapy. The etiology is not as important as the recognition of the symptoms of pulmonary congestion and prompt relief with diuretics, vasodilators, and/or inotropic agents.

The first item above should be easily recognized by the onset of dyspnea during, or very shortly after, the transfusion of whole or packed cells. The second item is more difficult since it may result in the insidious onset of dyspnea associated with a diffuse interstitial pattern on x-ray which could be misinterpreted as infection or tumor. The cancer patient may have multisystem failure resulting in obfuscation of the usual clues to the status of the intravascular volume.

The final cause of circulatory overload has become more important as new therapies are being tested. Some agents are now being used in doses or schedules which require prior or simultaneous hydration, either for pharmaceutical or toxicologic reasons. Continuous infusion of drugs over several days may obligate several liters of IV fluids per day. Platinum therapy requires aggressive hydration to avoid renal toxicity. Similarly, methotrexate when used in very high dosage requires hydration and alkalinization (with large quantities of sodium) to avoid renal, as well as systemic, toxicity. These therapies are relatively contraindicated in patients with signs of congestive failure or circulatory overload.

Diffuse Bilateral Infiltrates in the Patient with Neoplasia

Diffuse bilateral infiltrates in cancer patients present a diagnostic and therapeutic dilemma. A wide variety of unrelated causes can result in a similar roentographic picture.[75,76] Table 1 divides the causes into infection, toxic, and mechanical categories.

Approximately 5–20 percent of patients with diffuse bilateral infiltrates have a bacterial infection.[8,77,78] The organisms responsible are primarily gram-negative and gram-positive bacteria, especially streptococcus, although *Mycoplasma pneumonia*, *Legionella pneumophilia*, and mycobacteria have been reported.[78,79] Conversely, diffuse bilateral infiltrates were present in 15 percent of patients with gram-negative pneumonia in one series.[6] Fungal infections and *Pneumocystis carinii* are particularly common in patients with heavily treated hematologic malignancies or those receiving steroids. *Pneumocystis carinii* has a reported frequency between 10 and 80 percent in patients with these diseases and is associated with significant mortality.[80,81] Among the fungal infections, *Asper-*

Table 1
Major Causes of Diffuse Bilateral Infiltrates
in Patients with Cancer

Infectious	*Toxic*
Bacteria	Busulfan
Gram-negative bacteria	Methotrexate
Gram-positive bacteria	Bleomycin
Mycoplasma pneumoniae	BCNU
Legionella pneumophila	
Mycobacteria	*Mechanical/Tumor*
Fungi	Leukostasis
Aspergillus ssp.	Tumor infiltrates
Candida ssp.	Pulmonary edema
Cryptococcus neoformans	Pulmonary hemorrhage
Histoplasma capsulatum	
Coccidioides immitis	
Parasites	
Pneumocystis carinii	
Viral	
Cytomegalovirus	
Herpes simplex	
Influenza viruses	

gillus and *Candida* sp. are the most common organisms found.[3,77] *C. immitis* and *H. capsulatum* have also been reported in certain areas of the country.[78,81] Viral infections have been reported less frequently, although cytomegalovirus appears to occur in about 5–10 percent of patients.[8,77]

Diffuse interstitial changes have been noted following a variety of chemotherapeutic agents. Busulfan was the first reported agent to cause this problem. It has now been associated with cyclophosphamide, methotrexate, bleomycin, BCNU, 6-mercaptopurine, procarbazine, chlorambucil, azathioprine, and melphalan.[82-84] Bleomycin appears to be particularly toxic to the lungs. Fibrosis can occur with small doses, although there is increasing risk of pulmonary injury with an increasing dosage and pulmonary radiation.[85,86] Metastatic disease to the lungs can complicate the differential diagnosis (see above).

A diagnosis of nonspecific inflammation is also frequently reported in biopsy and autopsy series in patients with diffuse bilateral infiltrates. Many of these cases are associated with treatment with bleomycin but other causes, such as viral infections, are difficult to exclude.[87]

The patient with diffuse bilateral infiltrates may present with acute respiratory failure, hypoxemia, fever, cough, and sputum production. Alternatively, the history may be one of a slow, insidious decrease in exercise tolerance, with or without cough and fever. Patients with solid tumors and slowly progressive lesions more likely do not represent medical emergencies and diagnostic intervention may be less urgent. Patients with rapidly progressive respiratory distress and severe systemic symptoms such as fever, cardiovascular compromise, or dyspnea at rest should be considered for immediate diagnostic studies and therapy. This is more likely to occur in heavily treated patients with hematologic malignancies. Additional laboratory tests to be obtained in both groups of patients include blood cultures, sputum culture and gram stain, and evaluation for mycobacterial infection. In the more chronic presentation pulmonary function tests to assess the degree of impairment are indicated and can be used as a measure of response to therapy. If the picture is complicated by previous chemotherapy or progressive pulmonary infiltration in the face of tumor regression elsewhere, invasive diagnostic procedures should be considered. Nasal and stool cultures are helpful. *Candida* in the urine or stool may suggest systemic candidal infection. Positive nasal cultures for *Aspergillus* correlate with pulmonary infection.[88] Unless there is bacteriologic or pathologic evidence for fungal infection the initial approach to a patient with diffuse bilateral pneumonitis and fever is broad-spectrum antibiotics. In the presence of suggestive clinical findings or histologic confirmation of *Pneumocystis carinii* treatment can be started with Trimethoprim–sulfamethaxazole.

Failure to improve on empirical therapy is an indication for transbronchial or open-lung biopsy. We would advocate the use of this procedure in acutely ill patients if the course has been stable or there has been deterioration over 48 hours and other diagnostic studies have been unrevealing. Open-lung biopsies rather than transbronchial biopsies should be performed in thrombocytopenic patients for localized disease, or in patients in poor clinical condition. In patients with a normal platelet count and no other contraindications transbronchial biopsy with brushings may be sufficient. The latter procedure provides adequate diagnosis in 60 percent of patients with diffuse infiltrates. The value of performing a transbronchial biopsy is to identify conditions for which there is a specific therapy, such as *Pneumocystis*, fungus, or tumor. Complications from open-lung biopsy or transbronchial biopsy in the hands of experienced physicians are minimal. Bleeding can be prevented by avoiding transbronchial biopsy in patients with uncorrectable platelet counts of < 50,000.[9,78]

The pathologist should be alerted to an open-lung biopsy or

transbronchial biopsy since a methenamine silver stain can be quickly applied to fresh tissue for the diagnosis of *Pneumocystis*. In addition, other organisms such as fungi or mycobacteria can be quickly identified.[8,75]

Diagnosis of a treatable lesion by means of an open-lung biopsy or transbronchial biopsy is made in approximately 50 percent of patients who have diffuse bilateral infiltrates.[8,75,78]

The most common histopathologic picture following cytotoxic drug administration is that of a nonspecific pneumonitis, and has been noted with bleomycin and alkylating agents such as BCNU.[89] The use of steroids in these patients is controversial. Patients who develop an acute respiratory syndrome associated with bleomycin, BCNU, or methotrexate appear to have benefited from steroid treatment, whereas with the more chronic presentations the use of steroids has been less satisfactory.[89,90]

Occasionally, patients will present with symptoms suggestive of diffuse interstitial disease and a negative chest x-ray. In this special situation, gallium scanning has proved to be a useful means of identifying an incipient inflammatory lesion in the lung and may assist in localizing lesions for biopsy. Increased uptake has been reported in certain forms of toxic lung injury, including that from bleomycin pneumonitis and in *Pneumocystis carinii* infection.[91-93] In addition, positive gallium scans may be seen in certain tumors with a propensity for lung involvement such as lymphoma and melanoma.[94] A follow-up gallium scan may be used to assess disease activity or response.

References

1. Ingaki J, Rodriguez V, Rodey GP: Causes of death in cancer patients. Cancer 33:568–573, 1974
2. Klatersky J, Daneau D, Verhest A: Causes of death in patients with cancer. Europ J Cancer 8:149–154, 1972
3. Bodey GP, Powell RD, Hersh, EM, et al: Pulmonary complications of acute leukemia. Cancer 19:781–793, 1966
4. Goodell B, Jacobs JB, Pwell RD, et al: Pneumocystis carinii: The spectrum of diffuse interstitial pneumonia with neoplastic disease. Ann Intern Med 72:337–340, 1970
5. Orbals DW, Marr JJ: A comparative study of tuberculosis and other mycobacterial infections and their association with malignancy. Am Rev Resp Dis 117:39–45, 1978
6. Bode FR, Paré JAP, Fraser RG: Pulmonary diseases in the compromised host. Medicine 53:255–293, 1974

7. Valdivieso M, Gil-Extremera B, Zornoza J, et al: Gram-negative bacillary pneumonia in the compromised host. Medicine 56:241–254, 1977
8. Singer C, Armstrong D, Rosen PP, et al: Diffuse pulmonary infiltrates in immunosuppressed patients. Prospective study of 80 cases. Am J Med 66:110–120, 1979
9. Pennington JE, Feldman MT: Pulmonary infiltrates and fever in patients with hematologic malignancy. Assessment of transbronchial biopsy. Am J Med 62:581–587, 1977
10. Jones ME, Saleem A: Acute promyelocytic leukemia. Am J Med 65:673–677, 1978
11. Crocco JA, Rooney JJ, Fankushen DS, et al: Massive hemoptysis. Arch Intern Med 121:495–498, 1968
12. Robboy SJ, Minna JD, Colman RW: Pulmonary hemorrhage syndrome as a manifestation of disseminated intravascular coagulation: Analysis of ten cases. Chest 63:718–721, 1973
13. Relt RJ, Leite C, Hass CD, et al: Incidence of hemorrhagic complications in patients with cancer. JAMA 239:2571–2574, 1978
14. Golde DW, Drew WL, Klein HZ, et al: Occult pulmonary haemorrhage in leukemia. Br Med J 2:166–168, 1975
15. Palmer PES, Finley TN, Drew WL, et al: Radiographic aspects of occult pulmonary hemorrhage. Clin Radiol 29:139–143, 1978
16. Crocco JA, Rooney JJ, Fankushen DS, et al: Massive hemoptysis. Arch Intern Med 121:495–498, 1968
17. Smiddy JF, Elliot RC: The evaluation of hemoptysis with fiberoptic bronchoscopy. Chest 64:158–162, 1973
18. Bookstein JJ, Moser KM, Kalafer ME, et al: The role of bronchial arteriography and therapeutic embolization in hemoptysis. Chest 72:658–661, 1977
19. Bredin GP, Richardson PR, Kink TKC, et al: Treatment of massive hemoptysis by combined occlusion of pulmonary and bronchial arteries. Am Rev Resp Dis 117:969–973, 1978
20. Catovsky D, Ikoku NB, Pitney WR, et al: Thromboembolic complications in myelomatosis. Br Med J 2:438–439, 1970
21. Bruganolas A, Mink IB, Elias EG, et al: Correlation of hyperfibrinogenemia with major thromboembolism in patients with cancer. Surg Gyn Obstet 136:75–77, 1973
22. Rohner RF, Prior JT, Sipple JH: Mucinous malignancies, venous thrombosis and terminal endocarditis with emboli. A syndrome. Cancer 19:1805–1812, 1966
23. Lieberman JS, Borrero J, Urdaneta E, et al: Thrombophlebitis and cancer. JAMA 177:542–545, 1961

24. Sack GH, Levin J, Gell WR: Trousseau's syndrome and other mainte-
    nance of chronic disseminated coagulopathy in patients with neo-
    plasms: Clinical, pathophysiologic and therapeutic features. Medi-
    cine 56:1–37, 1977

25. Wiernik PH, Serpick AA: Pulmonary embolus in acute myelocytic
    leukemia. Cancer 24:581–584, 1969

26. Rasche H, Dietrich M: Hemostatic abnormalities associated with ma-
    lignant diseases. Europ J Cancer 13:1053–1064, 1977

27. Moser KM: Pulmonary embolism. Am Rev Resp Dis 115:829–860,
    1977

28. Murray HW, Ellis GC, Blumental DS, Sos TA: Fever and pulmonary
    thromboembolism. Am J Med 67:232–235, 1979

29. Vernant JP, Brun B, Mannoni P, et al: Respiratory distress of hyper-
    leukocytic granulocytic leukemias. Cancer 44:264–268, 1979

30. Schwartz JH, Canellos GP: Hydroxyurea in the management of the
    hematologic complications of CGL. Blood 46:11–16, 1975

31. Harris AL: Leukocytosis associated with blood transfusion in acute
    myeloid leukemia. Br Med J 1:1169–1171, 1978

32. Friedman MA, Slater E: Malignant pleural effusions. Cancer Treat
    Rep 5:49–66, 1978

33. Levallen EC, Carr DT: Pleural effusion: A statistical study of 436 pa-
    tients. N Engl J Med 252:79–83, 1955

34. Black LF: The pleural space and pleural fluid. Mayo Clin Proc 47:493–
    506, 1972

35. Adams FV, Galati U: M-mode ultrasonic localization of pleural effu-
    sion: Use in patients with non-diagnostic physical and roentgeno-
    graphic examinations. JAMA 299:1761–1764, 1978

36. Lambert CJ, Shah HH, Urschel HC, et al: The treatment of malignant
    pleural effusions by closed trocar tube drainage. Ann Thoracic Surg
    3:1–5, 1967

37. Light RW, Ball WC: Pleural effusions: The diagnostic separation of
    transudates and exudates. Ann Intern Med 77:507–513, 1972

38. Rudman D: Orosomucoid content of pleural and peritoneal effu-
    sions. J Clin Invest 54:147–155, 1974

39. Light RW, Ball WC: Glucose and amylase in pleural effusions. JAMA
    225:257–260, 1973

40. Light RW, Ball WC: Lactate dehydrogenase isoenzymes in pleural
    effusions. Am Rev Resp Dis 108:660–664, 1973

41. Light RW, Ball WC: Diagnostic significance of pleural fluid pH and
    pCO_2. Chest 64:591–596, 1973

42. Yam LT: Diagnosis significance of lymphocytes in pleural effusions. Ann Intern Med 66:972–982, 1967

43. Bower G: Eosinophilic pleural effusions. Am Rev Resp Dis 95:746–751, 1967

44. Light RW, Ball WC: Cells in the pleural fluid: Their value in differential diagnosis. Arch Intern Med 132:854–860, 1973

45. Storey DD, Dines DE, Coles DT: Pleural effusion. A diagnostic dilemma. JAMA 236:2183–2186, 1976

46. Griner PF: Bloody pleural fluid following pulmonary infarction. JAMA 202:947–949, 1968

47. Rosato FE, Wallach MW, Rosato EF: The management of malignant effusions for breast cancer. J Surg Oncol 6:441–449, 1974

48. Leff A, Hopewell PC, Costello J: Pleural effusion from malignancy. Ann Intern Med 88:532–537, 1978

49. Bayly TC, Kisner DL, Sybert A, et al: Tetracycline and quinacrine in the control of malignant pleural effusions: A randomized trial. Cancer 41:1188–1892, 1978

50. Dollinger MR, Krakoff IH, Kranofsky DA: Quinacrine in the treatment of neoplastic effusions. Ann Intern Med 66:249–257, 1967

51. Paladine W, Cunningham TJ, Sponzo R, et al: Intracavitary bleomycin in the management of malignant effusions. Cancer 38:1903–1908, 1976

52. Sutton ML: The management of malignant pleural effusion. Postgrad Med J 49:729–730, 1973

53. Martini H, Bains MS, Beattle EJ: Indications for pleurectomy in malignant effusions. Cancer 35:734–738, 1975

54. Cornwell GG, Pajak TF, McIntyre OR: Hypersensitivity reactions to IV melphalan during treatment of multiple myeloma: Cancer and leukemia Group B experience. Cancer Treat Rep 63:399–403, 1979

55. Khan A, Hill JM, Grater W, et al: Atopic hypersensitivity to cis-dichlorodiammineplatinum (II) and other platinum complexes. Cancer Res 35:2766–2770, 1975

56. Wiesenfeld M, Reinders E, Corder M, et al: Successful retreatment with cis-dichlorodiammineplatinum (II) after apparent allergic reactions. Cancer Treat Rep 63:219–221, 1979

57. Karchmer RK, Hansen VL: Possible anaphylactic reaction to intravenous cyclophosphamide. Report of a case. JAMA 237:475, 1977

58. Killander D, Dohlwitz A, Enstedt L, et al: Hypersensitivity reactions and antibody formation during L-asparaginase treatment of children and adults with acute leukemia. Cancer 37:220–228, 1976

59. Blum RH, Carter SK, Agre K: A clinical review of bleomycin—a new antineoplastic agent. Cancer 31:903–914, 1973
60. Libshitz HI, Brosof AB, Southard ME: Radiographic appearance of the chest following extended field radiation therapy for Hodgkin's disease. Cancer 32:206–215, 1973
61. Kaplan HS, Stewart JR: Complications of intensive megavoltage radiotherapy for Hodgkin's disease. Nat Cancer Inst Monogr 36:439–444, 1973
62. Wara WM, Phillips TL, Margolis LW, et al: Radiation pneumonitis: A new approach to the determination of time–dose factors. Cancer 32:547–552, 1973
63. Gross NJ: Pulmonary effects of radiation therapy. Ann Intern Med 86:81–92, 1977
64. Phillips TL, Margolis L: Radiation pathology and the clinical response of lung and esophagus. Radiat Therap Oncol 6:254–273, 1972
65. Einhorn L, Krause M, Hornback N, et al: Enhanced pulmonary toxicity with bleomycin and radiotherapy in oat cell lung cancer. Cancer 37:2414–2416, 1976
66. Nygaard K, Smith-Erichsen N, Hatlevoll R, et al: Pulmonary complications after bleomycin, irradiation and surgery for esophageal cancer. Cancer 41:17–22, 1978
67. Castellino RA, Glatstein E, Turbow MM, et al: Latent radiation injury of lungs or heart activated by steroid withdrawal. Ann Intern Med 80:593–599, 1974
68. Bennett DE, Million RR, Ackerman LV: Bilateral radiation pneumonitis, a complication of the radiotherapy of bronchogenic carcinoma. Cancer 23:1001–1018, 1969
69. Rubin P, Casarett GW: Clinical Radiation Pathology. Philadelphia, W. B. Saunders Co., 1968
70. Ward HN: Pulmonary infiltrates associated with leukoagglutinin transfusion reactions. Ann Intern Med 73:689–694, 1970
71. Thompson JS, Severson CD, Parmely MS, et al: Pulmonary "hypersensitivity" reactions induced by transfusion of non-HLA leukoagglutinins. N Engl J Med 284:1120–1125, 1971
72. Ward HN, Lipscomb TS, Cawley LP: Pulmonary hypersensitivity reaction after blood transfusion. Arch Intern Med 122:362–366, 1968
73. Byrne JP, Dixon JA: Pulmonary edema following blood transfusion reaction. Arch Surg 102:91–94, 1971
74. Wammerschmidt DE, Craddock PR, McCullough J, et al: Complement activities and pulmonary leukostasis during nylon fiber filtration leukapheresis. Blood 51:721–730, 1978

75. Armstrong D: Interstitial pneumonia in the immunosuppressed patient. Trans Proc 8:657–661, 1976
76. Schwartz MI, Whitecomb ME, Goldman AL: The spectrum of diffuse pulmonary infiltration in malignant disease. Chest 64:88–93, 1973
77. Greenman RL, Goodall PT, King D: Lung biopsy in immunocompromised hosts. Am J Med 59:488–496, 1975
78. Lauver GL, Hasan FM, Morgan RB, et al: The usefulness of fiberoptic bronchoscopy in evaluating new pulmonary lesions in the compromised host. Am J Med 66:580–585, 1979
79. Reaty HN, Miller AA, Broome CV, et al: Legionnaires' disease in Vermont, May to October, 1977. JAMA 240:127–131, 1978
80. Rosen PP, Martini N, Armstrong D: Pneumocystis carinii pneumonia. Diagnosis by lung biopsy. Am J Med 58:704–802, 1975
81. Wolff IJ, Bartlett MS, Baehner RL, et al: The causes of interstitial pneumonitis in immunocompromised children: An aggressive systematic approach to diagnosis. Pediatrics 60:41–45, 1977
82. Rosenow EC: The spectrum of drug-induced pulmonary disease. Ann Intern Med 77:977–991, 1972
83. Wilson JKV: Pulmonary toxicity of antineoplastic drugs. Cancer Treat Rep 62:2003–2008, 1978
84. Sostman HD, Matthay RA, Putnam CE: Cytotoxic drug-induced lung disease. Am J Med 62:608–615, 1977
85. Samuels ML, Johnson ED, Holoye PY, et al: Large-dose bleomycin therapy and pulmonary toxicity. A possible role of prior radiotherapy. JAMA 235:1117–1120, 1976
86. Holoye PY, Luna MS, MacKay B, et al: Bleomycin hypersensitivity pneumonitis. Ann Intern Med 88:47–49, 1978
87. Poe RW, Utell MJ, Israel RH, et al: Sensitivity and specificity of the non-specific transbronchial biopsy. Am Rev Resp Dis 119:25–31, 1979
88. Aisner J, Marillo J, Schimpff SC, et al: Invasive aspergillosis in acute leukemia: Correlation with nose cultures and antibiotic use. Ann Intern Med 90:4–9, 1978
89. Brown WG, Hasan FM, Barbee RA: Reversibility of severe bleomycin-induced pneumonitis. JAMA 239:2012–2014, 1978
90. Richter JE, Hastedt R, Dalton JF, et al: Pulmonary toxicity of bischloronitrosourea. Report of a case with transient response to corticosteroid therapy. Cancer 43:1607–1612, 1979
91. Richman SD, Levenson SM, Bunn PA, et al: ^{67}Ga accumulation in pulmonary lesions associated with bleomycin toxicity. Cancer 36:1966–1972, 1975

92. Turbiner EH, Yeh SDJ, Rosen PP, et al: Abnormal gallium scintigraphy in pneumocystis carinii pneumonia with a normal chest radiograph. Radiology 127:437–438, 1978
93. Levenson SM, Warren RD, Richman SD, et al: Abnormal and pulmonary gallium accumulation in P. carinii pneumonia. Radiology 119:395–398, 1976
94. Siemsen JK, Grebe SF, Waxman AD: The use of gallium-67 in pulmonary disorders. Sem Nucl Med 8:235–249, 1978

13

SUPPORTIVE CARE OF THE SERIOUSLY ILL CANCER PATIENT: PLATELET AND GRANULOCYTE TRANSFUSION THERAPY

Donald J. Higby
Edward S. Henderson

The treatment of advanced malignant disease often involves the administration of therapy which suppresses bone marrow function. Clinically significant thrombocytopenia and neutropenia are expected during the management of the acute leukemias, and in autologous and allogeneic marrow transplant procedures, which are finding wider application in the management of neoplastic disease.[1] Pancytopenic complications occur frequently as inadvertent side effects of therapy, especially in elderly patients and in those who have been exposed to multiple courses of radiotherapy or chemotherapy. Dangerous neutropenia and granulocytopenia can, of course, occur as side effects of the malignancy itself. In late-stage multiple myeloma and lymphoma, and in bone-marrow-seeking tumors of extramedullary origin, definitive treatment may require the administration of significantly myelosuppressive therapy in patients with

This study was supported in part by USPHS Grant CA-5834 from the National Cancer Institute and Grant #CH-146 from the American Cancer Society.

Without the dedicated services of Doris Burnett, Karen Ruppert, Ruth Johnson, Kathy Winkey, and the Roswell Park Memorial Institute plateletpheresis center, our transfusion studies could not have been performed; without the secretarial assistance of Ms. Corrine Cesari, this manuscript would have remained a personal communication.

marginal granulocyte and platelet counts. Myelofibrosis and myelosclerosis may complicate the chronic leukemias and late-stage lymphomas. Platelet consumption may occur, due to splenomegaly or the vascular properties of large tumors.[2] Certain malignancies (promyelocytic leukemia,[3] some monocytic leukemias,[4] prostatic carcinoma and pancreatic carcinoma[5]) are prone to disturb the coagulation system; rapid lysis of tumor tissue as a consequence of therapy[6,7] or septicemia occurring in the compromised host[8] may also produce disseminated intravascular coagulation. When this occurs, thrombocytopenia, resulting from platelet consumption is the rule. Occasionally, when septicemia occurs in the patient with a marginal marrow reserve, consumption of granulocytes in excess of production may cause a neutropenia.[9] Finally, autoimmune neutropenia and thrombocytopenia can exist in cancer patients with a prolonged transfusion history.

Before replacement of platelets or granuloyctes is contemplated in a cancer patient, it is important for the physician to ascertain the general cause of the problem. In some situations, simply replacing the blood components will not help, and may in fact convert a merely serious situation to one that is life-threatening. Other sections of this volume deal with some of these issues.

The purpose of this article is to describe an approach to granulocyte and platelet support, based upon the experience of the authors in a large medical oncology service.

Platelet Support

The procurement of platelets from normal donors is now a routine function of most large blood banking facilities, and platelets are readily available. This easy availability results in occasional thoughtless use of the product. Attention to the following observations and suggestions should alleviate this problem and maximize the utility of platelet transfusions.

Prophylactic Platelet Support

Indications

Several studies have indicated that platelet transfusions are beneficial in thrombocytopenic patients who are not bleeding.[10-12] The likelihood of bleeding has been clearly correlated with the level of thrombocytopenia.[13] At the same time, these studies indicate that in the individual who is merely thrombocytopenic, the risk of *serious* spontaneous bleeding is extremely small when the platelet count is above 20,000/mm³. Although the likelihood of spontaneous bleeding rises as the platelet count decreases below this level, it is often possible to manage normally active, afebrile patients who have low but *stable* platelet counts (i.e., patients with drug- or radiation-induced chronic thrombocytopenia) without platelet transfusions for long periods of time.[14] Of course frequent observation and careful instruction of the patient to avoid trauma and to report petechiae, spontaneous bruising or other bleeding, or fever is necessary. This course of action is advantageous in the patient where thrombocytopenia as an isolated problem is expected for a prolonged period, since restricting transfusions will reduce the risk of sensitization to platelets and other blood products.

Platelets should be administered prophylactically when thrombocytopenia is complicated by other factors which increase the risk of spontaneous hemorrhage. When petechiae in dependent areas or spontaneous ecchymosis exist, the likelihood of more serious bleeding is increased. In the patient who has a falling platelet count after a course of chemotherapy, platelets should be administered prophylactically.[13] Patients who are in addition markedly neutropenic (absolute granulocyte count less than 500/mm³) are more likely to develop fever (see below) and there is evidence[15,16] that fever increases the risk of spontaneous hemorrhage in thrombocytopenic patients. Finally, it should be kept in mind that the thrombocytopenic patient with chronic cough, frequent vomiting, or other conditions resulting in transient increases in intravascular pressure is at increased risk for developing serious or even fatal hemorrhage due to rupture of microvasculature.

In summary, platelet support is rarely required when the platelet count is above 20,000/mm³; below this level, the decision must be based upon the above-mentioned considerations.

Strategy

The object of prophylactic platelet transfusions is to prevent bleeding and not necessarily to raise the platelet count. At very low platelet levels, the degree of error in platelet enumeration rises, whether counts are performed by hand or by using automated systems.[17] Although the transfusion of 10^{11} platelets can be expected to raise the count by 10,000–20,000 per mm³ in the uncomplicated situation, in practice the increment is often lower due to the presence of fever, some degree of sensitization to blood products, or other factors resulting in increased platelet consumption.

Thus, clinical considerations are more important than the actual increments achieved when prophylaxis is desired.

In most situations, the platelets obtained from 3 to 4 units of fresh whole blood ($2-4 \times 10^{11}$ platelets) are administered every third day and the clinical response assessed. If the patient develops fresh dependent petechiae or spontaneous bleeding or bruising, the frequency (but not the dose) of platelets is increased. In the presence of fever or when febrile reactions routinely accompany platelet transfusions, the frequency is also increased to every other day or daily transfusions. Increasing the actual dose of platelets should be reserved for situations where daily transfusions of the above magnitude are not sufficient to prevent minor bleeding.

Prophylaxis for Surgery

In the patient with thrombocytopenia who requires surgery, even technically extensive procedures can be tolerated without platelet transfusions if the platelet count is greater than 30,000/mm³ if there are no complicating features.[18] Five to 10 units of platelets should be available in such situations, however. When counts are less than 30,000/mm³ or when complicating features exist, our approach is to transfuse the patient with 5 units of platelets immediately before surgery, and infuse 5 additional units during the procedure. If intraoperative hemostasis was particularly difficult, further doses of platelets (3–4 units) should be administered during the first 24 hours postoperatively. If hemostasis has been achieved at that point, further management should be as for standard prophylaxis. Our own observations and reports from others[19,20] suggest that this approach reduces the frequency of postoperative and intraoperative hemorrhage to that noted in surgical procedures in normal individuals.

Therapeutic Platelet Transfusions

The patient who is thrombocytopenic and bleeding (other than dependent area petechiae and minor ecchymoses) should be considered an emergency. The assessment must determine whether the coagulation abnormality depends upon factors other than bone marrow failure, such as sepsis, disseminated intravascular coagulation, or liver function abnormalities, all of which might be present in patients with malignancy. Similarly, an enlarged spleen or large, bulky tumor masses may contribute to the management problem by increasing sequestration and destruction of platelets. In such patients, a full coagulation workup is indicated at the time bleeding becomes evident.

Serious hemorrhage in thrombocytopenic patients is unusual in the absence of local lesions, such as peptic ulceration, bleeding hemorrhoids, endometritis, and cystitis. Pneumonia is doubtless the commonest underlying cause of pulmonary hemorrhage in platelet-deficient patients. Such local disorders must be corrected simultaneously with platelet replacement in order to adequately control bleeding.

Thus control of hemorrhage in thrombocytopenic patients should be approached in the same manner as hemorrhage in a normal individual, with the added therapeutic intervention of platelet transfusions.

Platelet replacement in these patients must take into account the fact that active bleeding results in platelet consumption, and thus more frequent (but not necessarily larger) doses of platelets are required. Our policy is to give 4–6 units of platelets every 6 hours until bleeding is controlled; following this, platelets are given daily for an additional 5–7 days, at which time, if bleeding has not recurred, the patient is placed on a prophylactic regimen until endogenous platelet production is sufficient to maintain safe platelet levels.

If bleeding is not sufficiently controlled with the above regimen, and if other problems contributing to the bleeding problem are controlled or ruled out, much higher doses of platelets are administered (8–20 units per transfusion) every 4–6 hours until bleeding is controlled.

Side Effects

Platelet transfusions are in general safe and associated with minimal complications. The most frequent complication noted is the development of febrile reactions during or shortly after the transfusion. If the reaction is mild, our policy is simply to slow the rate of platelet infusion. In the presence of fever greater than 38°C and/or chills, the transfusion may be temporarily stopped and the patient given hydrocortisone 50 mg intravenously. After 15–30 minutes, the infusion is resumed and further reactions are usually not noted. In the presence of severe rigors, meperidine 25 mg may be given intravenously[21]; this usually aborts the chills, but has no effect on the fever.

Hives may be associated with platelet transfusions. This implies some degree of alloimmunization; we have usually not noted hives until the entire transfusion has been administered, but it is probably reasonable to discontinue the transfusion of that particular platelet concentrate when hives occur before the material is entirely infused. Antihistamines are usually successful in ameliorating this reaction.

Pulmonary reactions have been noted in an occasional patient, manifested by tachypnea, shortness of breath, and occasionally the presence of diffuse infiltrates on the chest x-ray. These reactions are managed as described below (under Granulocyte Transfusion Therapy). If the platelet dose has not been completely administered, it is discontinued at once.

Platelet transfusions may also transmit blood-borne diseases such as hepatitis, syphilis, cytomegalovirus, etc. In platelet preparations which have been accidentally contaminated and stored for several hours at room temperature, the possibility of producing sepsis may occur. Careful screening of donors and proper storage and transfer techniques as practiced in major blood centers and hospitals reduces the frequency of these problems to minimal levels.

Graft-versus-host disease may occur in patients who have received platelet transfusions. This problem is considered below in the section on granulocyte transfusions.

Other Considerations

1. Routinely, platelets are prepared as "platelet-rich plasma" and the platelets prepared from several units of whole blood are combined; in certain circumstances, a platelet concentrate ("superpak") preparation may be desired to provide much larger doses of platelets with minimal extra volume. Platelet concentrates require an additional centrifugation step, at much higher G forces, and extra manipulation. As such, they are less effective, platelet for platelet, than the platelet-rich plasma preparations.[22] However, this decrease in effectiveness is variable and is overshadowed by the markedly increased numbers of platelets which can safely be obtained from an individual donor and administered to an individual recipient.

2. Platelet storage (noncryogenic), in controlled situations, can extend the effectiveness of a dose of platelets over 2–4 days.[23] However, since monitoring of platelet function is difficult and the slight risk of bacterial contamination becomes very much more serious with liquid storage, it is probably reasonable to use freshly drawn platelets to manage active hemorrhage.

3. In most patients not previously exposed to blood products, there are few, if any, circulating antibodies to "foreign" platelets. For this reason and for economical reasons, short-term platelet support (2–4 weeks) can be accomplished with platelets obtained from random donors. However, alloimmunization becomes a significant problem in about 50 percent of patients who have been exposed to random platelets in the past.[24] The diagnosis of significant alloimmunization is frequently difficult. It cannot be assumed that such is the case on the basis of an unexpectedly low post-

transfusion increment, until other causes have been ruled out. These include fever and sepsis, increased sequestration by the spleen, tumor tissue, or an occult bleeding lesion and drug-related antiplatelet antibodies (e.g., diuretics, quinidine, penicillin analogues, acetominophen).

Alloimmunization may be directed against HL-A antigens, specific platelet antigens, red-cell antigens presumed to be shared by the platelet, or other antigens not clearly defined. In a study performed by Duquesnoy,[25] improvement in platelet increments in alloimmunized patients could *usually* be accomplished with platelets from donors who were HL-A identical to the patient or who shared cross-reactive HL-A specificities with the patient. He also noted that alloimmunized patients lacking the HLA-A2 antigen could often be transfused successfully with mismatched donors who also lacked this specificity, suggesting that antibodies directed against HLA-A2 might be more significant than others with respect to clinically important alloimmunization. Likewise, matching of donor and recipient for the BW4/BW6 allele could in many cases avoid the necessity to find an HL-A matched donor. These important studies hold the hope that finding donors for alloimmunized patients may not require detailed tissue typing in most situations, an extremely expensive proposition.

Many centers, in view of the high frequency of alloimmunization, seek to delay this event by using single-donor platelets from the initiation of transfusion in the hopes that alloimmunization will be directed against a much smaller number of antigens than if multiple donors were used at the onset. Schiffer, in reviewing this approach, objects on the grounds that (1) there is greater expense; (2) there is increased risk to single donors from multiple and frequent pheresis procedures; and (3) there is no good evidence that the procedure really delays alloimmunization. In fact, his data would suggest that patients exposed to serial single donors develop clinically important alloimmunization at about the same frequency as those exposed to multiple donors.[24]

Schiffer points out that attempts to limit exposure of patients to HL-A specificities by restricting their exposure to donors may in fact selectively sensitize them to less well-defined non-HL-A antigens, making further selection of donors more difficult.[24]

Although all the evidence is not in, we do not feel that a sufficiently valid case has been made to *begin* platelet transfusions using a restricted donor pool or using donors who are "partially" compatible, and concur with Schiffer's analysis. Perhaps what will surmount some of the difficulties in selecting platelets for alloimmunized donors will be the development of procedures analogous to cross-matching whole blood. To this end, Duqesnoy has demonstrated that the lymphocytotoxicity assay is fairly predictive of platelet survival in the circulation of the recipient.[25]

In the significantly alloimmunized patient, donors with some degree of HL-A compatibility may be sought from a random donor pool or from relatives of the patient, as improvements in post-transfusion increments are seen even when only two antigens are shared[26]; where possible, more sophisticated approaches to matching might be attempted. Where HLA typing is not practical, siblings, parents, and children of the patient represent a pool of potential donors where the likelihood of their sharing some specificities with the recipient are high. Where neither is possible, another approach is to premedicate the patient with glucocorticoids and administer much larger doses of platelets than those described above. Under these circumstances, the initial rate of infusion should be slow and the patient carefully observed for adverse reactions. In the alloimmunized patient, it is worthwhile to obtain 1-hour post-transfusion platelet counts to determine whether the thrombocytopenia is being adequately corrected.

It should be noted that when a patient might eventually undergo allogeneic marrow transplantation, it is important to prevent his exposure to blood products from donors with HL-A antigens shared with the marrow donor. If the patient becomes sensitized to HL-A and non-HL-A determinants possessed by the potential marrow donor, the likelihood of graft rejection increases.[1] In practical terms, this end is accomplished by avoiding the use of blood relatives as platelet donors.

Cryopreserved Platelets

Schiffer has demonstrated that platelet concentrates can be preserved indefinitely in liquid nitrogen storage.[27] While there is some loss of platelets in such situations, those platelets surviving freezing and thawing appear to behave normally in terms of post-transfusion increments, survival, and hemostatic activity. Because of the expense and expertise needed in applying this technology, the indications for cryopreserved platelets are presently limited. Probably the major use would be in patients who had achieved a complete remission from acute leukemia but who had become highly alloimmunized during the initial remission induction. In these individuals, platelets could be collected and stored in anticipation of eventual relapse. Likewise, "banking" of platelets from histocompatible donors might be feasible in preparation for marrow transplant procedures, when it is impractical to keep the donor in the area during the time at risk.

It is theoretically possible that platelets obtained from patients in remission from acute leukemia may contain clonogenic leukemia cells.

Thus, it is not unreasonable to treat such platelets with radiation prior to their administration to the patient after therapeutic marrow aplasia has been achieved (see below under Graft versus Host Disease).

Granulocyte Transfusion Therapy

In contrast to transfusions of platelets or red blood cells, the indications for granulocyte transfusions are still being evolved. A number of randomized prospective studies have been performed in febrile, neutropenic patients, and a clear conclusion from these studies is that patients with bacteremia who receive granulocytes in addition to conventional antibiotics have significantly increased short-term survival compared to those who have received conventional antibiotics alone.[28-34] With other infections, the advantages of granulocyte transfusions are not so clear. Studies have insufficiently examined morbidity, duration of infection, or other "soft" parameters. Given the heterogeneity of infected neutropenic patients, a proper study of the effects of granulocyte transfusions on morbidity is currently difficult to perform.

Normal Granulocyte Behavior

In the average adult, about 2 percent of all granulocytes are circulating at any point in time. The transit time of granulocytes through the circulation is about 7 hours. Approximately 10^{11} mature granulocytes are produced daily. Under the stress of infection, this production rate may rise six- or seven-fold.[35,36]

Bodey has demonstrated that there is a quantitative relationship between the degree and duration of neutropenia and the frequency and severity of bacterial infection.[37] Analysis of his data suggests that a circulating granulocyte count of $1,500-2,000/mm^3$ is only slightly less effective in terms of protection against infection than a normal granulocyte count; below this level, the risk of infection increased rapidly. Also, the frequency of infection is greater with a falling versus a rising granulocyte count. Patients with granulocytopenia who present with early infection symptoms may rapidly progress to shock and death if untreated.[38]

In the absence of adequate granulocytes, the patient with infection has other defenses against progressive infection. The study performed by the EROTC[34] as well as other smaller studies[40-42] indicate that antibiotics in themselves are efficacious in the majority of patients. In addition, some 38 percent of patients with clinical signs and symptoms of infection never have a site or organism demonstrated, and of those who do, only 13 percent are documented to have septicemia. This implies that defenses other than granulocytes are serving to limit the infection. Most likely, the major element in this defense is the tissue macrophage system, which has been shown to persist for long periods of time following the production of aplasia in the marrow.[43]

Thus, the exogenous (systemic antibiotics) and endogenous defenses, together with the "pathogenicity" of the offending organism, may be such as to permit the patient to live in an admittedly precarious coexistence with his infection until granulocyte production returns to safe levels.

McCullough has described the different modes of granulocyte procurement.[44] It is not the purpose of this article to discuss them in depth. The clinician should be familiar with the method used in his local blood bank, the yields obtained, the handling and storage, and how the quality of the product is being controlled.

Centrifugal systems of granulocyte procurement are used in the majority of facilities. Specially designed equipment permits in-line continuous or intermittent collection of granulocytes from a normal donor. Many investigators augment the yields of granulocytes by the administration of glucocorticoids to the donors according to varying schedules.[45-47] In addition, the efficiency of separation can be increased markedly by adding hydroxyethyl starch to the blood prior to its entry into the centrifugation chamber. This material, which has an extremely high safety record, is not allergenic, and is probably metabolized completely by the donor, increases the rate of red-cell sedimentation by causing roleaux formation, and consequently more of the granulocytes appear in the buffy coat.[48]

Centrifugally collected granulocytes have been found by most investigators to show no abnormalities in function, and their transfusion into recipients is associated with a very low reaction rate.[49] Reactions occurring are almost always attributable to recipient sensitization.

Under standard conditions, yields of granulocytes from centrifugal methods, given a 3–4-hour collection period, approach 2.5×10^{10} cells. Many donor centers, however, produce mean yields of 10^{10} cells or less when HES and steroid augmentation are not used. Centrifugally procured granulocytes are heavily contaminated with lymphocytes, a fact which should be kept in mind in patients who are at risk for developing graft-versus-host disease.

Filtration leukapheresis depends on the fact that granulocytes adhere avidly to nylon fiber.[50] Blood from heparinized donors is propelled through nylon wool filters; red cells, plasma, platelets, and lymphocytes pass through the filters without significant adhesion and are returned to the donor. Granulocytes (and monocytes) initially adhere to the fibers, and subsequently preferentially adhere to granulocytes already attached. Since the process of adherence begins a sequence of changes in the granulocyte which involve enzyme release, cell vacuolization, and eventually cell death, the cells which adhere to the fibers first undergo the most damage, whereas those which adhered later are progressively less damaged at the time of recovery.[51]

Following the passage of 3–5 liters of blood through each filter in the system, the blood remaining in the system is returned to the donor by flushing the system with saline, and the filters eluted. Elution involves the passage of a calcium-chelating solution (acid-citrate-dextrose, sodium citrate, EDTA) which has been buffered with electrolytes, and which (in most cases) contains plasma protein. The buffering and the protein serve to protect the recovered granulocytes from further injury.[52,53]

Because of the potential for injury to granulocytes produced with filtration leukapheresis, and because damaged granulocytes, in addition to being ineffective, may harm the recipient, centers using filter-procured material should carefully monitor the quality of granulocytes obtained.

Clinical Use of Granulocyte Transfusions

Prophylactic Granulocyte Support

Several studies have been performed which indicate that granulocyte transfusions given prophylactically are effective in preventing or delaying the onset of infection in neutropenic patients. The study performed by Ford would suggest that giving such transfusions every other day is ineffective,[54] whereas those performed by the Seattle transplant group[55] and the Baltimore Cancer Research Center[56] suggest that daily transfusions may delay the onset and decrease the severity of the infection. These studies, however, do not demonstrate that mortality was affected. The Baltimore study also noted a high incidence of sensitization to blood products in the recipients of prophylactic transfusions.

It is our feeling that, given the expense, possible complications, and the higher probability of alloimmunization inherent in granulocyte transfusions, the extremely small increments which can be produced by standard doses of granulocytes, and, most pertinent, the lack of evidence that prophylactic transfusions actually alter mortality or even shorten hospital stay in patients, prophylactic support with granulocyte transfusions should be restricted to experimental studies.

Therapeutic Support

Background

Conventional granulocyte transfusions (1–2.5 × 10^{10} cells) produce 1-hour post-transfusion increments in the recipient of about 200–500 cells/μl.[44] As mentioned above, the circulation of these granulocytes in the blood is extremely brief and is further shortened in patients with fever, bacteremia, and alloimmunization. When the levels and kinetics of transfused granulocytes are contrasted with those of granulocytes in normal individuals faced with an infection, it seems unlikely that the efficacy of PMN transfusions can be explained solely by postulating that transfused granulocytes "substitute" for endogenous granulocytes. Furthermore, clinical studies usually report gradual improvement in signs and symptoms of infection following transfusion, with only occasional dramatic responses.

Epstein has demonstrated that dogs made aplastic by radiation, when injected with pathogenic organisms, go through an initial phase of bacteremia followed by a latent phase during which organisms cannot be cultured from blood, and finally a second phase of bacteremia terminating in shock and death.[57] The latent phase can be significantly prolonged with a single small dose of granulocytes administered 2 hours after the bacterial challenge. In nontransfused dogs, the median latent phase was about 18 hours, whereas in the animals receiving granulocytes, progressive bacteremia reappeared at a median of 72 hours.

One explanation which could account for all the above observations is that the *usual* benefit of granulocyte transfusions is to bolster the normal blood clearing effect of the tissue defense system (i.e., macrophages, fixed monocytes, Kupffer cells, etc.). Since this benefit occurs both clinically and in the dog experiments for a period of time and to a degree in excess of that predicted by the circulation kinetics of the transfused cells, we postulate that standard doses of granulocytes rapidly become fixed to tissue and continue to exert a clearing effect long after their disappearance from the circulation.

This hypothesis can explain a number of puzzling clinical observations. For example, the benefit of PMN transfusions in neutropenic patients with organ infections is disappointing when contrasted to the dramatic response to granulocytes in septicemic, neutropenic recipients. Furthermore, in many studies, the observed post-transfusion increments do not correlate with clinical results in most cases, and despite good PMN recoveries, the benefits from granulocyte transfusions are frequently gradual and incomplete. Finally, the hypothesis may account for the benefit noted in early studies of filtration-procured cells, which showed PMNs to be effective despite their impaired circulation kinetics and functional defects such as increased adherence, loss of specific granules, vacuolization, and decreased chemotaxis.[51,58]

Indirect support for the hypothesis is provided by the study of Ambinder[59] and our recent study,[60] both of which have defined serologic parameters which predict the outcome of anti-infective therapy in neutropenic patients. Ambinder found that low levels of circulating complement were associated with treatment failure. Our studies confirmed this observation, but noted a stronger association between a high chemotactic activity in the serum of such patients and mortality from infection. We further found a relationship between changes in chemotactic activity and the results of therapy. When chemotactic activity was initially high and returned to normal after the institution of anti-infective therapy, survival was the rule; when the reverse was true or when an initial low chemotaxis score rose despite the therapy, death from infection followed. Elevations in chemotactic activity and decreases in hemolytic complement levels probably reflect the presence of circulating organisms or bacterial products such as endotoxins, which in turn would suggest a breakdown in blood-clearing mechanisms. The fact that initially high chemotactic activity is seen to return to normal with successful anti-infection therapy which includes granulocytes strengthens the hypothesis derived from the above observations.

The above speculation precedes a discussion of the therapeutic use of granulocytes, since it sets limits on what can be expected from such transfusions and establishes an hypothesis upon which total management of the infected, neutropenic patient can proceed rationally.

Selection of Recipients

In general, infected patients with absolute granulocyte counts of 500/mm^3 or less are candidates for granulocyte support. Our policy is to begin broad-spectrum antibiotic coverage, e.g., tobramycin and carbenicillin. If the patient is deteriorating after 2 days of antibiotic therapy, granulocyte transfusions are begun while continuing the antibiotics. Persistence of fever per se is not reason to begin granulocytes if the patient is clinically stable, eating, having no fevers over 39°C, and if there is no evidence of shock.

Once a decision to begin granulocytes is made, they are administered from random or family donors initially, at the rate of $1-2.5 \times 10^{10}$ cells per day. Since such transfusions commonly contain red blood cells, donors compatible for red-cell antigens should be sought. Granulocytes are administered daily until there is evidence of return of endogenous granulocyte production or until 5–7 transfusions have been administered. In the latter case, we customarily reevaluate the infection and the clinical condition of the patient and reassess prognosis. If the patient has definitely improved despite continuing fever, we may choose to withhold granulocytes and continue antibiotics alone, and in most cases this is sufficient to tide the patient over until marrow regeneration becomes evident. On the other hand, if the patient has progressively deteriorated despite granulocyte support, we may add other antibiotics (chloramphenicol, miconazole, amphotericin B) to the regimen while granulocyte transfusions are continued. Unless the patient has suffered organ damage incompatible with recovery, we continue such therapy indefinitely. Some patients have received such regimens in excess of 30 days and eventually recovered from their infection.

In patients who continue to deteriorate despite such measures, and who still do not have a demonstrable organism or site of infection, we may choose to add high doses of steroids to other agents. A significant fraction of such patients have circulating endotoxins or disturbances in complement activity or other serologic phenomena which have been described in patients with clinical septic shock. Based upon the studies of Jacobs,[61] our suspicion is that neutropenic patients might not develop the full-blown shock syndrome because of an absence of circulating granulocytes; consequently, they have attenuated development of those intravascular reactions which result in hypotension, vascular damage, etc.

In some patients, the addition of steroids has appeared to improve the clinical syndrome sufficiently to reverse life-threatening disease.

Administration of Granulocyte Transfusions

Granulocyte transfusions should be administered as soon as possible after procurement. Under optimal conditions, granulocytes obtained by centrifugation leukapheresis remain sufficiently intact to permit their storage in carefully defined conditions for 24–48 hours, but even then, decreases in some functional parameters have been described.[62,63] Filtration-procured cells should not be stored at all because of a more rapid rate of deterioration.[62] The clinician administering granulocytes should explicitly instruct the blood receiving center and the floor personnel to expedite the transfusion of granulocytes into the patient. Too often, we have observed delays of several hours between the time the transfusion is received on the floor and the time it is actually infused.

Pulmonary complications, fevers, chills, and other adverse effects sometimes accompany the rapid infusion of granulocytes, especially those procured by filtration. It is important to assure that such transfusions are administered relatively slowly; our practice is to infuse them at a rate of 10^{10} cells over 30 minutes or more. If fever and chills occur during the transfusion, it should be stopped and the patient medicated with 100 mg of hydrocortisone or other intravenous glucocorticoid, and if chills are sufficiently severe, an injection of meperidine (25 mg) given intravenously. After the symptoms have lessened, the infusion can be resumed at half the previous rate, and the patient observed carefully. Usually second reactions do not occur.

In the patient with a history of reactions to blood products, highly alloimmunized patients, or patients who have reacted adversely to previous granulocyte transfusions, premedication with a glucocorticoid and an antihistamine should be given prophylactically. If available, histocompatible granulocytes may reduce reaction rates in patients previously reactive to randomly obtained granulocytes,[64,65] although it should be noted that most reactions are not apparently related to histocompatibility factors.[66,67]

Complications of Granulocyte Transfusions

Fever and chills.   About 5 percent of patients receiving centrifuge-procured cells and 15 percent or more of those receiving filtration cells develop fever, often accompanied by chilling.[49] Usually this is attributed to alloimmunization of the recipient, although this is seldom if ever proven. In the case of filtration leukapheresis, chills and fever may also be related to the infusion of cells which are partially damaged or of intracellular enzymes, etc., which have exuded into the solution suspending the cells. In small children where the cell dose per square meter of body surface area was particularly large, we have observed extremely high posttransfusion fevers and prolonged chilling, followed by defervescence and apparent resolution of the infection. This unusual reaction may be the result of complete destruction of the infecting organisms associated with granulocyte breakdown; thus, endotoxins and granulocyte contents may cause the pyrogenic reaction.

Febrile reactions can in general be managed according to the scheme described above, but extremely high fevers accompanied by rigors should probably also be managed with physical cooling of the patient and the infusion of extra platelets if the patient is also thrombocytopenic. If reactions cannot easily be controlled, the remaining granulocytes should be discarded.

Hypersensitivity reactions.   In our experience, these are exceedingly rare and almost always manifest only by hives. Usually the administration of an antihistamine is sufficient to control this problem.

Pulmonary reactions.   The development of shortness of breath, wheezing, and other signs of pulmonary distress during a granulocyte transfusion should be considered an emergency. This sort of reaction is rare, and in our experience occurs in approximately 1 percent of patients when the protocol of slow administration of the granulocyte transfusion is followed. Assessment of the patient is necessary, since more than one cause is possible.

Fluid overload should be considered in the patient with compromised cardiovascular status who does not have an accompanying febrile reaction. Such patients clinically appear to be in pulmonary edema and respond to appropriate management.

In the patient with high levels of circulating leukoagglutinins, aggregation of granulocytes may take place in the pulmonary bed, and this is detectable by the appearance of fluffy infiltrates bilaterally on chest x-ray.[68] Aggregation of granulocytes may also take place in the vasculature prior to the cells' migration to the pulmonary bed, and microembolization may occur. This reaction probably occurs because of damage to the cells during collection or storage, and increased aggregation after dilution of the anticoagulant by the plasma. The actual infusion of cell aggregates may also occur and the fluid path of the granulocyte transfusion should be inspected to rule this out.

In individuals who have pneumonia and in some in whom the source of infection is unknown, the infusion of granulocytes may result in sequestration in the site of infection, subsequent edema, and other accompaniments of an inflammatory reaction in the lungs.[69] This reaction clinically and roentgenologically resembles a segmental or lobar pneumonia, and may be associated with the development of a productive cough when this has not been present before.

Most reactions do not fall into the above identifiable categories, and respiratory distress is mild and unaccompanied by physical and roentgenological findings. It is possible that these represent a forme fruste of the "shock lung" syndrome, caused by complement activation and subsequent mild endothelial damage due to the intravascular materials.[61] Alternatively, such reactions may be due to alloimmunization not detectable by current methods.

The management of pulmonary reactions is straightforward and usually successful. The granulocyte transfusion should be stopped, a blood sample drawn for measurement of leukoagglutinins (if the test is available), the patient quickly assessed to rule out fluid overload as a cause, and a bolus of 100 mg hydrocortisone administered. We usually also administer diphenhydramine, 30 mg. Nasal oxygen may be given if distress is moderate. If the reaction does not rapidly subside, a chest x-ray should be obtained and further treatment predicated on this basis.

Patients who have had pulmonary reactions should not have granulocyte transfusion support discontinued. Rather, future transfusions should be administered after premedication with steroids, at a very slow rate, while under careful observation. Rarely, it may be necessary to search for a histocompatible donor if alloimmunization is felt to be the etiology of the problem.

Transfusion compatibility.   It is known that post-transfusion increments of granulocytes in the circulation correlate directly with the degree to which donor and recipient are histocompatible.[64,65] On the other hand, the degree to which this is clinically meaningful is not known. Most centers, out of necessity, continue to rely on random donors for most granulocyte transfusions.

Parenthetically, it should be noted that patients in whom the possibility of a future marrow transplant exists should not be exposed to blood products from family members in order to prevent sensitization of the patient to minor histocompatibility antigens shared by the donor.[1]

Antileukocyte antibodies are detectable by a variety of means in some patients who have previously been exposed to blood products. Whether the presence of such affects the outcome of granulocyte transfusions and reactions to such transfusions is in question, and Ungerleider was not able to correlate clinical events or post-transfusion increments with the presence or levels of such antibodies.[70]

Except in unusual circumstances, therefore, the donor of granulocytes needs only to be screened insofar as the major ABO group and a major and minor cross-match with the recipient performed.

Graft-versus-host disease. The transfusion of granulocytes (especially those procured with centrifugation procedures which are contaminated heavily with lymphocytes), like the transfusion of platelets and fresh whole blood, carries the potential of inducing graft-versus-host disease in a compromised recipient.[71,72] In the past 10 years on the medical oncology service at Roswell Park Memorial Institute, we have suspected graft-versus-host disease attributable to blood products in 12 patients. Nine of these had advanced lymphomas and had previously been exposed to radiation and chemotherapy in the management of their diseases. Two patients with blastic transformation of chronic myelocytic leukemia developed the syndrome. Although the heaviest use of platelets and granulocyte transfusions is in patients with acute myelocytic leukemia, only one individual with this disorder developed clinical graft-versus-host disease, and this patient had received previous intensive chemotherapy and radiotherapy for another malignancy.

The diagnosis of graft-versus-host disease is often obscured in patients receiving cytotoxic chemotherapy. Skin rashes suggesting that the syndrome may be caused by reactions to allopurinol or antibiotics, and jaundice and diarrhea may result from both antibiotics and cytostatics. Even histopathological examination may fail to distinguish the syndrome from the more reversible side effects of drugs. Nonetheless, this disease can be a fatal complication of otherwise curative therapy. For this reason, all blood products given to immunosuppressed individuals should be irradiated to 1000–3000 rads.[44]

Chronic myelocytic leukemia cells as a source of granulocyte transfusions. Patients with chronic myelocytic leukemia (CML) who consent to leukapheresis are excellent sources for extremely high doses of granulocytes for transfusion. If anti-CML therapy can be delayed safely for a reasonable length of time, and if the patient is willing, we leukapherese these individuals as frequently as possible using intermittent-flow centrifugation. Since the doses of cells which can be transfused are several-fold higher, better clinical results can be expected. We recommend that clinicians attempt to arrange with their local blood bank a cooperative effort to make available granulocytes from such individuals.

Prospects for the Future

1. Cryopreservation of granulocytes has not yet become clinically feasible. It appears that small aliquots can be cryopreserved under exacting conditions with partial recovery of function.[73,74] Recently, some success, on a larger scale, has been achieved in dogs.[75]

2. Better definition of the mode of action of granulocyte transfusions, and more intensive study of factors in the recipient which promote and retard granulocyte function, should permit more rational use of this expensive resource. In addition, more careful definition of indications are needed, since it is obvious that a fairly large fraction of patients probably do not need such transfusions to survive their infections, whereas in others, standard doses together with antibiotics are not sufficient to salvage the patient.

3. While cryopreservation of granulocytes is still experimental and not yet adaptable to the clinical situation, the cryopreservation of granulocyte precursors is quite possible. Where buffy coats from patients with chronic myelocytic leukemia have been transfused, temporary but prolonged elevations in granulocyte counts have been observed in some recipients, occasionally accompanied by mild symptoms and signs of graft-versus-host disease.[73,76,77] The cryopreservation of immature myeloid precursors from patients with CML, and their use in establishing temporary grafts of myeloid cells, is an area worth exploring.

Conclusions

The use of platelet and granulocyte transfusions is widespread and well established. It is important that their limitations be recognized and that the responsible clinician use them with careful attention to the whole clinical picture.

References

1. Thomas ED, Storb R, Clift RA, et al: Bone marrow transplantation. N Engl J Med 292:16–17, 832–843, 895–902, 1975
2. Brodie GN, Bliss O, Firkin BG: Thrombocytopenia and carcinoma. Br Med J 1:540, 1970
3. Hillestadt LK: acute promyelocytic leukemia. Acta Medica Scandia 159:189, 1957
4. Rosner F, Dobbs JV, Ritz ND, et al: Disturbances of hemostasis in acute myeloblastic leukemia. Acta Haemat 43:65, 1970
5. Levin J, Conley CL: Thrombocytopenia associated with malignant disease. Arch Intern Med 114:497, 1964
6. Gralnick HR, Marchesi S, Givelber H: Intravascular coagulation in acute leukemia: Clinical and subclinical abnormalities. Blood 40:709, 1972

7. Ogston D, Dawson AA: The fibrinolytic enzyme system in malignant lymphomas. Acta Haematol 49:89, 1973

8. Lerner RG, Rapaport SI, Spitzer JM: Endotoxin-induced intravascular clotting: The need for granulocytes. Throm Diath Haemorrh 20:430, 1968

9. Marsh JC, Boggs DR, Cartwright GE, et al: Neutrophil kinetics in acute infections. J Clin Invest 46:1943, 1967

10. Han T, Stutzman L, Cohen E, et al: Effects of platelet transfusions on hemorrhage in patients with acute leukemia. Cancer 19:1937–1942, 1966

11. Higby D, Cohen E, Holland JF, et al: The prophylactic treatment of thrombocytopenic leukemic patients with platelets: A double-blind study. Transfusion 14(5):440–446, 1974

12. Simone JV: Use of fresh blood components during intensive combination therapy of childhood leukemia. Cancer 28:562, 1971

13. Gaydos LA, Freireich EJ, Mantel N: The quantitative relation between platelet count and hemorrhage in patients with acute leukemia. N Engl J Med 226:905–909, 1962

14. Solomon J, Beutler E, Bofenkamp T, et al: Indications for the administration of platelet transfusions during remission induction therapy of acute leukemia. Blood (Suppl) 50:210, 1977 (Abstract 408)

15. Cohen P, Gardner FH: Thrombocytopenia as a laboratory sign and complication of gram-negative bacteremic infection. Arch Intern Med 117:113, 1966

16. Wilson SJ, Dean CA: The pathogenesis of hemorrhage in artificially induced fever. Ann Intern Med 13:1214, 1940

17. Wintrobe, MM: The diagnostic approach to bleeding disorders, in Wintrobe MM, Lee RG, Boggs OR, et al (eds): Clinical Hematology, 7th Ed. Philadelphia, Lea and Febiger, 1974, pp 1051–1053

18. Mittelman A, Elias EG, Wieckowska W, et al: Splenectomy in patients with malignant lymphoma or chronic leukemia. Cancer Bull 22:10–13, 1970

19. Seligman B, Rosner F, Ritz ND: Major surgery in patients with acute leukemia. Am J Surg 124:629–633, 1972

20. Bjornsson S, Yates J, Mittelman A, et al: Major surgery in acute leukemia. Cancer 34(4):1272–1275, 1974

21. Djerassi I: Methotrexate infusions and intensive supportive care in the management of children with acute lymphocytic leukemia: Follow-up report. Cancer Res 27:2561–2564, 1967

22. Abelson NM: Blood components, in Abelson NM (ed): Topics in Blood Banking. Philadelphia, Lea and Febiger, 1974, pp 103–113

23. Becker GA, Aster RH: Short-term platelet preservation at 22°C and at 4°C. Blood 40:593, 1972

24. Schiffer CA, Aisner J, Wiernik PH: Platelet transfusion therapy for patients with leukemia, in Greenwalt TJ, Jamieson GA (eds): The Blood Platelet in Transfusion Therapy. Progr Clin Biol Res 28:267–280, 1978

25. Duquesnoy RJ: Donor selection in platelet transfusion therapy of alloimmunized patients, in Greenwalt TJ and Jamieson GA (eds): The Blood Platelet in Transfusion Therapy. Progr Clin Biol Res 28: 229–244, 1978

26. Hester JP, McCredie KB, Freireich EJ: Platelet replacement therapy: A clinical assessment, in Greenwalt TJ and Jamieson GA (eds): The Blood Platelet in Transfusion Therapy. Progr Clin Biol Res 28:281–292, 1978

27. Schiffer CA, Aisner J, Wiernik PH: Frozen autologous platelet transfusion for patients with leukemia. NEJM 299(1):7–11, 1978

28. McCredie KB, Freireich EJ, Hester JP, et al: Leukocyte transfusion therapy for patients with host-defense failure. Transplant Proc 5:1285, 1973

29. Graw RG, Herzig G, Perry S, et al: Normal granulocyte transfusion therapy: Treatment of septicemia due to gram-negative bacteria. N Engl J Med 287:367, 1962

30. Higby DJ, Yates J, Henderson ES, et al: Filtration leukapheresis for granulocyte transfusion therapy. Clinical and laboratory studies. NEJM 292:761, 1975

31. Vogler WR, Winton EF: A controlled study of the efficacy of granulocyte transfusions in patients with neutropenia. Am J Med 63:548, 1977

32. Alavi J, Root RK, Remischovsky J, et al: Leucocyte transfusions in acute leukemia. N Engl J Med 296:706–711, 1977

33. Herzig R, Herzig G, Bull M, et al: Efficacy of granulocyte transfusion therapy for gram-negative sepsis: A prospectively randomized controlled study. N Engl J Med 296:701–705, 1977

34. Schiffer CA, Buccholz DH, Aisner J, et al: Clinical experience with transfusion of granulocytes obtained by continuous flow filtration leukapheresis. Am J Med 58:373–381, 1975

35. Cartwright GE, Athens JW, Wintrobe MM: The kinetics of granulopoiesis in normal man. Blood 24:708–713, 1964

36. Craddock G, Perry S, Lawerence JS, et al: The dynamics of leukopenia and leukocytosis. Ann Intern Med 52:281–283, 1960

37. Bodey GP, Buckley M, Sathe YS, et al: Quantitative relationships be-

tween circulating leukocytes and infection in patients with acute leukemia. Ann Intern Med 64:328–336, 1966

38. Gaya H, Klastersky J, Schimpff S, et al: Prospective randomly controlled trial of three antibiotic combinations for empiric therapy of suspected sepsis in neutropenic cancer patients. Europ J Cancer 11(Suppl):5–8, 1975

39. The EORTC International Antimicrobial Therapy Project Group: Three antibiotic regimens in the treatment of infection in febrile granulocytopenic patients with cancer. J Infect Dis 137(1):14–29, 1978

40. Tattersall MN, Spiers AS, Darrel JH: Initial therapy with combination of five antibiotics in febrile patients with leukemia and neutropenia. Lancet:162–165, 1972 (January 22, 1972)

41. Rodriguez V, Burgess M, Bodey GP: Management of fever of unknown origin in patients with neoplasms and neutropenia. Cancer 32:1007–1912, 1973

42. Schimpff S, Satterlee W, Young VM, et al: Empiric therapy with carbenicillin and gentamycin for febrile patients with cancer and granulocytopenia. N Engl J Med 284(19):1061–1069, 1971

43. Van Furth R: Origin and kinetics of monocytes and macrophages Semin Hematol 7(2):125–141, 1970

44. McCullough J: Leukapheresis and granulocyte transfusion. Crit Rev Clin Lab Sci 10(3):275–327, 1979

45. MacPherson JL, Nusbacher J, Bennett JM: The acquisition of granulocytes by leukapheresis: A comparison of continuous flow centrifugation and filtration leukapheresis in normal and corticosteroid-stimulated donors. Transfusion 16:221, 1976

46. Shoji M, Vogler WR: Effects of hydrocortisone on the yield and bacterial function of granulocytes collected by continuous flow centrifugation. Blood 44:435–440, 1974

47. Higby DJ, Mishler JM, Rhomberg W, et al: The effect of a single or double dose of dexamethasone on granulocyte collection with the continuous flow centrifuge. Vox Sang 28:243–246, 1974

48. Mishler JM, Hadlock DC, Fortuny IE, et al: Increased efficacy of leukocyte collection by the addition of hydroxyethyl starch to the continuous flow centrifuge. Blood 44:571–579, 1974

49. Buchholz DH, Houx JL: Survey of filtration leukapheresis. Exp Hematol 7(Suppl 4):1–10, 1979

50. Djerassi I, Kim JS, Mitrakul C, et al: Filtration leukapheresis for separation and concentration of transfusable amounts of normal human granulocytes. J Med 1:358–362, 1970

51. Wright DG, Klock JC: Functional changes in neutrophils collected by

filtration leukapheresis and their relationship to cellular events that occur during adherence of neutrophils to nylon fibers. Exp Hematol 7(Suppl 4):11–23, 1979

52. Sanel FT, Aisner J, Tillman C, et al: Evaluation of granulocytes harvested by filtration leukapheresis: Functional histochemical and ultrastructural studies, in Goldman JM and Lowenthal RM (eds): Leucocytes: Separation, Collection & Transfusion. London, Academic Press, 1975, pp 236–242

53. Higby DJ, Salvatori V, Burnett D, et al: Improving the quality of granulocytes obtained by filtration leukapheresis. Exp Hematol 7(Suppl 4):36–42, 1979

54. Ford JM, Cullen M: Prophylactic granulocyte transfusions. Semin Hematol 5(Suppl 1):65–72, 1977

55. Clift RA, Sanders RE, Thomas ED, et al: Granulocyte transfusions for the prevention of infection in patients receiving bone marrow transplants. NEJM 298:1052–1057, 1978

56. Schiffer CA, Aisner J, Daly D, et al: Alloimmunization following prophylactic granulocyte transfusion. Blood (in press)

57. Epstein R, Clift RA, Thomas ED: The effect of leukocyte transfusions on experimental bacteremia in the dog. Blood 34:782–790, 1969

58. Herzig G, Root RK, Graw RG: Granulocyte collection by continuous flow filtration leukapheresis. Blood 39:554–567, 1972

59. Ambinder E, Keusch G, Kovacs I: Serum opsonins as a determinant of success in granulocyte transfusions. Proc AACR ASCO 19:350, 1978 (abstract)

60. Higby DJ, Salvatori V, Burnett D, et al: Serum factors affecting granulocytes are associated with outcome of infection in neutropenic patients. Proc AACR ASCO 21:442, 1980 (abstract)

61. Jacobs HS: Granulocyte complement interaction: A beneficial antimicrobial mechanism that can cause disease. Arch Intern Med 138:461–463, 1976

62. McCullogh J: Liquid preservation of granulocytes for transfusion, in Greenwalt TJ and Jamieson TA (eds): The Granulocyte: Function and Clinical Utilization. Vol 13, Progress in Clinical and Biological Research. New York, Alan R. Liss, 1977, pp 185–193

63. Price T, Dale DC: Neutrophil preservation. The effect of short term storage on in vivo kinetics. J Clin Invest 59:475–481, 1977

64. DeBruyere M, Moriau M, Bellenot C: Histocompatibility matching and results of granulocyte and platelet transfusions, in Goldman JM and Lowenthal RM (eds): Leucocytes: Separation, Collection and Transfusion. London, Academic Press, 1975, pp 450–455

65. Higby DJ, Mishler JM, Cohen E, et al: Increased elevation of peripheral leukocyte counts by infusion of histocompatible granulocytes. Vox Sang 27:186–189, 1974
66. Aisner J, Schiffer CA, Wiernik PH: Granulocyte transfusions: Evaluation of factors influencing results and a comparison of filtration and intermittent centrifugation leukapheresis. Br J Haematol 38:121–127, 1978
67. McCullogh J, Wood N, Wieblin BJ, et al: The role of histocompatibility testing in granulocyte infusions, in Greenwalt TJ and Jamieson JA (eds): The Granulocyte: Function and Clinical Utilization. Vol 13, Progress in Clinical and Biological Research. New York, Alan R. Liss, 1977, pp 321–328
68. Ward HN: Pulmonary infiltrates associated with leukoagglutinin transfusion reactions. Ann Intern Med 73:689–694, 1970
69. Higby DJ, Freeman AI, Henderson ES, et al: Granulocyte transfusions in children using filter-collected cells. Cancer 38(3):1407–1413, 1976
70. Ungerleider RS, Appelbaum FR, Trapani RJ, et al: Lack of predictive value of antileukocyte antibody screening in granulocyte transfusion therapy. Transfusion 19(1):90–94, 1974
71. Salfner B, Borberg H, Kruger G, et al: Graft versus host reaction following granulocyte transfusion from a normal donor. Blut 36:27–29, 1978
72. Cohen D, Weinstein H, Mihm M, et al: Nonfatal graft vs host disease occurring after transfusion with leukocytes and platelets obtained from normal donors. Blood 53(6):1053–1057, 1979
73. Lionetti FJ, Hunt SM, Gore JM, et al: Cryopreservation of human granulocytes. Cryobiology 12:181–191, 1975
74. Meryman HT, Howard J: Cryopreservation of granulocytes, in Greenwalt TJ and Jamieson GA (eds): The Granulocyte: Function and Clinical Utilization. Vol 13, Progress in Clinical and Biological Research. New York, Alan R. Liss, 1977, pp 193–202
75. French JE, Jemionek JF, Contreras TJ: Cryopreservation and dog polymorphonuclear leukocytes for transfusion. Exp Hematol 6(Suppl 3):107, 1978 (abstract)
76. Coltman CA, Uhl GS, Bearden JD, et al: Marrow engraftment with extreme leukocytosis in a patient with non-Hodgkin's lymphoma, in Goldman JM and Lowenthal RM (eds): Leucocytes: Separation, Collection and Transfusion. London, Academic Press, 1975, pp 385–394
77. Buskard NA, Kaur J, Goldman JM, et al: Chronic granulocytic leukemia engraftment in acute myeloid leukemia. Ann Roy Coll Phys Surg Cancer 10:59, 1977 (abstract)

14

SUPPORTIVE CARE OF THE SERIOUSLY ILL CANCER PATIENT: INTRAVENOUS HYPERALIMENTATION

Ezra Steiger
Janet M. Blanchard

Metabolic and nutritional consequences of cachexia and malnutrition can lead to a multitude of multisystem abberations in the cancer patient. It has been well documented that the single entity responsible for the greatest morbidity and mortality of cancer patients is malnutrition.[1-4] This entity has been given its own definitive term in "cancer cachexia."

Recent advances in oral food supplements and specialized tube feeding diets have enlarged the armamentarium of nutritional support modalities available to the clinician for the support of the patient with cancer. However, successful application of the enteral feeding regimens require well-motivated patients and a normally functioning gastrointestinal tract. The nausea, vomiting, and diarrhea present in cancer patients receiving active antineoplastic therapy often precludes the use of the intestinal tract. Intravenous hyperalimentation (IVH) or total parenteral nutrition (TPN) has allowed for the restoration and maintenance of normal nutritional status in a variety of conditions usually associated with inadequate gastrointestinal tract function, weight loss, malnutrition, and clinical deterioration of the patient. TPN has also been used to support the patient with

The authors would like to express their appreciation to Ms. Ruth Hooley for her contribution to this paper.

347

cancer in preparation for major surgery, postoperatively and during periods of chemotherapy or radiation therapy. In this chapter, the consequences of cancer on nutritional status will be reviewed and techniques of TPN in the management of the patient with cancer will be presented.

Metabolism in Cancer

The exact etiology of the increased energy requirements of the patient with cancer has not been fully delineated. In 1914, Wallersteiner, as reviewed by Fenninger et al.,[5] demonstrated that 15 of 33 patients with carcinoma of the stomach had an increased basal metabolic rate. Although tumor growth utilizes energy from aerobic and anaerobic metabolism, the majority comes from anaerobic glycolysis due to limited oxygen supply and enzyme content of the tumor tissue. The anaerobic metabolism of glucose by the tumor consumes a significant amount of energy in the form of ATP and thus accelerates the energy expenditure of the host.

Fenninger[5] showed that both exogenous and endogenous nitrogen is used for tumor growth in patients with lymphoma and leukemia. Steiger et al.[6] showed that diet did influence tumor growth rate and that the amino acids in the diet were the primary stimulants of tumor growth. Protein synthesis in skeletal muscle of tumor-bearing rats was noted to be decreased by Clark.[7] Recently, Schein et al.[8] proposed that perhaps the abnormal glucose tolerance curve seen in some patients with cancer is probably related to a marked increase in resistance to insulin. Studies on 7 cachetic patients given continuous glucose and exogenous insulin infusion with epinephrine and propranolol resulted in a mean glucose concentration of 119 mg% (60–170 percent of normal) in cachectic patients as compared to 50 mg% for 10 controls, plasma insulin levels being equivalent and receptor sites on monocytes being the same. They postulated that the possible mechanisms for increased protein breakdown in cancer patients was due to an increase in gluconeogenesis.

Impaired utilization by normal tissues of dietary protein and amino acids and their enhanced utilization by tumor tissue, as demonstrated by enhanced breakdown of protein by the tumor bearing host, accentuates the malnutrition that occurs in the cancer patient.

Although considerable controversy exists concerning alterations in the metabolic responses in the cancer patient, the clinical end result is a widely known and, again, poorly understood syndrome, "cancer cachexia". Costa[9] defines this syndrome, which is again reinforced by more recent articles,[10,11] as weakness, anorexia, depletion and redistribution of host components, hormonal aberrations, and progressive alterations of vital function, in addition to anemia. The patients often appear chronically ill, emaciated, pale, and progressively fading. The degree of cachexia bears no relation to the cell type of the tumor, tumor burden, anatomical site, or caloric intake. Costa[9] enumerated the possible causes of anorexia leading to cachexia; these are defined as being alteration of taste and/or smell perception, production of lactate and ketone bodies, "tumor toxins," effect on appetite center, and psychologic factors.

Equally important and yet probably not emphasized enough were the psychological aspects of the malnourished cachectic cancer patient who neither is hungry nor has the desire to eat. Dewys[12] suggested selection of foods with flavors and odors that appeal to altered chemoreceptors and minimize mechanical digestive activity.

Nutritional Assessment of the Cancer Patient

Nutritional assessment can provide objective measurements of the cancer patient's nutritional status. This is important in assessing whether or not intensive nutritional support is indicated and also to assess the effects of nutritional support used.

In the clinical setting, evaluation of protein/calorie nutrition consists of three general types of information: anthropometric, laboratory data, and nutritional history. Clinical interrelationships between the patient and the various nutritional parameters utilized for assessment purposes, and also patient-specific nutrition/cancer interactions which affect the selection of nutritional support, are also evaluated.

Anthropometric Measurements

Anthropometric measurements utilized for the evaluation of protein/calorie status are listed in Table 1. These parameters include: weight, weight/height, recent involuntary weight losses, triceps skin fold thickness, and mid-upper-arm muscle circumference.

Laboratory Tests

Laboratory tests and laboratory values used in nutritional assessment are delineated in Table 2. Those most commonly used include hemoglobin, hematocrit, serum albumin, serum transferrin, nitrogen balance (as measured by 24-hour urinary urea nitrogen excretion), creatinine–height

Table 1
Anthropometric Measurements

1. Usual weight
2. Weight/height (ideal body weight)
3. Recent weight losses
   % Weight Loss
   Conditions: (a) weight loss, involuntary
                   (b) weight loss within 6 mos.

$$\frac{\text{Usual Weight } - \text{ Current Weight}}{\text{Usual Weight}} \times 100 = \% \text{ Wt. Loss}$$

4. Triceps skinfold thickness[13] (TSF) (50th percentile values)

Male—age	TSF (mm)	Female—age	TSF (mm)
25–34	11	25–34	19*
35–44	12	35–44	22

5. Arm circumference/arm muscle circumference[13] (AMC) (50th percentile values)

$$\text{AMC} = \text{arm circumference (cm)} - [\text{TSF (mm)} \times 0.314]$$

Male—age	AMC (cm)	Female—age	AMC (cm)
25–34	27.0	25–34	21.3*
35–44	27.0	35–44	21.6

*For those patients over 44 years in age, use the standards for 35–44 age group.

index, peripheral lymphocyte count, and cell-mediated immunocompetence (as evaluated by delayed hypersensitivity response to common recall antigens).

Nutritional History

A nutritional history includes food tolerances/intolerances, dietary habits and patterns, gastrointestinal symptoms associated with oral food intake, socioeconomic and psychosocial influences, and food intake data. Food intake data is obtained by asking the patient to recall the types and amounts of food normally consumed during 24 hours. Nutritional history information is used to (1) generate enough estimations of past nutrient intake in terms of quantity and quality (it also may alert one to other potential nutrient deficiencies which merit further investigation), (2) establish individualized enteral nutritional support programs in a patient with normal gastrointestinal function, and (3) form the data base for patient education pertaining to diet and nutrition.

The final assessment of protein–calorie status may be evaluated in a

Table 2
Laboratory Parameters

1. Serum albumin
2. Serum transferrin (measured by single radial immuno-diffusion)
3. Nitrogen balance (using 24-hr urinary urea excretion)[14]
4. Creatinine–height index[15] (CHI)
    Conditions: 1. Adult
    2. Normal renal and excretory function (continence or foley)

$$\frac{\text{Urine creatinine (mg)}}{\text{Reference creatinine (mg)}} = \text{CHI}$$

Reference creatinine:

$$\text{Males} = \text{IBW* (kg)} \times 23$$
$$\text{Females} = \text{IBW (kg)} \times 18$$

5. Peripheral lymphocyte count (total lymphocyte count)[16]

$$\frac{\text{White Blood Count} \times \% \text{ Lymphocytes}}{100}$$

Abnormal = < 1000
6. Delayed hypersensitivity skin tests[17]
    Conditions: Positive = 5 mm or greater induration or erythema per
                manufacturer's instructions
    Antigens (concentration/0.1 ml.)
    Candida albicans (1:100)
    Trichophyton (1:100)
    Mumps (undiluted)
    Tuberculin PPD (5 units)
    Streptokinase/Streptodornase (10 units kinase)
    (Varidase)   (2.5 units dornase)
7. Hemoglobin[18]
8. Hematocrit[18]

*IBW = ideal body weight.

number of ways.[19–23] At the Cleveland Clinic Foundation, a point system consisting of parameters which have been correlated with increased postoperative morbidity and mortality has been developed and is currently being used for the purpose of objectively determining somatic and visceral protein status. Table 3 illustrates this point system. In this system, individual point values (serum albumin, serum transferrin, percent weight loss, creatinine–height index, and delayed hypersensitivity skin tests) are summed to arrive at three basic categories: normal, moderately depleted, or severely depleted. Efficacy of nutritional support may be measured by serial assessments of protein–calorie status at 2-week intervals. In any institution, skin testing, serum albumin levels, and weight

Table 3
Objective Measurement Standards[24,25]

---

1. % weight loss:

$$0-\ 5\% = 0 \text{ points (normal)}$$
$$6-15\% = 1 \text{ point\ \ (depleted)}$$
$$> 15\% = 2 \text{ points (severely depleted)}$$

2. Creatinine–height index:

$$0.75 = 0 \text{ points}$$
$$0.50-0.75 = 1 \text{ point}$$
$$< 0.50 = 2 \text{ points}$$

3. Serum albumin:

$$3.5 = 0 \text{ points}$$
$$3.0-3.5 = 1 \text{ point}$$
$$< 3.0 = 2 \text{ points}$$

4. Serum tranferrin:

$$190 = 0 \text{ points}$$
$$100-190 = 1 \text{ point}$$
$$< 100 = 2 \text{ points}$$

5. Delayed hypersensitivity skin tests:

$$\text{2 or more positive skin tests} = 0 \text{ points}$$
$$\text{one positive skin test} = 1 \text{ point}$$
$$\text{zero positive skin tests} = 2 \text{ points}$$

6. Overall assessment of protein nutritional status:

$$\text{normal} = 0-\ 2 \text{ points}$$
$$\text{moderate depletion} = 3-\ 5 \text{ points}$$
$$\text{severe depletion} = 6-10 \text{ points}$$

---

loss can be used to reflect the potential nutritional status in a more simplified form.

Nutritional Repletion with Total Parenteral Nutrition

All of the above parameters of nutritional assessment alert the physician and supportive personnel into directing their attention to the nutritional status of the cancer patient. Once assessment is completed, decisions regarding nutritional repletion are necessary. The most natural and practical methods of nutrition are by the oral route; however, as previously noted, this may be completely impractical. The next most feasible route is by nasogastric, gastrostomy, or jejunostomy feeding tubes. However, when the gastrointestinal tract cannot be used in the malnourished patient, total parenteral nutrition (TPN) should be considered. The relative indications for TPN in the patient with cancer are (1) malnutrition or suspected deprivation of adequate oral nutrition for 7 or more days, (2) inability to adequately use the gastrointestinal tract, and (3) a patient who is a candidate for continuing treatment of his or her neoplastic disease.

The concept of total intravenous feeding was advanced experimentally in 1949 when Rhodes et al.[26] used a catheter in the superior vena cava of dogs to infuse a 50-percent solution of dextrose and protein hydrolysate and were able to achieve positive nitrogen balance in these dogs. Further progress was made by Dudrick et al. in 1966[27] when they infused 30-percent dextrose, protein hydrolysate, vitamins, minerals, and trace elements into beagle puppies and were able to demonstrate normal growth and development. This was successfully applied by Dudrick et al.[28] for infants and adults with a wide variety of clinical states characterized by malnutrition and gastrointestinal tract dysfunction. This was further applied in the treatment of cancer patients at the M.D. Anderson Hospital in 1975 when Copeland et al.[29] reported results of the use of TPN in 58 patients with mostly solid tumors and demonstrated a decreased morbidity and enhanced ability to respond to chemotherapy when these patients were supported with intravenous hyperalimentation.

To meet basic caloric needs and food requirements in adults (see Refs. 30–32 for pediatric patients) most commercially available intravenous nutrient solutions have been formulated so that 3 liters per day provides 2,700 nonprotein kilocalories and 105–150 grams of amino acids. The usual caloric requirements for hospitalized patients are 25 kilocalories/kg/day at basic levels to 45 kilocalories/kg/day in the hypermetabolic state. The usual adult patient in the hospital weighing 70 kg needs approximately 2,700 kilocalories per day. Amino acid requirements are usually 1–2 g/kg/day or 70–140 g/day for the usual 70-kg adult patient. Each liter of nutrient solution is prepared in a central additive area of the hospital pharmacy under a laminar-air-flow hood by mixing 500 ml of a 7–10-percent amino acid solution into a liter bottle half filled with 500 ml of 50-percent dextrose. Table 4 shows the typical additives that are placed in each of 3 liters for the usual patient each day.

All solutions should be used within 24 hours and no single bottle should hang longer than 12 hours. Each bottle should be inspected for clarity, cracks, and particulate matter. If any of these are found, the bottle should be discarded and/or sent back to the pharmacy.

The liter solution provides approximately 900 kilocalories per liter and 30–50 grams of amino acids and has an osmolality of 1,800–2,400 mOsm. The requirements for sodium in TPN are not different than the usual requirements of patients on standard 5-percent dextrose intravenous infusion. Sodium acetate is added to one of the 3 liters each day to prevent the development of metabolic acidosis that occurs as a result of metabolism of the infused amino acids. Serum carbon dioxide levels are monitored to assess if more (low carbon dioxide levels) or less (high carbon dioxide levels) acetate should be added. If sodium additives need to be restricted, potassium acetate might be used in its place.

More potassium than normal may need to be added, as glucose, under the influence of insulin, moves into the cell and is associated with intracellular movement of potassium and amino acids. Also, Copeland[2] points out that in cachectic patients, an increase in the need for calcium, magnesium, and phosphorus will parallel the increased need for potassium. Phosphorus is added to prevent hypophosphatemia which is associated with decreased levels of 2–3 DPG and a left-shifted oxyhemoglobin dissociation curve. Perioral and fingertip paresthesias, numbness, and/or difficulty with respiration have also occurred.[33] If phosphorus were added without an additional amount of calcium, symptomatic hypocalcemia may occur. Both water- and fat-soluble vitamins must be added to 1 liter of intravenous hyperalimentation solution daily. Five millimeters of a multivitamin infusion (USV Lab, Division of USV Pharmaceutical Corporation, Tuckahoe, New Jersey) delivers water-soluble B-complex vitamins and fat-soluble A, D, and E. No parenteral mixture contains vitamin B_{12}, folate, or vitamin K, and these should be given intramuscularly as follows: IM doses of 500 μg of vitamin B_{12} every 2 weeks, 5 mg of folic acid every week, and 10 mg of vitamin K weekly or more often as the prothrombin time is determined. Optional additives may include (1) 1,000 units of heparin to each liter, which has been shown to decrease the incidence of thrombosis and peripheral intravenous infusions and may be of value in central venous infections,[34] (b) insulin, if the patient is unable to handle the glucose load and the blood sugar level is over 150 mg%, and (c) trace elements: the exact requirements for these are not precisely known but have been the subject of a recent review.[35] Alterations in the amounts of the above fluids have to be made for the patient with renal failure.[36–47] Intravenous fat emulsions are routinely given through a separate peripheral IV to prevent essential fatty acid deficiency.[48–50] Usually one 500-ml bottle of 10-percent fat emulsion given 3 times weekly is sufficient to prevent essential fatty acid deficiency states.

Catheter Placement

Delivery of the hypertonic intravenous hyperalimentation solution necessitates the use of a large-caliber vein. Access is gained to the superior vena cava through the subclavian vein. Approaches to the subclavian vein may either be supraclavicular or infraclavicular; however, the most common site is infraclavicular because the supraclavicular avenue usually is uncomfortable to the patient and the dressing is cumbersome and more difficult to manage. Therefore, percutaneous infraclavicular subclavian catheterization remains the preferred venous access route for TPN.

The patient should be well informed about the procedure and then be placed in the Trendelenburg position with the head turned away from the side of the cannulation side. Strict sterile conditions should be maintained at all times. The area is defatted with acetone or adhesive remover and then prepped with povidone iodine solution and draped with towels leaving the lower neck, medial two thirds of the clavicle, and sternal notch exposed. The area to be cannulated (the medial one third of the inferior border of the clavicle) should be anesthetized with 1-percent Xylocaine, first making a wheal with a 25-gauge needle and then starting infiltration of the deeper tissues toward the sternal notch, making sure not to give intravenous anesthesia. The 14-gauge, 2-inch-long, large intracath needle is placed on a non-luer-lock 5-ml glass syringe. Then using the sternal notch as a guide; the needle, with the bevel pointed down and the barrel of the syringe parallel to the chest, is directed through the skin, beneath the clavicle, and toward the anterior margin of the trachea and the sternal notch. Continuous gentle suction is placed on the syringe so when the vein is cannulated, a flash-back of blood will appear immediately. When blood appears, the patient is asked, when possible, to hold his breath or perform a Valsalva maneuver. The syringe is then removed, the gloved thumb placed over the hub of the needle to prevent air embolism, and the plastic radio-opaque catheter is placed through the needle to the catheter hub. If the bevel of the needle is pointed toward the feet, this will minimize the chance of the catheter being directed up into the internal jugular vein. The catheter should thread *easily;* if there is any resistance, the needle and catheter should be removed as a unit, as any forced manipulation of the catheter in the needle may cause a portion of the catheter to be sheared off. Once the catheter is in the superior vena cava, the needle and catheter as a unit are pulled back so that the needle is entirely out of the skin and the needle guard is placed in position. The tubing from the bottle of 5-percent or 10-percent dextrose is then placed into the catheter and the bottle lowered below the patient's head. A bottle return through the catheter should be observed; this insures that the catheter is in the proper site. The catheter is then secured with a nonabsorbable suture.

The catheter exit site, junction of the catheter hub, and IV tubing are then cleansed with iodine ointment. An uncomplicated but adequate dressing should be applied; i.e., paint the skin with a tincture of benzoin and cover the catheter exit tip with gauze and tape. Then the catheter hub and IV junction should be taped with a narrow strip of tape and gauze placed over it so that it is accessible for an IV tubing change without disturbing the main catheter dressing. The IV tubing should be looped over the dressing to prevent dislodging the catheter with inadvertent traction.

To assure proper placement in the superior vena cava and to make sure that there is no pneumothorax or hemothorax, a chest x-ray should be obtained. Auscultation of the chest should be performed immediately after insertion of the catheter and dressing placement. If the catheter is not positioned correctly or if it is in the internal or external jugular vein, it should be removed and repositioned.

Fastidious care of the catheter is a must and the dressing is changed 3 times a week; usually Monday, Wednesday, and Friday, preferably by the same person. This will help prevent most infectious complications. When the dressing is changed, the skin should be cleansed with acetone, followed by the povidone iodine, and the catheter site covered with a povidone iodine ointment and taped. The IV tubing is changed daily. Strict adherence to the following rules should be enforced without any deviation:

1. No blood should be aspirated through the catheter.
2. No piggyback tubing should be applied, as this serves as an avenue for microorganisms.
3. No other medication should be given through the tubing and especially no blood.
4. No central venous pressure monitoring should be performed through the catheter.

If possible, there should be a single bottle connected to a drip chamber and IV tubing which connects directly to the catheter. Infusion pumps are ideal, as they deliver solutions at a constant rate and prevent accidental infusions of large amounts of hypertonic solution.

Recognition of catheter sepsis is the key to reducing the morbidity of long-term intravenous hyperalimentation. Other sources of temperature elevation should be searched thoroughly. If no source of the fever is found, then the bottle containing the hyperalimentation should be taken down and sent for culture, replacing it with another. If the temperature still does not go down promptly, then the catheter should be removed in the following manner:

1. Start a peripheral infusion of 5-percent or 10-percent dextrose to avoid hypoglycemia.
2. Blood cultures should be drawn through the catheter before removal.
3. After removal, the catheter tip should be cultured.

If the catheter was the source of the fever, it usually subsides within hours and no further therapy is required. If the fever persists, antibiotics should be started.

There may be instances when long-term chemotherapy and/or intravenous hyperalimentation may be needed in the treatment of the cancer patient. For this purpose, Broviac et al. described a silastic catheter in 1973.[51] This catheter is approximately 90 cm long and is made up of silicone rubber with two parts: (1) intravascular; this portion is thin and flexible so that it will flow freely in the superior vena cava; and (2) extravascular; this portion is thicker and has an attached Dacron cuff. This latter portion lies in the subcutaneous tunnel where the Dacron cuff allows for ingrowth of fibrous tissue which helps to anchor and minimize the secondary infection from skin contaminants.

This catheter should be inserted in an operating room that has fluoroscopy available, and bilateral venograms should be performed preoperatively.

Successful use of total parenteral nutrition requires careful monitoring. Prior to the initiation of the intravenous feeding, baseline laboratory studies should be ordered and fluid and electrolyte abnormalities corrected. Initial baseline studies should include the following: (1) complete blood count, (2) glucose, (3) creatinine and blood urea nitrogen, (4) electrolyte determinations, (5) SGOT, SGPT, alkaline phosphatase, and bilirubin, (6) total protein and albumin, (7) calcium, (8) phosphorus, and (9) magnesium determination.

After intravenous hyperalimentation has been initiated, there are a number of parameters that must be monitored. Laboratory monitoring of the TPN patients at the Cleveland Clinic includes glucose, BUN, and electrolytes 3 times a week; complete blood count, magnesium, calcium, phosphorus, liver function, and prothrombin time are performed weekly. Initially, the glucose may have to be measured every day. Continuous administration of the hypertonic solution may cause hyperglycemia and/or glycosuria. Insulin added to each bottle may be needed to maintain blood sugar levels below 150 mg%.

If a patient demonstrates an electrolyte imbalance, it may be necessary to order electrolytes daily. If it is necessary, pH, arterial blood gases, osmolarity, and ammonia may be ordered to help in diagnosing metabolic abnormalities.

Nursing monitoring of the patient includes the following: vital signs every 4 hours; any change in temperature reported immediately and sources investigated; intake and output charting to help assure proper fluid management; and daily weighing should be performed on the same metabolic scale and preferably at the same time each day. If the patient is gaining weight in excess of ½ pound per day, this is probably due to excess fluid retention. Physical findings such as rales, gallop, and presacral and peripheral edema aid in diagnosing fluid excess. Proper management includes decreasing the hyperalimentation infusion rate or instituting diuretics; urine reductions are done every 6 hours. Test tapes should be used to monitor glycosuria as the tablets may cause a false positive reaction.

Intravenous Hyperalimentation in Cancer

There are a number of questions that need to be answered by randomized prospective studies regarding the use of TPN in patients with cancer. These include what effect nutrition has on tumor growth, what effect TPN has on postoperative morbidity and mortality when given perioperatively to patients with cancer, and what effect TPN has on the tolerance and response to chemotherapy. There is some information available that addresses these issues in the form of laboratory animal experiments and also in the form of retrospective analysis of clinical data.

To help answer the first question regarding nutrition–tumor growth interactions, Steiger et al.[6] studied an implantable nonmetastasizing rat mammary tumor in groups of rats receiving intravenous 5-percent dextrose and 5-percent amino acids, or 30-percent dextrose and 5-percent amino acids (TPN regimen). Tumors grew significantly larger in the rats receiving TPN fluid as compared to the ones with 5-percent dextrose. The tumor weight to nontumor carcass weight ratio was approximately 0.1 in both groups. Of considerable interest was that rats who received only 5-percent amino acids had carcass weights similar to the group receiving 5-percent dextrose, yet their tumors were significantly larger, as large as the rats receiving the TPN regimen. The tumor weight to nontumor carcass weight in this group was 0.2. The authors concluded that the different types of intravenous nutritional support did influence the rate of tumor growth and that it was the amino acid content of the diet that exerted this influence. The authors further hypothesized that by using intravenous hyperalimentation or amino acid infusions clinically, tumor growth might be enhanced and that the use of cell-cycle-specific chemotherapeutic agents might be more efficacious. Cameron and Rozer[52] subsequently showed that when rats with a Morris hepatoma were given chemotherapy with hydroxyurea, those rats receiving intravenous hyperalimentation had a significantly greater reduction in tumor weight compared to rats who were ad libitum orally fed with a much-reduced nutrient intake. On the other hand, working with sarcoma-bearing rats, Lowry et al.[53] investigated the effect of oral diet on tumor growth and carcass protein. They concluded that dietary protein restriction with a low-protein diet did not affect growth characteristics or composition of the sarcomas. Analysis of their data at the end of the 21-day experiment, however, showed that although total tumor DNA was not affected by a protein-free diet, tumor weight and tumor nitrogen content were significantly reduced by the low-protein diet. Daly et al.[54] also noted that rats given intravenous hyperalimentation had larger tumors than rats getting oral protein-free diets.

Despite these animal observations that nutrition can affect tumor growth, there have been no clinical reports of enhanced tumor growth occurring secondary to intravenous hyperalimentation or nutritional support in humans. This might be due to the concomitant usage of chemotherapy, radiation therapy, or surgery. In addition, the tumor growth in humans is relatively slow, and measurable increases in growth over a few weeks may be difficult to measure, especially using retrospective analysis of data. It is our policy to avoid the prolonged administration of intensive nutritional support to patients with tumor in the absence of a specific antitumor therapy such as surgery or chemotherapy.

There have been few studies to assess the effects of nutritional support preoperatively in patients with cancer. Holter and Fisher[55] randomized 84 patients into a control group with minimal or no weight loss, and those patients who lost 10 or more pounds were randomized into TPN or no TPN groups for 72 hours preoperatively and continued postoperatively. Although weight loss in the postoperative period was largely avoided in the group receiving intravenous hyperalimentation, there was no significant difference in major or minor complications or mortality rates when comparing the two groups with and without hyperalimentation. A longer period of preoperative nutritional support, perhaps long enough to improve nutritional assessment status, might have demonstrated a clear benefit for the use of perioperative TPN. Daly et al.[56] retrospectively analyzed 36 malnourished patients who underwent perioperative TPN. Those patients who were skin-test negative at the start of TPN demonstrated a higher incidence of postoperative complications compared to the skin-test positive group. Although TPN was administered to both skin-test negative and skin-test positive groups, the pre-TPN skin testing predicted that the group that was skin-test negative would have a greater number of complications; administration of TPN did not appear to prevent the complications. This analysis suffers from a lack of a control group and careful documentation of the type and degree of postoperative complications.

Malnutrition does lead to increased postoperative complications, and TPN can reverse malnutrition. It stands to reason that TPN should improve postoperative convalescence. It has been shown to enhance wound healing experimentally,[57] but a more defined randomized prospective clinical study still needs to be finished to document its efficacy preoperatively in humans.

Intravenous hyperalimentation can be given safely to patients receiving chemotherapy,[58,59] even in the presence of episodes of neutropenia. Most studies on the use of TPN in patients receiving chemotherapy are retrospective and do not compare in a randomized prospective way the efficacy of TPN in patients receiving chemotherapy. The gastrointestinal side effects of chemotherapy are minimized by placing the intestinal tract at rest and giving patients TPN both experimentally[60] and clinically.[61] Marrow toxicity of chemotherapeutic agents was not prevented experimentally by the concomitant use of intensive and nutritional support, however.[6]

Copeland et al.[62] noted that those patients on TPN who maintained or converted to normal reactions, when delayed hypersensitivity skin testing was measured, responded better to chemotherapy than patients who were skin-test negative. Immunosuppression previously thought to be due to chemotherapy may, in many instances, be due to malnutrition. The correction of malnutrition can restore delayed hypersensitivity skin testing to normal and may allow the patient to be more responsive to chemotherapy.

Conclusions

Intravenous hyperalimentation or total parenteral nutrition can be a very useful tool in the management of the critically ill patient with cancer. It can reverse the malnutrition in the cancer patient who is unable to use his or her own intestinal tract. Clinically, the effects on tumor growth seem to be negligible, especially when used in combination with other antineoplastic therapy. There are a number of precautions relating to catheter insertion, catheter care, proper preparation and delivery of the nutrient solution, and proper monitoring of the patient that will assure the relative safety of the use of intravenous hyperalimentation in the patient with cancer. Malnutrition need no longer be a contraindication to the use of surgery, radiation therapy, or chemotherapy in the management of patients with cancer, even when the gastrointestinal tract cannot be adequately utilized. With proper diligence in its application, total parenteral nutrition can be a life-saving modality in the management of patients with cancer.

References

1. Brennan MF: Uncomplicated starvation versus cancer cachexia. Cancer Res 37:2359–2364, 1977
2. Copeland EM, Dudrick SJ: Current Prob Cancer 1(3):4, 1976
3. Ohnuma T, Holland JF: Nutritional consequences of cancer chemotherapy and immunotherapy. Cancer Res 37:2396, 1977
4. Theologides A: The anorexia–cachexia syndrome: A new hypothesis. Ann NY Acad Sci 230:14–22, 1974
5. Fenninger LD, Mider GB: Energy and nitrogen metabolism in cancer. Adv Cancer Res 2:229–253, 1954
6. Steiger E, Smith-Oram J, Miller J, et al: Effects of nutrition on tumor growth and tolerance to chemotherapy. J Surg Res 18:455–461, 1975
7. Clark CM, Goodlad GA: Muscle protein biosynthesis in the tumor bearing rat. A defect in the post-initiation stage of translation. Biochem Biophys Acta 378:230–240, 1975
8. Schein PS, Kisner D, Haller D, et al: Cachexia in malignancy. Cancer (Suppl) 43(5):2070–2076, 1979
9. Costa G: Cachexia, the metabolic component of neoplastic. Cancer Res 37:2327–2335, 1977
10. Costa G, Donaldson SS: Current concepts in cancer; effects of cancer treatment on the nutrition of the host. N Engl J Med 300(22):1471–1473, 1979
11. DeWys WD: Anorexia in cancer patients. Cancer Res 37:2354–2358, 1977
12. DeWys WD: Anorexia as a general effect of cancer. Cancer (Suppl) 43(5):2013–2019, 1979
13. Frisancho AR: Triceps skinfold and upper arm muscle size norms for assessment of nutritional status. Am J Clin Nutr 27:1052, 1974
14. MacKenzie TA, Blackburn GL, Flatt JP: Clinical assessment of nutritional status using nitrogen balance. Fed Proc 33:683, 1974
15. Bistrian BR, Blackburn GL, Sherman M, et al: Therapeutic index of nutritional depletion in hospitalized patients. Surg Gynecol Obstet 141:152, 1975
16. Lewis RT, Klein H: Risk factors in post-operative sepsis. J Surg Res 26:365, 1979
17. MacLean LD: Host resistance in surgical patients. J Trauma 19:297, 1979
18. Canstakis G: Nutritional assessment in health programs. Am J Pub Health 63:Part 2, 1973
19. Copeland EM, Daly JM, Dudrick SJ: Nutritional concepts in the treat-

ment of head and neck malignancies. Head Neck Surg 1:350–363, 1979

20. Sobol SM, Conoyer JM, Zill R, et al: Nutritional concepts in the management of the head and neck cancer patient. I. Basic concepts. The Laryngoscope 89:794–803, 1979

21. Dwyer JT: Dietetic assessment of ambulatory cancer patient: With special attention to problems of patients suffering from head–neck cancers undergoing radiation therapy. Cancer (Suppl) 43(5):2077–2086, 1979

22. Blackburn GL, Bistrian BR, Maini BS, et al: Nutritional and metabolic assessment of the hospitalized patient. J Parenteral Enteral Nutr 1:11–22, 1977

23. Shils ME: Principles of nutritional therapy. Cancer (Suppl) 43 (5):2093–2101, 1979

24. Studley HO: Percentage of weight loss: A basic indicator of surgical risk in patients with chronic peptic ulcer. JAMA 106:458, 1936

25. Harvey, KB, Bothe A, Blackburn GL: Nutritional assessment and patient outcome during oncological therapy. Cancer 43:2065, 1979

26. Rhodes CM, Parkins W, Vars HM: Nitrogen balances of dogs continuously infused with 50% glucose and protein preparations. Am J Physiol 159:415–425, 1949

27. Dudrick SJ, Vars HM, Rhoads JE: Growth of puppies receiving all nutritional requirements by vein. Fortschritte der parenter Ernahr, in Symposium of the International Society of Parenteral Nutrition, 1966. Fortschr. Parenter Ernahr, 1967, p 2

28. Dudrick SJ, Wilmore DW, Vars HM, et al: Long-term total parenteral nutrition with growth, development and positive nitrogen balance. Surgery 64:134–142, 1968

29. Copeland EM, MacFadyen BV, Lanzotti VJ, et al: Intravenous hyperalimentation as an adjunct to cancer chemotherapy. Am J Surg 129:167–173, 1975

30. Dudrick SJ, MacFadyen BV, Souchon EA, et al: Parenteral nutrition techniques in cancer patients. Cancer Res 37:2440–2450, 1977

31. Heird WC, MacMillan RW, Winters RW: Total parenteral nutrition in the pediatric patient, in Fischer J (ed): Total Parenteral Nutrition, 1976, pp 263–284

32. Filler RM, Deitz W, Suskind RM: Parenteral feeding in the management of children with cancer. Cancer (Suppl) 43(5):2117–2120, 1979

33. Steiger E, Fazio VW: Total parenteral nutrition: A clinical manual of principles and techniques. Cleveland, Cleveland Clinic Press, 1976, p 12

34. Peters WR, Bush WH, McIntyrne RD, et al: The development of fi-

brin sheath on indwelling venous catheters. Surg Gynecol Obstet 137:43, 1973

35. American Medical Association Department of Foods and Nutrition: Guidelines for essential trace element preparations for parenteral use. JAMA 241:2051–2054, 1979

36. Abel RM, Beck CH, Abbott WM, et al: Improved survival from acute renal failure after treatment with intravenous essential L-amino acids and glucose. N Engl J Med 288:695, 1973

37. Abel RM, Shih VE, Abbott WM, et al: Amino acid metabolism in acute renal failure: Influence of intravenous essential L-amino acid hyperalimentation therapy. Ann Surg 180:350, 1974

38. Baek SM, Makabali GG, Bryan-Grown CW, et al: The influence of parenteral nutrition on the course of acute renal failure. Surg Gynecol Obstet 141:405, 1975

39. Bergstrom J, Furst J, Hultman E, et al: Parenteral nutrition in uremia. Acta Anarth Scand 55:147, 1974

40. Dudrick SJ, Steiger E, Long JM: Renal failure in surgical patients. Treatment with intravenous essential amino acids and hypertonic glucose. Surgery 68:180, 1970

41. Jeejeebhoy KN: Nutritional support of the azotemic patient. Urol Clin North Am 1:345, 1974

42. Kaminski MV, Light JA, Briggs WA: Parenteral nutrition with essential amino acids in pretransplantation anephrics. JPEN 2:1, 1978, pp 22–27

43. Leonard CD, Luke RG, Siegel RR: Parenteral essential amino acids in acute renal failure. Urology 6:154, 1975

44. Maddock RK, Bloomer HA, De St. Jeor SW: Low protein diets in the management of renal failure. Ann Intern Med 69:1003, 1968

45. Wilmore DW, Dudrick SJ: Treatment of acute renal failure with intravenous essential L-amino acids. Arch Surg 99:669, 1969

46. Long JM, Dudrick SJ, Steiger E, et al: Use of intravenous hyperalimentation in patients with renal or liver failure, in Cowan and Scheetz (eds): Intravenous Hyperalimentation. Philadelphia, Lea and Febiger, 1972, pp 147–151

47. Able RM: Parenteral nutrition in the treatment of renal failure, in Fischer J (ed): Total Parenteral Nutrition. 1976, pp 143–170

48. MacFadyen BV Jr, Dudrick SJ, Tagudar EP, et al: Triglyceride and free fatty acid clearances in patients receiving complete parenteral nutrition using a 10% soybean oil emulsion. Surg Gynecol Obstet 137:813, 1973

49. Meng HC: Fat emulsions in parenteral nutrition, in Fischer J (ed): Total Parenteral Nutrition. 1976, pp 305–334

50. Grotte G, Jacobson S, Wretlend A: Lipid emulsions and technique of peripheral administration in parenteral nutrition. In Fischer (ed): Total Parenteral Nutrition. 1976, pp 335–362

51. Broviac JW, Cole JJ, Scribner BH: A silicone rubber atrial catheter for prolonged parenteral alimentation. Surg Gynecol Obstet 136:602, 1973

52. Cameron IL, Roger W: Total intravenous hyperalimentation and hydroxyurea chemotherapy in hepatoma-bearing rats. J Surg Res 23:279–288, 1977

53. Lowry SF, Goodgame JT, Norton JA, et al: Effect of chronic protein malnutrition on host-tumor composition and growth. J Surg Res 26:79–86, 1979

54. Daly JM, Copeland E, Guinn E, et al: Relationship of protein nutrition to tumor growth and host immunocompetence. Surgical Forum 27:113, 1976

55. Holter AR, Fischer JE: The effects of perioperative hyperalimentation on complications in patients with carcinoma and weight loss. J Surg Res 23:31–34, 1977

56. Daly JM, Dudrick SJ, Copeland EM: Evaluation of nutritional indices as prognostic indicators in the cancer patient. Cancer 43:925–931, 1979

57. Steiger E, Daly JM, Allen TR, et al: Post-operative intravenous nutrition effects on body weight, protein regeneration, wound healing and liver morphology. Surgery 73:686–691, 1973

58. Summers JE, Zee, P, Hughes WT: Intravenous alimentation in patients with cancer and neutropenia. J Pediat 83:288–290, 1973

59. Copeland EM, MacFadyen BV, McGowan C, et al: The use of hyperalimentation in patients with potential sepsis. Surg Gynecol Obstet 138:377–380, 1974

60. Souchon EA, Copeland EM, Watson P, et al: Intravenous hyperalimentation as an adjunct to cancer chemotherapy with 5-fluorouracil. J Surg Res 18:451–454, 1975

61. Schwartz GF, Green HC, Bendon ML, et al: Combined parenteral hyperalimentation and chemotherapy in the treatment of disseminated solid tumors. Am J Surg 121:169, 1971

62. Copeland EM, MacFadyen BV, Dudrick SJ: Effect of intravenous hyperalimentation on established delayed hypersensitivity in the cancer patient. Ann Surg 184:60–64, 1976

15

SUPPORTIVE CARE OF THE SERIOUSLY ILL CANCER PATIENT: CONTROL OF PAIN

Robert B. Catalano

Acute pain is a common complaint of patients seeking medical care. It can serve a useful purpose if it is evaluated and treated for what it represents, a symptom, and not a primary disease. Initially, all complaints obtained should be viewed as an indicator of underlying disease. Primary efforts to control pain symptomatology should then be directed towards the elimination of the cause of the noxious stimuli rather than suppression of the symptoms. This general concept also applies to the management of the pain associated with malignant diseases. Unfortunately, the pain that complicates cancer is often a difficult and frustrating clinical problem. The complexity of pain problems in patients with cancer is of particular importance, since treatment available for controlling the primary malignant process is often palliative and noncurative in nature. While the incidence of severe intractable pain in advanced cancer is relatively low, there are many instances when pain becomes a major problem because of its refractoriness to specific antineoplastic therapy, thus necessitating the use of symptomatic treatment with analgesics.

Chronic pain differs from acute pain in that it no longer serves as a protective or warning function but has become an end unto itself. Although there are no data from large-scale national epidemiologic studies on the incidence and severity of cancer pain, the data from several surveys of small groups of patients in specific institutions suggest that moderate to

Table 1
Incidence of Cancer-Related Pain

Investigator	Number of Patients	Incidence of Pain
Wilkes	300	58%
Turgcross	500	80%
Foley	540	52–85%
Bonica	387	Early Disease—38%
		Terminal Phase—80%
Pannuti	290	64%
Parker	400	Inpatients—59%
		Outpatients—71%

severe pain is experienced in about one-third of patients with the intermediate stages of the disease, and by 60–80 percent of patients with advanced cancer (see Table 1).

Oster et al.[42] evaluated the degree of pain experienced by dying patients, with and without cancer, at a large medical center. Patterns of analgesic administration and physician and nurse progress notes demonstrated that patients dying with cancer had significantly higher preterminal daily pain ratings and significantly fewer pain-free days than patients dying without cancer. Of the 90 patients he studied, 75 percent of those with cancer endure various degrees of pain in their last days alive.

General Considerations

Evaluating Pain

Despite the poor prognosis associated with recurrent or advanced malignancies, the evaluation and ultimate control of pain is an important and complex clinical problem that deserves an intelligent appraisal of the patient's physical, mental, and moral resources, as well as his or her social usefulness. In each case, selection of appropriate therapy can be accomplished only after thorough consideration of several parameters.[1,2] These include (1) the location of the pain; (2) the mechanism of the pain; (3) the nature of the cause of the disease; (4) the physical and mental condition of the patient; and (5) the availability and practicality of the various methods of pain relief available.

A physician unfamiliar with the complexity of problems in cancer patients may be prone to attribute all complaints of pain to his disease. It is important to evaluate each new complaint, each time determining the etiology of the pain. Because of the conception of cancer in our society, as always fatal, as always painful and usually prolonged, the nonmalignant causes of pain are often overlooked. In many cases, pain symptomatology is debilitating, and, since definitive therapy is dependent upon correct diagnosis, the need for detailed history and complete diagnostic workup is obvious.

The first principle to remember in pain management is that a diag-

Table 2
Pain Syndromes in Patients with Cancer

I. Pain Associated with Direct Tumor Involvement
    A. Tumor infiltration of bone
        1. Base-of-skull metastases
            A. Jugular foramen
            B. Clivus
            C. Sphenoid sinus
        2. Vertebral-body metastases
            A. Subluxation of the atlas
            B. C-7–T-1 metastases
            C. L-1 metastases
            D. Sacral metastases
    B. Tumor infiltration of nerve
        1. Peripheral neuropathy
        2. Brachial, lumbar, sacral plexopathy
        3. Meningeal carcinomatosis
        4. Epidural spinal-cord compression
    C. Tumor infiltration of hollow viscus
II. Pain Associated with Cancer Therapy
    A. Pain occurring postsurgery
        1. Postthoracotomy pain
        2. Postmastectomy pain
        3. Postradical neck pain
        4. Phantom-limb pain
    B. Pain occurring postchemotherapy
        1. Peripheral neuropathy
        2. Postherpetic neuralgia
        3. Steroid pseudorheumatism
        4. Aseptic necrosis of bone
    C. Pain occurring postradiation
        1. Radiation fibrosis of the brachial plexus and lumbar plexus
        2. Radiation myelopathy
        3. Radiation-induced peripheral-nerve tumors
III. Pain Unrelated to Cancer or Cancer Therapy
    A. Diabetetic neuropathy
    B. Cervical- and lumbar-disc disease
    C. Rheumatoid arthritis

nosis of cancer does not necessarily mean that the malignant process is responsible for a particular episode of pain. As described by Foley,[43] the etiology of cancer pain may be classified into one of three major categories: (1) pain associated with direct tumor involvement; (2) pain associated with cancer therapy; and (3) pain unrelated to cancer or cancer therapy. In the average cancer hospital population, pain is caused by direct tumor involvement in approximately 75 percent of the patients. Twenty percent of the complaints of pain can be directly attributed to patient's cancer therapy and about 5 percent of the pain complaints will be unrelated to the patient's malignant disease (see Table 2).

Psychological Aspects of Pain

Psychologic variables, as well as sensory input, play an important role in the production of pain. Pain is a subjective emotional experience, and patient reaction to it varies tremendously from person to person, and even in the same person from time to time. Depending upon the emotional state of a patient, the perception of pain may vary considerably. Most patients who know or suspect that their pain may be due to cancer manifest emotional factors such as fear, apprehension, anxiety, and depression, which accentuate painful stimuli. Long-standing pain may eventually affect every aspect of patients' lives, with gradual but complete alteration in their attitudes toward their environment. If allowed to continue, the pain becomes an overwhelming problem that completely dominates a patient's life. Patients with chronic pain often do not become tolerant or accustomed to it, but rather seem to become increasingly more sensitive, and to suffer more as their disease progresses.

The physician's approach to this aspect of pain is critical for the success of any treatment plan. An attitude of helplessness or apparent lack of concern on the part of the physician is keenly sensed by most patients and may contribute to the patient's fears of death, or feelings of hopelessness and rejection. For these reasons, the ability to listen, discuss, and gain the confidence of the patient are necessary qualities in the good physician who manages patients with pain. Attempts to manage pain without considering the underlying emotional aspects will probably result in failure to relieve pain, and possibly lead to narcotic addiction or indirectly forcing the patient to seek costly, ineffective, and even dangerous quackery.

Mechanisms of Cancer-Related Pain

Host as well as tumor factors are involved in many situations characterized by pain. The pain associated with cancer presents no new or different physiologic problems concerning the cause and perception of pain.

It is usually caused, either directly or indirectly, by one or more of the following mechanisms:[3]

1. Compression of nerve roots, trunks, or plexus by tumor or by metastatic fractures of bones adjacent to nerves, which causes radiculopathy or neuropathy with sharp, well-localized, projected pain typical of neuralgia
2. Infiltration of the nerves and blood vessels by tumor cells, which results in perivascular and perineural lymphangitis with irritation of the sensory nerve endings and diffuse burning pain—the so-called sympathetic pain
3. Obstruction of a viscus, particularly the gastrointestinal or genitourinary tract, which produces true visceral pain that is characteristically described as dull, diffuse, and poorly localized
4. Partial or complete occlusion of blood vessels by an adjacent tumor that causes venous engorgement or arterial ischemia or both, and pain
5. Infiltration and tumefaction in tissue invested snugly by fascia, periosteum, or other pain-sensitive structures
6. Necrosis, infection, and inflammation of pain-sensitive structures produced by contiguous tumors, which can cause excruciating pain.

Principles of Pain Control

The management of cancer-related pain can be separated into two distinct approaches:[4] primary control or reversal of specific pathophysiologic events causing the noxious stimulation, and symptomatic control by alteration of the perception of pain in the central nervous system (see Table 3).

Primary Control

Obviously, the best treatment for any symptom is the treatment of the disease itself. When dealing with malignant disease, primary efforts to control pain involve, if at all possible, surgical, chemical, or radiotherapeutic removal of the pain-producing tumor. Even in cases beyond hope of cure, appropriate antitumor therapy often provides dramatic relief of pain and should always be tried, when indicated, before resorting solely to symptomatic control. Such palliative antitumor therapy should only be attempted at an intensity that is proportional to the expected benefit. In certain situations, the appropriate combination of primary and sympto-

Table 3
Analgesics and Other Drugs for Relief of Pain

Mechanisms of Interference With Pain	Drug Type
Reversal of specific pathophysiologic events, such as	
Infection	Antibiotics
Inflammation	Anti-inflammatory agents
Gout	Antihyperuricemic agents
Interference with specific chemical substance involved in pain reception peripherally	Antipyretic analgesics
Interference with conduction of pain away from affected site	Local anesthetics
Interference with central nervous system perception of pain and development of affective responses	Narcotic analgesics
Interference with anxiety, tension, or depression	Sedatives and hypnotics Phenothiazine tranquilizers Skeletal muscle relaxants Antidepressants
Interference with consciousness	Anesthetics

Reprinted, with permission, from Catalano RB: The medical approach to management of pain caused by cancer. Sem Oncol 2(4):380, 1975.

matic therapy may convert what appears to be a hopelessly advanced tumor in a patient with intractable pain into a treatable cancer and a comfortable patient.

An in-depth review of the primary methods of cancer control is beyond the scope of this discussion. However, mention of several general concepts of primary cancer therapy and how it relates to the management of pain seems appropriate.

Surgery

Certain cancer-related pain may be controlled with surgical intervention and should be considered independent of its potential for cure. Operations considered palliative in nature are commonly performed for known incurable cases. Examples of indications for this approach are bypass operations of tumors causing obstruction of a hollow viscus or large vein or artery. Pain due to this process is often severe and persistent and is usually not adequately relieved by systemic analgesics or neurosurgical interruption of the ascending pain pathways.

Ablation of endocrine glands by surgical castration not only has caused regression of advanced carcinoma of the breast and of the prostate[10,11] but also has often produced dramatic relief of pain and general improvement. Adrenalectomy and hypophysectomy have similar effects, particularly in certain tumors suspected of being hormone dependent, such as breast carcinoma.[12]

Irradiation

When the problem of pain due to metastatic tumor can be localized, the relief produced by palliative radiation therapy, while being sometimes unpredictable, is sufficiently striking in many situations to warrant consideration. In addition to producing somewhat rapid pain relief, irradiation introduces a local cytotoxic effect and retardation of neoplastic spread in the area of treatment.

The type of patients most likely to benefit from irradiation in regards to pain relief are those with metastatic bone disease from primary tumors of the glandular organs. Subjective pain relief has been reported in up to 90 percent of patients with bony metastasis from breast carcinoma and 65–75 percent of those with metastasis from primary prostate, thyroid, or renal carcinoma.[5]

In the management of the severe headaches associated with metastatic cancer to the brain the concomitant use of relatively high doses of corticosteroids for acute relief of symptoms coupled with palliative radiotherapy to the contents of the calvarium can improve or completely control the painful symptoms in over 85 percent of the patients.[6,7]

Chemotherapy

Control of the painful symptoms of cancer with the use of systemic cytotoxic agents is usually a consequence of objective response with shrinkage of the tumor mass. As a result, this method of control is often slow and unpredictable. However, certain methods of administration of chemotherapy have been developed using pain symptomatology as one of the primary indications for implementation. An example of this is control of liver pain caused by hepatic metastases by the use of regional intrahepatic arterial infusion chemotherapy. Administration of the antineoplastic agent via the hepatic artery permits a higher tissue-dose concentration into tumorous tissue while minimizing the potential systemic toxicity. This method of chemotherapy has been reported to produce symptomatic relief in up to 70 percent of those patients treated.[8,9]

Symptomatic Control

When the disease responsible for pain can no longer be treated specifically, the symptomatic treatment of the pain becomes essential. This approach involves the use of agents or procedures that modify or interrupt the painful stimuli without affecting the primary cause of the pain. Usually, attempts at symptomatic control require the use of systemic analgesics, psychologic techniques, neurosurgery, or nerve blocks.

Cancer pain is often controlled with systemic analgesics. Generally, the least potent analgesic capable of producing adequate relief should be used. Mild to moderate cancer pain can usually be controlled with nonnarcotic analgesics, alone or in combination. While the efficacy of narcotic analgesics for the severe pain of terminal malignancy is well known, premature use leads to early tolerance so that in the later stages of the disease massive doses of narcotics will not relieve the pain.

Nonnarcotic Analgesics

The most significant factor in the field of nonnarcotic analgesia is the failure of any of the newer nonnarcotic analgesics to displace aspirin as the agent of choice. Recent studies by Moertel,[13,14] comparing the relative effectiveness of 9 analgesics given by the oral route to relieve cancer pain, seem to confirm this. The first study was performed utilizing 57 ambulatory patients who had definite pain resulting from nonresectable cancer and compared the analgesic effect in a double-blind crossover study (Table 4). Of the 9 agents studied, aspirin 650 mg was superior to all agents tested. Mefenamic acid (Ponstel) 250 mg, pentazocine (Talwin) 50 mg, acetaminophen (Tylenol) 650 mg, phenacetin 650 mg, and codeine 65 mg also showed significant advantage over placebo. Propoxyphene (Darvon) 65 mg, ethoheptazine (Zactane) 75 mg, and promazine (Sparine) 25 mg gave no significant evidence of therapeutic activity, and each of these agents was significantly inferior to aspirin in analgesic effects.

Pentazocine produced sufficient gastrointestinal and central nervous system side effects to make this agent of dubious value for ambulatory patients. All other agents tested in the single-dose study did not produce significantly greater side effects than a placebo. It is also of interest to note the cost comparison included by the authors shows a several hundred percent higher cost of agents proven to be less effective than aspirin.

In a follow-up comparison of analgesics given in combination to 100 patients with pain due to cancer, the results were similar (Fig. 1). The

Table 4

Relative Therapeutic Effect of Oral Analgesics According to Mean
Percentage of Relief of Pain Achieved in 57 Patients

Analgesic Agent	Dose (mg)	Relief of Pain (%)	
Aspirin	650	62	Significantly superior to placebo ($p < 0.05$)
Pentazocine	50	54	
Acetaminophen	650	50	
Phenacetin	650	48	
Mefenamic acid	250	47	
Codiene	65	46	
Propoxyphene	65	43	Significantly inferior to aspirin ($p < 0.05$)
Ethoheptazine	75	38	
Promazine	25	37	
Placebo	—	32	

From Moertel.[13] Reprinted, with permission, from Catalano RB: The medical approach to management of pain caused by cancer. Sem Oncol 2(4):382, 1975.

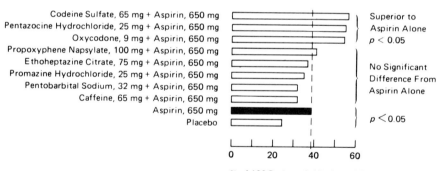

% of 100 Patients Achieving > 50% Relief

Fig. 1. *Comparative therapeutic effects of placebo, aspirin alone, and aspirin combinations according to percentage of patients achieving significant (i.e., more than 50%) relief of pain. (From Moertel[14] and reprinted, with permission from Catalano RB: The medical approach to the management of pain caused by cancer. Sem Oncol 2(4):382, 1975.)*

combination of aspirin 650 mg, plus either codeine 65 mg, oxycodone 9.76 mg, or pentazocine 25 mg, produced significantly greater pain relief than aspirin alone. The combination of aspirin 650 mg, plus either caffeine 65 mg, pentobarbital 32 mg, promazine 25 mg, ethoheptazine 75 mg, or propoxyphene napsylate 100 mg did not show significant advantage in analgesic effect over aspirin alone. The side effects for a single dose of the effective combinations were essentially equal and clinically tolerable.

It has never been demonstrated that aspirin, phenacetin, and caffeine formulations (APC) are superior to aspirin alone in providing relief from pain of any etiology.[15] There is much evidence that persons who over-use this type of combination are at risk of developing what is now called "analgesic nephropathy" characterized by papillary necrosis and interstitial nephritis.[16]

There are, of course, conditions that preclude the use of aspirin despite its superiority to other agents. Among these are preexisting histories of gastrointestinal ulceration or hemorrhage, hypersensitivity reactions, and certain asthmatic conditions. Increasing emphasis is being given to aspirin as a major cause of hospital admissions due to gastrointestinal bleeding. Most reports on the incidence of aspirin-induced gastrointestinal hemorrhage conclude that at least 50 percent and up to 94 percent of patients admitted with that diagnosis have a positive history of recent salicylate ingestion. Perry[17] stated that almost 100 percent of patients admitted to hospitals bleeding from acute gastric erosions and with no radiologically demonstrable lesion have given a history of prior consumption of aspirin.

Intolerance to aspirin can also manifest itself in the form of an allergic response.[18] This is particularly important in evaluating a patient with a history of asthma. Signs and symptoms of allergic response observed when patients allergic to aspirin were challenged with other commonly used analgesics make clear the need for caution in prescribing analgesic agents to patients sensitive to aspirin.[19]

The clinical signs of aspirin allergy are usually first seen in the third or fourth decade of life. Watery nasal discharge and, later, nasal polypi are generally the first signs. Bronchial asthma develops after a variable interval of weeks to years; it is often precipitated by nasal polypectomy or by ingestion of aspirin. Thereafter, persistent wheezing occurs with severe— even life-threatening—attacks of asthma after aspirin is taken. Avoiding aspirin does not abolish the asthma, but it is usually well controlled by small regular doses of corticosteroids. Alcohol, indomethacin, amidopyrine, and other drugs and chemicals may precipitate asthmatic attacks in patients with this condition.

Five patients who had a clear history of asthmatic attacks after taking aspirin were challenged with the following drugs: paracetamol, 500 mg; mefenamic acid, 250 mg; indomethacin, 25 mg; dextropropoxyphene, 65 mg; phenylbutazone, 100 mg; and inert white lactose tablets. Aspirin itself was not used, for fear of producing a dangerous attack. The forced expiratory volume (in 1 second) was measured every 30 minutes on a spirometer.

Marked decreases in forced expiratory volume, accompanied in some cases by asthma and rhinitis, were observed after administration of most of these analgesics. Paracetamol, indomethacin, and mefenamic acid caused the most severe and frequent rhinitis reactions. Dextropropoxyphene caused a severe reaction in one case. Phenylbutazone did not have any untoward effects in any of the patients tested.

The results of the study underline the need for great caution when prescribing analgesic drugs to patients sensitive to aspirin. Exacerbations of asthma or increases in steroid requirements in patients with conditions requiring analgesics should be evaluated in the light of evidence that analgesics may cause severe bronchoconstriction.

Aspirin has also demonstrated an ability to inhibit collagen-induced release of adenine diphosphate (ADP) from platelets, resulting in impaired aggregation of platelets.[20] This effect may prove to be therapeutically beneficial in patients with ischemic heart disease; however, it may well be detrimental if used concomitantly with other agents known to affect the clotting mechanisms. Physicians desiring not to prescribe aspirin or to warn patients to avoid aspirin-containing products will find over 500 products available on the market with at least one of many salicylate derivatives as their active ingredient.

Acetaminophen, although devoid of any substantial anti-inflammatory action, runs a close second to aspirin as an effective nonnarcotic analgesic–antipyretic agent.[21] It possesses the advantage of not causing the gastritis associated with aspirin ingestion. It also lacks the platelet inhibitory powers of aspirin. Chronic high-dose abuse of acetaminophen has been associated with production of hepatotoxicity and also the analgesic nephropathy described previously.

The propoxyphene series of prescription drugs (Darvon, Dolene) remains one of the most prescribed agents of any class in the United States despite eight known controlled prospective studies disputing their effectiveness.[13,14,22–27] Much of the popularity is based on claims of less adverse effects when compared to equal doses of codeine, but this may not be true for equianalgesic potency.

Usual adverse effects noted with the use of therapeutic doses of propoxyphene include nausea, vomiting, constipation, dizziness, and drowsiness. While the addiction potential of propoxyphene is low as compared to the opioids, it is important to note the increasing incidence of overdosage and subsequent death due to propoxyphene abuse. Young, in 1972,[28] reported nine deaths due to propoxyphene overdosage; the probable cause for death being apnea followed by convulsions. Due to the structural similarity between propoxyphene and methadone, the prompt use of the narcotic antagonist naloxone (Narcan) can effectively reverse the respiratory depression and avoid most deaths.

Pentazocine (Talwin) is a benzomorphan derivative which possesses a weak morphine antagonist action. In early clinical studies 30 mg of pentazocine was found to have an analgesic activity equivalent to 75–100 mg of meperidine or 10 mg of morphine. After intramuscular administration of pentazocine the onset of analgesia is noticeable after 20 minutes. The duration of analgesic effect is only about 3 hours.

The disadvantages of pentazocine as an analgesic are its irritative effect at the site of injection and its relatively short duration of action. The analgesia produced by oral administration of pentazocine is not dependable, possibly because of the poor absorption of the drug in the gastrointestinal tract and its extensive metabolism when given orally.

Beaver et al.[29] showed that it required 90 mg of oral pentazocine to produce analgesia equivalent to that produced with 30 mg of parenteral pentazocine for cancer patients with chronic pain. The same investigators had previously shown that it required 30 mg of pentazocine intramuscularly, to produce an equianalgesic effect of 5 mg of morphine in the same type of patients.[30]

The most common side effects of pentazocine consist of sedation, drowsiness, nausea, vomiting, and blurring of vision. Side effects that have occurred at times include hallucinations, fever, urinary retention, euphoria, changes in mood, constipation, dry mouth, and respiratory depression. The propensity for producing central nervous system side effects, particularly vertigo, reduces substantially the value of this drug in ambulatory patients.

The original claims that pentazocine was nonaddicting has proved incorrect. Its dependence potential is substantially less than that of morphine or meperidine. At this point, however, no conclusion may be drawn as to whether pentazocine has less addiction potential than codeine, the drug to which it is frequently compared in the commercial literature. Dependence on parenteral pentazocine has been reported by several investigators.[31] Doses exceeding 180 mg daily for at least 1 month predispose susceptible individuals to morphine-like dependence. To date there are no reports of dependence on the oral form of the drug.

The final limiting factor in the use of pentazocine is in respect to the respiratory depressant effects produced by this agent. Bellville[32] found that pentazocine produced the same amount of respiratory depression as morphine when each was given in equianalgesic doses. Reichenber,[33] in reporting a case of pentazocine-induced respiratory depression, suggested that the problems seen with morphine when used in patients with limited respiratory function are also seen with pentazocine.

Narcotic Analgesics

Narcotic analgesics or opiates are terms intended to denote a group of naturally occurring, semisynthetic, and synthetic drugs which effectively relieve pain without producing loss of consciousness and which have the potential to produce physical dependence. Although the narcotic analgesics may vary with one another in quantitative effects and even in some qualitative effects, the similarity of the pharmacologic and therapeutic properties of these drugs permits their discussion as a class. The relative differences of the available agents are summarized in Table 5.

Chemically, narcotic analgesics may be classified as phenanthrene, phenylpiperidine, or diphenylheptane derivatives (see Table 6). Modifications of the parent structure produces changes in the pharmacologic activity that may alter or eliminate the analgesic potential but increase its antitussive, antidiarrheal, or antagonistic properties.

Pharmacologic Actions

Central Nervous System Effects

Narcotic analgesics exert their primary effect on the central nervous system.[34] The precise biochemical mechanism by which they produce their effects is not known. It has been suggested that opiates may act on the diencephalon and frontal lobes of the brain to cause modification of the central nervous system response to pain,[36] or may affect the patient's emotional response (perception) to pain.[34]

In addition to analgesia, the central nervous system response to the administration of an opiate may produce a broad spectrum of effects. The type and degree of response seems to be attributed largely to the condi-

Table 5
Pharmacologic Activity of Analgesics

Drugs	Analgesic[a]	Antitussive	Sedation	Emesis	Respiratory Depressant	Constipation	Addictive	Equianalgesic Dose[b] (mg)	Average Adult Dose[c] (mg)
Morphine	V++	++	++	++	++	++	++	10	10–15
Diacetylmorphine (Heroin)	V++	++	++	+	++	+	+++	4	Illegal
Ethylmorphine (Dionin)	V+	+++	++		++		?		15–60
Nalorphine (Nalline)	V++	+	+or 0	+	++	+		8	15–10[d]
Codeine	V+	+++	+	+	+	++	+	120	15–60 (8–20)
Hydromorphone (Dilaudid)	V++	++	+	+	++	+	++	1	1–2
Methyldihydromorphinone (Metopon)	V+++	++	++	++	+++	+	+	3	3–9
Hydrocodone (Dicodid, etc.)	V++	+++				?	++		(5–10)
Dihydrocodeine (Paracodin, etc).	V++	+++		+	+		+	60	30–60
Dihydrodesoxymorphine-D (Desomorphine)	V+++					+	+++	1	
Oxymorphone (Numorphan)	V++	+		+++	+++	+++	+++	1	0.5–1

Oxycodone (Percodan)	V++	+++	++	++	++	++	++	10	10–15 (3–5)
Nalmexone (EN-1620A)	V++		++	+	++		?		70–90
Levorphanol (Levo-Dromoran)	V++	++	++	+	++	+			
Racemorphan (Dromoran)	V++	++	++	+	++	?	++	2	2–4
Dextrorphan (Dromoran)	V++	++	+	+	++	+	++	2.5	1–5
Dextromethorphan (Romilar)		+++	?	?	++				(10–20)
Levallorphan (Lorfan)	V++	+	+	+	++			2	1d
Pentazocine (Talwin)	V++		++ or 0	++	++	+	+	30	20–30
Naloxone (Narcan)					++	+	+		0.5–1d
Naltrexone (EN-1639A)					++		+		0.5d
Methadone (Dolophine, etc.)	V++	++	+	+	++	+	+	8	5–15
Propoxyphene (Darvon)	V+		+	+	+	?	+	130	32–65
Levopropoxyphene (Novrad)		+++	++	++	++				(50–100)
Noracymethadol	V++	++	+	++	++		+	10	8–30
Dextromoramide (Palfium, etc.)	V++	++	+	++	++	+	+	5	5–10
Meperidine (Demerol, etc.)	V++	+	+	?	++	+	++	100	30–75

(continued)

Table 5 (*continued*)
Pharmacologic Activity of Analgesics

Drugs	Analgesic[a]	Antitussive	Sedation	Emesis	Respiratory Depressant	Constipation	Addictive	Equianalgesic Dose[b] (mg)	Average Adult Dose[c] (mg)
Alphaprodine (Nisentil)	V++		++	+	++	+	++	40	25–60
Anileridine (Leritine)	V++	+	++	?	++	+	++	30	25–50
Piminodine (Alvodine)	V++		+	+	++	+	++	7.5	10–20
Ethoheptazine (Zactane)	V+				++		+	200	100

From Morris.[35] Reprinted, with permission, from Catalano RB: The medical approach to management of pain caused by cancer. Sem Oncol 2(4):384–385, 1975.

[a]V = Visceral and deep traumatic pain in contrast to somatic and joint pains.
+ = Degree of activity from the least (+) to the greatest (+++) activity.
O = Produces the opposite effect.
? = Questionable activity.
    Blank space indicates that no such activity has been reported for this compound.
[b]Equianalgesic to morphine sulfate, 10 mg SC.
[c]Oral antitussive dose in parenthesis.
[d]Used solely as narcotic antagonist and not as analgesic.

380

Table 6
Chemical Classification of Narcotic Analgesics

Phenanthrene Derivatives
  Codeine
  Hydromorphone (Dilaudid)
  Levorphanol tartrate (Levo-Dromoran)
  Morphine sulfate
  Opium alkaloids, concentrated (Pantopon)
  Oxycodone
  Oxymorphone (Numorphan)
Phenylpiperidine Derivatives
  Alphaprodine (Nisentil)
  Anileridine (Leritine)
  Fentanyl (Sublimaze)
  Meperidine (Demerol)
Diphenylheptane Derivatives
  Methadone (Dolophine)

Reprinted, with permission, from Catalano RB: The medical approach to management of pain caused by cancer. Sem Oncol 2(4):386, 1975.

tions under which an opiate was administered.[37] In the presence of significant pain, the narcotic-induced analgesia is accompanied by sedation and alteration of mood characterized by euphoria. In this case, the sedative action and sleep may be an incidental occurrence resulting from the relief of pain and from its accompanying mental and physical exhaustion. When a narcotic is given in the absence of pain, the resultant effect may be one of dysphoria, apprehension, apathy, or mental confusion, and rarely hallucinations and delirium. In certain patients, especially those with a history of seizure disorders, administration of a narcotic analgesic produces a stimulating effect in the motor sphere, causing a lowering of the seizure threshold which may precipitate convulsions in a previously controlled patient.

Other centrally mediated effects of narcotic analgesics will be discussed in relation to their importance on end-organ function.

Respiratory Effects

Opiates produce respiratory depression by a direct effect on the chemoreceptors of the respiratory centers in the brain stem. This effect seems to result from a decreased sensitivity and responsiveness to increases in serum carbon dioxide tension (pCO_2). The narcotic analgesics also depress the pontine medullary centers responsible for regulation of the rate of respiration, thereby altering voluntary control of respiration. Initially, there is a depression of tidal volume followed by a decreased respiratory rate. Clinically, the narcotic-induced respiratory depression is characterized by slow, irregular, periodic respiration.

Since both primary and metastatic malignant involvement of the pulmonary system is a common situation, the importance of determining the extent of any respiratory insufficiency prior to treatment becomes evident. The additional carbon dioxide retention induced by the administration of opiates may be sufficient to precipitate coma.

The diagnostic and treatment dilemmas may be further complicated by the fact that the patient may continue to breathe, despite the coma, through the hypoxic drive mechanism regulated by the carotid and aortic chemoreceptors. If the responsible physician is not aware of this situation, the impulse to support the patient with administration of oxygen without assisted or controlled ventilation will eliminate the hypoxic drive and rapidly produce apnea. Additional problems relating to the hazards of the respiratory suppression induced by opiates arise in the evaluation of patients with suspected intracranial malignancies. The increased arterial pCO_2 will result in a cerebrovascular dilatation with a consequent rise in cerebral blood flow and cerebrospinal fluid pressure. In this case, administration of a narcotic analgesic ma j cause what seems to be a paradoxical increase in the pain.

A second action of the opiates on the respiratory system is worth mentioning here, despite the fact it is not directly related to pain control. This is the ability of opiates to suppress the cough reflex. The antitussive action is a consequence of the direct effect on the cough centers in the medulla. This may occur with doses lower than those required for analgesia. Therapeutic suppression of the cough reflex has been accomplished with opiate cogeners devoid of significant analgesic activity (i.e., dextromethorphan). In the treatment of pain this action could theoretically become an adverse effect that may need to be considered in the final choice of agents. The cough reflex is one of the body's natural defense mechanisms against invasion by foreign substances via the respiratory tract. Administration of certain narcotics nulifies this mechanism. Considering the fact that malignant disease may well be an expression of a compromised host response system, or that a patient may receive immunosuppressive agents as part of his or her therapy, suppresison of cough mechanisms becomes an undesirable effect.

Gastrointestinal Effects

Therapeutic doses of narcotic analgesics produce a variety of effects on the gastrointestinal system as a result of both direct and centrally mediated mechanisms. Gastric, biliary, and pancreatic secretions are decreased by opiates, causing delay in digestion. Smooth muscle tone of the bowel is decreased in intensity and frequency of propulsive contractions. The ultimate result is constipation. Usually, the morphine cogeners, meperidine and its cogeners, and methadone are less constipating than morphine. The smooth muscle tone in the biliary tract, especially at the sphincter of Oddi, is increased. This may cause a rise in the common bile duct pressure from 20 ml to as high as 200–300 ml of water and precipitate biliary colic. Such spasm may result in plasma amylase and lipase levels as much as 2–15 times the normal values. Because of this effect, plasma amylase and lipase determinations should not be performed within 24 hours after a narcotic analgesic has been given.

Nausea and vomiting is a common occurrence with the initial administration of a narcotic analgesic. This effect may indirectly result from a central stimulation of the chemoreceptor trigger zone in the medulla oblongata. With continued administration, however, the narcotic analgesics depress the vomiting center; therefore, subsequent doses of these agents are unlikely to produce vomiting by this mechanism. Ambulatory patients and those patients not experiencing severe pain seem to have a higher incidence of nausea and vomiting than those who are in a supine position due to an enhanced vestibular sensitivity induced by narcotic analgesics.

Urinary Tract Effects

Narcotic analgesics increase smooth muscle tone in the urinary tract and may induce spasms. Although the response of the ureters is quite variable, these drugs may increase the tone and amplitude of contractions, especially of the lower third of the ureter. In the urinary bladder, tone of the detrusor muscle is increased, possibly resulting in urinary urgency. There is also an increase in the tone of the vesical sphincter, which may make urination difficult. Patients with prostatic hypertrophy or urethral stricture may be prone to urinary retention and oliguria when narcotic analgesics are used.

The initial decresae in urinary excretion usually seen following administration of narcotics may be an indirect effect of a central action causing an increased secretion of antidiuretic hormone (ADH). Results of one study,[38] however, suggest that decreased urine output may occur without any apparent release of excess ADH and may be attributed to decreased renal plasma flow or increased reabsorption from the renal tubules.

Cardiovascular Effects

The circulatory effects of narcotics are caused by their central action with depression of the vasomotor center and stimulation of medullary vagal nuclei, or by a histamine release and a direct effect on peripheral effector cells. When therapeutic doses are given to supine patients, narcotic analgesics have little cardiovascular effect. When the supine patient assumes a head-up position, however, orthostatic hypotension and fainting may occur as a result of peripheral vasodilatation. The myocardial tone and contractility is usually increased by small doses and decreased by large doses of narcotics.

The adverse circulatory effect of opiates are increased in the presence of reduced circulatory blood volume and with the concomitant use of drugs which have α-adrenergic blocking activity (e.g., phenothiazines).

With the exception of meperidine, which has anticholinergic effects, narcotics usually decrease heart rate. They may also cause sinus bradyarrhythmias that can be abolished by atropine.

Endocrine Effects

Opiates produce endocrinologic alterations, some of which may be related to central nervous system effects. In addition to the inappropriate ADH secretion previously mentioned, narcotic analgesics have been reported to inhibit the release of adrenocorticotropic and gonadotropic hormone from the pituitary. This results in decreased plasma and urinary 17-hydroxycorticosteroid and 17-ketosteroid levels. The secondary nature of the hypofunction has been demonstrated by the production of normal responses to administration of the appropriate tropic hormone.

Narcotic analgesics have also been associated with inhibition of release of thyroid-stimulating hormone, leading to a clinically detectable suppression of thyroid hormone production. Basal metabolism rates may be decreased by 10–20 percent in patients receiving narcotic analgesia.

Hyperglycemia may also occur in patients receiving opiates. This response is thought to be secondary to a direct action on the paraventricular receptor sites near the foramen of Monro, or as a result of stimulating the release of epinephrine.

Choice of Narcotic Analgesics

Although most of these drugs produce a similar quality of analgesia in equianalgesic doses, factors such as oral effectiveness, duration of action, degree of action on smooth muscle, route of metabolism, and most important, individual variation in patient response should be considered in the selection of a specific narcotic analgesic. No single drug or procedure is always or almost always best for every patient. The final criterion, as with any treatment of pain, is patient comfort.

The most effective analgesics thus far tested have been the morphine surrogates but, even though the range of relative potency of these drugs extends up to several hundred-fold, well controlled studies to date have failed to show appreciable differences in their "ceiling" effects. Relative potency is, of course, merely an expression of the ratio of doses to produce a given effect, and a more potent drug is not necessarily a more effective drug.

Among drugs of the same class, differences in side effect liability at equianalgesic doses tend to be insignificant. Among drugs of different classes, however, the spectra of side effects can be quite different and may be important considerations. With increasing doses, higher degrees of pain relief can be obtained before encountering limiting toxic effects with drugs of the morphine type than is possible with the narcotic-antagonist analgesics or methotrimeprazine (a phenothiazine), or drugs of the anti-pyretic analgesic type such as the salicylates, para-aminophenols, and phenyl pyrrazoles. Thus differences do exist among different classes of drugs as to their relative analgesic potentials which do not necessarily correlate with their relative analgesic potencies, or to any demonstrable decrease in increment of analgesic effect with dose. Most severe pain can generally be controlled only by drugs with high analgesic potentials, although other undesirable side effect considerations (such as drug dependence liability) often dictate the choice of a drug with a lower potential in individual situations.

The determination of equivalent analgesic doses is usually based upon a comparison of one drug with another, with the most frequently used standard drugs being either morphine or aspirin. Commonly, the relative potencies or equianalgesic doses are expressed either in terms of peak (zenith) or the time–effect curve, or in terms of total effect, i.e., the area under the time–effect curve. When the time–effect curves are not the same for two drugs, neither the peak nor the total effect parameters adequately express the equivalent analgesic doses. The peak effects of a short-acting drug such as alphaprodine or hydromorphone may be underestimated when compared in terms of equivalent total effect to a longer-acting drug such as morphine or methadone, and vice versa. Virtually all drugs are less potent and more variable in their analgesic effects when given orally than when given parenterally. When a drug is given orally, its time–effect curve also tends to be flatter and more extended than when it is administered parenterally, so that greater differences in potency are noted in peak rather than total effects. Appreciable differences exist in the relative oral–parenteral analgesic potencies of various narcotic drugs. Drugs such as morphine and oxymorphone have relatively low oral-to-parenteral potency ratios, whereas other drugs such as codeine, oxycodone, and methadone have relatively high oral-to-parenteral potency ratios. Select-

Table 7
Comparison of Time of Onset and Duration of Action
of Narcotic Analgesics

Drugs	Route of Administration	Time to Onset or Peak Effect (min)	Duration of Action (hr)
Anileridine	PO, IM, SC	15	2–3
Alphaprodine	SC	5–10	2
	IV	1–2	0.5–1
Codeine	PO, SC, IM	15–30	4–6
Fentanyl	IM	7–15	1–2
	IV	3–5	0.5–1
Hydromorphone	PO, SC, IM	15–30	4–5
Levorphanol	IV	20	4–6
	PO, IM, SC	60–90	6–8
Meperidine	PO	40–60	2–4
	SC	40–60	2–4
	IM	30–50	2–4
Methadone	PO	30–60	4–6
	IM	30–60	4–6
	SC	30–60	4–6
Morphine	SC	50–90	up to 7
	IM	30–60	up to 7
	IV	20	up to 7
Oxycodone	PO	10–15	3–6
Oxymorphone	Rectal	15–30	3–6
	SC	10–15	3–6
	IM	10–15	3–6
	IV	5–10	3–6

Reprinted, with permission, from Catalano RB: The medical approach to management of
pain caused by cancer. Sem Oncol 2(4):389, 1975.

ing the appropriate dose and route of administration can make the difference between effective and ineffective use of a drug (see Table 7).

Tolerance will develop on the repeated administration of drugs of the
narcotic class, and is associated with a parallel shift of the dose–effect
curves to the right such that a larger dose will be required to produce the
same effect that a small dose produced initially. Tolerance to one narcotic
drug has long been known to produce tolerance to other narcotics, but
recent evidence would seem to indicate that analgesic cross-tolerance is
not complete.[39] Tolerance to the respiratory depressant, emetic, hypnotic,
and other central nervous system effects of narcotics develops at essentially the same rate as tolerance to the analgesic effects, so that increasing
the dose of a narcotic to keep pace with the analgesic needs of the patient
carries with it little risk of increased toxicity.

Physical dependence to narcotics appears to develop at approximately the same rate as does tolerance, and characteristic narcotic abstinence signs can be precipitated in a tolerant patient if his narcotic is suddenly withdrawn.

Patients who have received therapeutic doses of morphine several times a day for 1–2 weeks will have only mild symptoms once the drug is stopped. These may even go entirely unnoticed.

Withdrawal symptoms can differ quantitatively according to which opiate the patient is physically dependent upon. A general rule is that opiates with a shorter duration of action, e.g., meperidine, anileridine, etc., tend to produce shorter but more intense symptoms.

Drugs that have a longer duration of action, e.g., methadone, will produce a milder but a more prolonged period of withdrawal symptoms. This general rule holds true only when the drugs are stopped abruptly; not if a narcotic antagonist is administered. For example, if a naloxzone were to be administered to a patient physically dependent on methadone, the withdrawal symptoms should be extremely severe.

The fear of producing drug addiction should never prevent the administration of morphine or other analgesics in patients with terminal malignant disease. Unfortunately, this effect of narcotic analgesics has been shown to be a major cause of underprescribing, even for patients with severe pain caused by a terminal malignant disease. Results of a study on narcotic use in two hospitals showed that 32 percent of the patients remained in severe distress and 41 percent were in moderate distress despite the administration of a narcotic, usually meperidine.[40] A review of the medication records showed that the dosage ordered for these patients was lower than that usually recommended, and that the amount they actually received was substantially less than ordered.

By surveying physicians to elicit their attitudes about the use of this narcotic analgesic, it was determined that the principle reasons for underprescribing were a misunderstanding of (1) the optimal effective dosages and the duration of the drug's action, and (2) the possible serious side effects, especially dependence-liability and withdrawal symptoms. These physicians underestimated the dosage requirements and overestimated the duration of action of the drug. Because they had misconceptions concerning the danger of addiction, they indicated a reluctance to order an increase in the dosage or in the frequency of administration, even for patients with severe pain caused by a terminal malignant disease.

Actually, experience has demonstrated that the likelihood of a hospitalized patient becoming "addicted" to meperidine is very slight. A report points out that "Ironically, under-treatment with analgesic medication may also encourage craving for the drug."[40] This might be misinterpreted to suggest that the patient is developing a degree of dependence, which, in turn, may cause the physician to reduce the dose when it actually should be increased to ease the patient's discomfort. Moreover, it should be kept in mind that severe pain can best be relieved by morphine or its potent cogeners, and that it may be necessary to prescribe a more potent agent in place of an intermediately acting one in order to provide adequate relief. Most patients who are given a morphine-like drug for relief of pain, especially in a hospital, are able to discontinue its use without difficulty even though they have developed mild degrees of dependence; only a small percentage become compulsive abusers.

Addiction and tolerance may possibly be delayed with use of a dose adequate to control the pain. Narcotics should be offered at regular intervals. This recommendation is based upon principles of operant conditioning.[41] The traditional method of giving narcotics when the patient complains of pain makes the administration of the drug contingent on the patient's complaint of pain. Thus, the pharmacologic and psychologic effects of the drug administration become a positive reinforcer for chronic pain behavior and may facilitate addiction. Using the operant conditioning strategy, it is first necessary to determine the average duration of pain relief produced by the chosen drug given in response to a patient's request during a period of a couple of days. Once the time duration of relief is ascertained, the drug is given at fixed intervals which are just short of the predetermined period of relief. This strategy makes the administration of the narcotic not contingent on pain, but rather on "nonpain" or well behavior.

Combining the narcotic with barbiturates, chloropromazine, or amphetamine may also help by reducing the patient's fear of the pain. Fear may escalate pain and lead to greater need for the narcotic.

Brompton's Cocktail

Brompton's cocktail is an oral, liquid analgesic mixture which has been used in Great Britain and Canada for a number of years. There are numerous variations of this mixture appearing in probably as many pharmacies throughout the country. The official preparation according to the British National Formulary is morphine 10 mg, cocaine 10 mg, ethol alcohol 95 percent 5 ml, cherry syrup 5 ml, chloroform water qs 20 ml. It appeared from the literature that Brompton's cocktail may be more effective in the treatment of pain because of interaction between its various ingredients: narcotics plus alcohol equals potentiation; narcotics plus phenothiazines equals potentiation; alcohol plus phenothiazines equals potentiation. In actuality, Brompton's cocktail is no more than a traditional British way of administering oral morphine to cancer patients in pain. The value of the cocaine and alcoholic base of the mixture is questioned.

Recent studies by Forest et al.[44] have demonstrated that the addition of amphetamines to the morphine administration may well potentiate the analgesic activity. In a double-blind study of 450 patients, each receiving morphine sulfate alone or morphine sulfate with 5–10 mg of dextroamphetamine, the combinations of dextroamphetamine 10 mg with morphine was twice as effective as morphine alone, and the combination with 5 mg was 1½ times as potent as morphine alone. In simple performance tests and in measures of side effects, dextroamphetamine generally offsets the undesirable effects of morphine (sedation and loss of alertness) while increasing the analgesia. The effects on blood pressure, pulse, and respiration were insignificant.

Based upon this observation, as well as the desire to maintain patients in a pain-free state on oral preparations, we recently have developed a modification of Brompton's mixture with significant success in achieving complete analgesia. This modified formulation consists of morphine sulfate 30 mg and dextroamphetamine 5 mg, in an aromatic elixir base of 10 ml. This is prescribed initially as a dose of 10 ml repeated every 6 hours with the exception of eliminating the dextroamphetamine from the preparation given at bedtime. This preparation has rendered many people pain-free but able to maintain mental alertness and to function properly.

New Methods of Morphine Administration

Several reports have appeared in the literature recently regarding attempts at the treatment of intractable pain by the use of the chronic intravenous infusion of morphine.[45-47] Doses of morphine ranging from 30 to 144 mg/hour have been administered relatively safely to terminal cancer patients with successful analgesia being achieved. Remarkably, the patients remained reasonably coherent and alert with this method of administering the morphine. Several points must be considered when placing a patient on this method of narcotic administration. These precautions are: (1) That the use of a narcotic antagonist is contraindicated; therefore, respiratory depression must be treated by mechanical means only. One must remember that narcotic antagonists reverse all of the effects of the narcotic, including morphine effects on neurotransmitters. Thus the administration of a narcotic antagonist may result in a sympathetic crisis and all of its subsequent ramifications. (2) Infusion must be administered through a controlled system (i.e., mechanical pumping device) that will signal the nursing staff if the infusion is obstructed in any way or running at an excessive rate of speed. This is critical consideration in a patient population because if the flow is interrupted for any length of time, the patient may undergo withdrawal. (3) Rate changes should only be carried out after evaluation of patient status by a trained clinical observer who is familiar with the objective and subjective effects of morphine in this select patient population. It is not surprising that most patients will be less lethargic and more coherent when receiving morphine by a constant intravenous infusion system since one avoids peaks and valleys in morphine blood levels. The result is a patient who does not fluctuate between toxic levels of the agent and subtherapeutic levels of the morphine. Not only does constant infusion eliminate the peaks and valleys, it also decreases the anxiety levels in these patients caused by the anticipation of their next pain injection.

Until more information becomes available it would not seem appropriate to advocate the use of continuous intravenous infusions of morphine in all terminal cancer patients. This mode of administration should be reserved for patients who failed to respond to conventional means of pain treatment. The long-term effects of narcotics on body homeostasis are unknown; therefore, one should approach this area with extreme caution.

Summary

Every physician must sometime manage pain associated with malignant disease. Despite the hopeless prognosis, the problem of pain deserves an intelligent appraisal and a systematic plan for relief to conserve the patient's physical, mental, and moral resources and social usefulness as long as possible. Keeping in mind that the major objective in treating the pain of advanced cancer is to keep the patient both free of pain and fully alert, the selection of a method of tumor therapy from an array of alternatives demands study of the individual patient and careful consideration of the appropriate measures, the possibilities for success, and the limitations, benefits, and risks involved. With comprehensive attention to the physical and personal needs of the patient and his or her family, the cancer patient's pain can be managed within a total framework of medical care. It is, therefore, only the rare cancer patient who will require referral to a psychiatric consultation for neurosurgical procedures as the only means of controlling their complaints of pain.

References

1. Bonica JJ; Fundamental considerations of chronic pain therapy. Postgrad Med 53:81–95, 1973
2. Murphy TM: Cancer pain. Postgrad Med 53;187–194, 1973
3. Bonica JJ: The Management of Pain. Philadelphia, Lea & Febiger, 1953
4. Halpern LM: Analgesics and other drugs for relief of pain. Postgrad Med 53:91–100, 1973
5. Parker RG: Pain relief for the cancer patients through selective radiation therapy. Northwest Med 69:1022–1025, 1968
6. Horton J, Barter OH, Olsen KB: The management of metastases to brain by irradiation and corticosteroids. Am J Roentgenol Radiat Ther Nucl Med 111:334–336, 1971
7. Weinstein EA: The effect of dexamethasone on brain edema in patients with metastatic brain tumors. Neurology 23:121–129, 1973
8. Cady B, Oberfield RA: Regional infusion chemotherapy of hepatic metastases from carcinoma of the colon. Am J Surg 127:220–226, 1974
9. Massey WH, Fletcher WS, Judkins MP, et al: Hepatic artery infusion for metastatic malignancy using precutaneous-placed catheters. Am J Surg 121:160–164, 1971
10. Kennedy BJ, Fortung IE: Therapeutic castration in the treatment of advanced breast cancer. Cancer 17:1197–1202, 1964
11. Scott WW: Rationale and results of primary endocrine therapy in patients with prostatic cancer. Cancer 32:1119–1125, 1973
12. Fracchia AA, Farrow JH, Miller TR: Hypophysectomy as compared to adrenalectomy in the treatment of advanced breast cancer. Surg Gynecol Obstet 133:241, 1971
13. Moertel CG, Ohmann DL, Taylor WF, et al: A comparative evaluation of marketed analgestic drugs. N Engl J Med 286:813–815, 1972
14. Moertel CG, Ohmann DL, Taylor WF, et al: Relief of pain by oral medications. JAMA 229:55–59, 1974
15. Beaver WT: Mild analgesics: A review of their clinical pharmacology, Part II. Am J Med Sci 251:576–599, 1966
16. Abels: Analgesic nephropathy. Clin Pharmacol Therap 12:583–587, 1971
17. Perry DJ, Wood PHN: Relationship between aspirin taking and gastrointestinal hemorrhage. Gut 8:301–308, 1967
18. Chafee FH: Aspirin intolerance. I. Frequency in an allergic population. J Allergy Clin Immunol—53:193–199, 1974

19. Smith AP: Response of aspirin-allergic patients to challenge by some analgesics in common use. Br Med J 2:494–496, 1971

20. Weiss HJ, Aledorf LM: Impaired platelet/connective tissue reaction in man after aspirin ingestion. Lancet 2:499, 1967

21. Ruter S, Montgomery WW: Aspirin vs. acetaminophen after tonsilectomy. Arch Otolaryngol 80:214–217, 1964

22. Cass LJ, Fredrich WS: Clinical comparison of the analgesic effects of dextropropoxyphene and other analgesics. Antibiot Med Clin Ther 6:362–370, 1959

23. Graber CM: The post-partum patients in evaluating analgesic drugs. Clin Pharmacol Ther 2:429–440, 1961

24. Procko LD: Evaluation of d-propoxyphene, codeine and aspirin. Obstet Gynecol 16:113–118, 1960

25. Berdon JK: The effectiveness of d-propoxyphene in the control of pain after peridontal surgery. J Periodont 39:106–111, 1964

26. Chilton NW: Double-blind evaluation of a new analgesic agent in post-extraction pain. Am J Med Sci 242:702–706, 1961

27. Hopkinson JH: Acetaminophen vs. propoxyphene for relief of pain in episiotomy patients. J Clin Pham 7:251–263, 1973

28. Young DJ: Propoxyphene suicides. Arch Intern Med 129:62–66, 1972

29. Beaver WT, Wallenstein SL, Houde RW: A clinical comparison of the effects of oral and intramuscular administration of analgesics: pentaxocine and phenazocine. Clin Pharmacol Ther 9:582–597, 1968

30. Beaver WT, Wallenstein SL, Houde RW: A comparison of the analgesic effects of pentazocine and morphine in patients with cancer. Clin Pharmacol Ther 7:740–751, 1966

31. Lewis JR: Misprescribing analgesics. JAMA 228:1155–1156, 1974

32. Bellville JW, Green J: The respiratory and subjective effects of pentazocine. Clin Pharmacol Ther 6:152, 1965

33. Reichenberg S, Pobers F: Severe respiratory depression following Talwin. Am Rev Resp Dis 107:280–282, 1973

34. Goodman LS, Gilman A (eds): The Pharmacologic Basis of Therapeutics, 4th ed. New York, Macmillan, 1970

35. Morris RW: Pharmindex, Vol. 14, No. 6, 1974, p 3

36. Swerdlow M: General analgesics used in pain relief: Pharmacology. Br J Anaesth 39:699–720, 1967

37. Vandam LD: Analgetic drugs—The potent analgetics. N Engl J Med 286:249–252, 1972

38. Papper S, Papper EM: The effects of preanesthetics, anesthetics and post-operative drugs on renal function. Clin Pharmacol Therap 5:205, 1964

39. House RW, Wallenstein SL, Beaver WT: Clinical measurement of pain, in de Stevens G (ed): Analgesics. New York, Academic Press, 1965, pp 75–122

40. Marks RM, Sachar EJ: Undertreatment of medical patients with narcotic analgesics. Ann Intern Med 78:173–181, 1973

41. Bonica JJ: The total management of the patient with chronic pain. Drug Therapy 3:33–47, 1973

42. Oster MW: Pain of terminal cancer patients. Arch Intern Med 138:1801–1803, 1978

43. Foley KM: Pain syndromes in patients with cancer, in Bonica JJ and Ventafridda, V: Advances in Pain Research and Therapy, Vol. 2. New York, Raven Press, 1979, pp 59–75

44. Forrest WH: Detroamphetamine with morphine for the treatment of postoperative pain. N Engl J Med 296:712–715, 1977

45. Holmes H: Morphine IV infusion for chronic pain. Drug Intell Clin Pharm 12:556, 1978

46. Ensworth S: Morphine IV infusion for chronic pain. Drug Intell Clin Pharm 13:297, 1979

47. Kowolenko M: Morphine IV infusion. Drug Intell Clin Pharm 14:296–297, 1980

16

PSYCHOLOGIC EXIGENCIES IN ONCOLOGY

Melvin J. Krant
Philip F. Roy

The word cancer connotes malevolence in its commonplace usage; the diagnosis of cancer as a disease entity evokes psychologic responses of considerable magnitude, often with resultant behaviors that can be judged as maladaptive or even self-destructive. The physician involved in cancer care is often central in both recognizing and inaugurating interventions in psychologic aberrant responses. This chapter is written not from a psychiatrist's viewpoint, but in respect to the oncologist's opportunities and responsibilities in this regard.

Denial and Delay

Delay in seeking medical care for a sign or symptom suggestive of cancer is usually posed as a patient problem, and not a physician's. The patient with an advanced ulcerating carcinoma of the breast who comes for medical care only after a relation or friend demands such action, but who insists that the lesion is no more than a week or two "old," is often cited as a problem in personal fault for delaying until opportunity for cure had vanished. The physician may also play a role in the overall picture of delay in appropriate action, however.

The physician's cognitive level of suspicion, and the psychologic processing of suspected reality, exert pressure in medical care-giving which may be influential in a patient's outcome. Older studies of delay criticized the physician's role in arriving at the diagnosis and implied that the physician was a significant factor in a number of instances of delay.[1,2] The suspicious patient may present with a lump, or mass, or another sign or symptom, but these complaints either fail to arouse appropriate diagnostic suspicion, or unconsciously, the physician seems to avoid investigating the presenting problems. Physicians are not immune from wishing to deny the potential implication of a sign or symptom, especially in a particular patient who arouses a set of psychologic responses such as identification. Education of the public may chip at a source of denial—failure to cognitively grasp the implication of a novel finding in the body. Education of the physician may reduce "mistakes" that result in delay. But the occasional presenting patient may still be subject to unnecessary delay by a physician who "cannot" think logically or "equitably" about a particular problem. Perhaps the only appropriate response of the physician in such circumstances is to back away from the responsibility and refer the patient to another colleague. When the physician is aware that he might have an emotional interaction with a particular patient, that physician should hesitate to become the investigator of a problem.

Secondly, the physician's response to a presenting patient may, on occasion, push the patient into a maladaptive response in order for the patient to maintain some sense of control over his or her destiny. An angry patient, and the diagnosis of cancer can evoke great anger in people, may provoke responsive anger in the physician, which then offers a patient justification for noncompliance with appropriate medical advice, much to the injury of that person. The excessively frightened patient, hesitant and clinging, may well arouse impatience and frustration in the physician, who then rejects or repudiates the patient, with the resultant failure of both the patient and the physician to follow through on necessary procedures. Poignant descriptions of such reactions can be found in the writings of patients. *Sunshine,* a biographic account of a young woman with osteogenic sarcoma, describes her refusal to accept amputation for the management of her localized disease in part through the "hurried" approach of her surgeon.[3] Neil Fiore,[4] in a recent article, similarly describes his reaction to the first physician that he consulted for a testicular mass. The physician's manner resulted in the feeling that Fiore "had little control over the decision" (for an exploratory operative procedure that could see the removal of a testicle), eventuating in "more delay" as he attempted to digest the result of this first examination. An understanding second physician who with considerable tact gained the patient's trust, helped Fiore accept the treatment program offered for his embryonal testicular cancer. The physician who does not grasp the fright that can be elicited by the potential diagnosis and treatment, whose ego requires instant compliance (in the name of "for the patient's own good"), or who responds with anger to the resentful (and frequently frightened) patient, may well promote maladaptive delaying that cannot be in the patient's best interests.

Throughout the trajectory of a course with cancer, the patient's psychologic responses can promote hostility, anger, frustration, and a sense of futility in the physician. The physician needs to be able to recognize his feelings, and to acknowledge that he or she might need help in sorting them out so that excessive havoc does not befall the patient.

Suicide and Suicidal-Ideation

The incidence of successfully completed suicide in both the early and the late stages of cancer is not really known, although a recent publication presents data that males have a rate 1.3 times higher than the general population, and that female cancer patients have a rate 1.9 times that of normal.[5] Leigh noted that medical reports of actual suicidal attempts by cancer patients are not common,[6] but added that he felt that the actual incidence was higher than recovered from medical literature. Farberow et al. reported 32 cancer-patient suicides[7] in a general Veteran's Administration Hospital in a 5-year period, and stated that suicide occurs disporportionately more often among cancer patients than among the general population.

Anecdotes about suicide abound. The New York Times recently carried the story of a 62-year-old woman who convened a party of friends some months after the diagnosis of breast cancer, and proceeded to overdose with sleeping pills at the conclusion of the affair.[8] The report is presented as an instance of an "ethical" decision, rather than a psychologic one. Ervin reported the successful suicides of 3 patients following mastectomy, supposedly as a consequence of spouse rejection.[9] Just how often a successful suicide occurs may be less critical than the realization that suicidal ideation is not at all uncommon as a response to the diagnosis, or treatment, or to the expectation of a cruel dying. Suicidal ideation, as part of the depressive reaction of cancer patients, may spontaneously resolve, may linger as a part of chronic reactive depression, or may manifest into an action, depending upon medical and psychosocial circumstances. The frequency of suicidal ideation is completely unknown, but a recent report by Jameson, Wellisch, and Pasnau[10] indicated that in postmastectomy breast cancer patients such ideation is not infrequent, and could be made apparent by direct questioning or by the careful listening of a concerned and suspicious investigator. Morris' work with breast cancer patients clearly demonstrates that depression may linger for at least 2 years following surgical breast amputation.[11]

Whether a society greets suicide as an ethical right of patients, or as a desparate response to despair, will result in what actions seem appropriate and supportable. For the purposes of this paper, we will treat suicidal ideation and behavior as acts of despair. As such, for this argument, we will hold that the physician's obligation is to both recognize the depressed patient who is apt to be suicidal, and to develop a comfortable sense of appropriate intervention.

Suicide appears seldomly as a spontaneous act. Rather, significant lengths of time in contemplation of the action seems to be the rule.[12] The depressed patient frequently signals to both family and to others around them that suicide is being considered as a way out of an intolerable situation.[13] Such signals include withdrawal from interaction in family or community affairs, the giving away of prized possessions, and the general behavior that indicates that the individual does not intend to be around much longer. Overt comments about suicide may be made. Similar signals are also given with considerably frequency to the attending physician. There is evidence that persons with suicidal thoughts will usually tell a physician if asked.[14] The elements of life's intolerability appear to relate to self-condemnation, feelings of radical loneliness and alienation, feelings of helplessness to control events in life, and sensing the loss of one's social roles and positions, eventuating into the feeling that a person is becoming an intolerable burden to others. Elements of rage and reprisal may also be entwined in the decision to act.

As stated, the patient may often signal dispair and depression to a physician. If the latter is sensitive to the signals, or can "read" depression or despair in the patient, open dialogue can ensue, with the patient being encouraged to voice feelings and share thoughts. Patients can be openly asked if they are considering, or have recently considered self-destruction. Unfortunately, in the hurried disease-oriented day of the surgical, or medical, oncologist, paying attention to depressive signals, and acting on them, usually with a rapid and direct referal to a psychiatric colleague, may not take place. In Murphy's study of 35 physicians involved in the care of suicidal patients, the majority were aware that the patient appeared depressed, or talked of a depressed mood, or acted in a depressed manner. But aware as they were, the diagnosis of a depressive syndrome with possible suicidal ideation was not made, and appropriate intervention was not taken.[12] DeRogatis has emphasized the significant tendency for physicians to underrate the distress the patient is experiencing.[15] Murphy[12] offers the following diagnostic symptoms to aid in the recognition of a depressive syndrome:

1. Insomnia
2. Poor appetite and weight loss
3. Fatigue or loss of energy
4. Loss of interest in previously enjoyable pursuits
5. Agitation or marked retardation
6. Feelings of guilt or self-reproach
7. Diminished ability to think or concentrate
8. The presence of thoughts of death or suicide.

Clearly, some of these features overlap with physiological responses to advanced cancer, making the diagnosis of depression somewhat difficult to secure.

The treatment of depression and suicidal ideation may require electroconvulsive therapy and/or antidepressive medication in an atmosphere of support and family counseling. Referral to appropriate mental health workers is clearly indicated once recognition of the clinical situation occurs. An important element in suicide prevention is physician self-examination. Some physicians become angry when confronted by a suicidal patient feeling, in part, that they are being manipulated. An angry response to a patient is rarely helpful. The physician who can recognize his personal feelings may avoid antagonizing a patient further.

Is there ever a place for acceptable suicide? The issue is critical in its ethical questioning of right conduct in befitting circumstances, but we will not carry the issue further in this paper. If there is a role for the physician in aiding, abetting, or not interfering, society and the law will need to examine the consequence of such medical behavior with a fine lens.

Anxiety

States of anxiety are synonomous with great personal discomfort without necessarily leading to suicide. Cancer may arouse great anxiety in patients and families, but there are several specific moments in the course of illness when high, and sometimes overwhelming, levels of anxiousness may appear.

The first of these is in the diagnostic period, especially that time between the discovery of an abnormality and the appearance at the physician's office. Patients should be seen immediately once they have called for an appointment, for any delay greatly compounds anxious uncertainty. Office personnel should be especially trained to respond rapidly to a request for an appointment when a suspicion of cancer has been raised. The finding, by a woman, of a lump in the breast, can be extremely panic-inducing.

A second time of great stress is the interval between a specific diagnostic maneuver and communication of the findings. Biopsy is most to the point; waiting to be told is a time of crisis-dimension anxiety. "For many women, waiting for a possible diagnosis of breast cancer (or any other cancer) is a traumatic experience. Fear of cancer, breast loss, and death can be overwhelming during this period."[16] The implication of this quote is clear—the actual diagnosis of cancer is less traumatic to many patients, especially if a therapeutic plan comfortably accompanies the diagnosis, than is the uncertain time of waiting. The shorter that time is made between definitive diagnosis and communication (a comfortable, face-to-face environment, sometimes, although not always, with a loved-one nearby adds to the patient's sense of feeling supported), the easier it all is on the patient.

Cancer patients do not always feel a sense of closure that the disease is over with, even after a definitive surgical or radiotherapeutic procedure. The months post-op may be a time of significant anxiety, signaled by any bodily ache or pain which may be immediately interpreted as recurrence. A great deal of reassurance is often necessary, offered accurately after investigation of the complaint. For some patients, a continuous search for reassurance is a signal of underlying depression requiring specific psychiatric consultation. Scars that do not heal provoke great anxiety and depression, and as Quint demonstrated, the slowly healing scar is often interpreted as cancer and a failed operation.[17] The more the patient is encouraged to speak of her or his anxieties and the more an accurate and sympathetic review of the situation is offered, the more the patient feels reassured, and the less the level of anxiety. Such reassurance may be repetitively required. This is far from a trivial situation, for desparate actions, such as marital break-up, can result from an anxiety that is given no respite.

A terrible anxiety and depression may ensue when the diagnosis of recurrence is made. The outcome of that anxiety is dependent upon both the depth of relationship to the physician, and the sense of trust, as well as the sense of open communication within the family. Recurrence is frequently seen as the death-knoll, setting into motion a number of psychologic postures and defenses that need understanding and at times psychologic interventions. Intervention is required principally when emotional responses, or defenses, interfere with appropriate therapeutic plans or interpersonal relationships.

Delerium (Confusional State)

The onset of a confusional state is an indication for a careful diagnostic evaluation. There are three major causes for the sudden onset of a confusional state in the cancer patient, namely, alteration in disease states, toxic reactions to chemotherapeutic drugs, and toxic reactions to other medications. The acute confusional syndrome, known also as acute delirium, or as acute brain syndrome, is characterized by the clouding and disorganization of conscious awareness. This alteration may fluctuate from time to time, may be at its worst either upon awakening from sleep or late in the day, and can vary in degree, from minimal lapses in attention or problems in concentration to major disturbances in which affect is usually altered, and agitation, a sense of terror, or motions to "escape" may be apparent. In the major varients of the syndrome, hallucinations are frequent, and a delusional system on the basis of abnormal or distorted sensory experiences and interpretations may emerge. The patient can appear psychotic, with rambling and incoherent patterns of speech. When questioned, patients exhibit poor concentration and a fluctuating state of disorientation; impairment of short-term memory is not infrequent. Acute confusional states are more common in the elderly than in the young.[18]

It is usually possible to distinguish acute confusional states from a chronic brain syndrome, both from the temporal appearance of the deranged state and from the clinical characteristics of the disorder. However, a patient with minimal chronic dementia, compensating in a familiar surrounding, may break down acutely when admitted to a hospital.

Common medical causes of the acute confusional state in the cancer patient include the following:

1. Infections (in the elderly, confusion may appear as the first and sometimes the only early manifestation of sepsis; pyrexia may be minimal)
2. Dehydration (secondary to vomiting and/or decreased fluid intake, especially in the elderly)
3. Rapidly advancing renal or liver failure
4. Electrolyte abnormalities, such as acute hypercalcemia or inappropriate antidiuretic hormone secretion
5. Metastases to the cerebrum (psychiatric symptoms may appear even in the absence of neurological findings)

6. Hypoxic states (secondary to lymphangitic pulmonary metastatic involvement, multiple pulmonary emboli, pulmonary infections)
7. Trauma (especially subdural hematomas).

Appropriate resolution of the underlying medical problem may result in a rapid reversal of the confusional state. But since several days may elapse before specific disease-oriented treatment is effective, symptomatic management is important.

Drugs commonly employed for a variety of problems, such as sleeplessness, anxiety, depression, and pain, may produce a confusional state, especially in the elderly. A review of the drug intake is critical in assessing the onset of the syndrome. Barbituates, diazepam, the tricyclics, and the narcotics are all potentially causative, or contributory, agents to acute confusional states. Withdrawal of the offending agent(s) usually results in abatement of the delerious state.

Certain antineoplastic agents have been associated with the development of an acute confusional disorder. Chief among these appears to be L-asparaginase.[19]

L-Asparaginase

Cerebral dysfunction is one of the more common, and often striking, side effects of this agent. Lethargy, somnolence, and confusion were observed in 48 of 147 trials of L-asparaginase in children, and in 46 percent of 156 trials in adults.[20] Other reports have confirmed this toxic manifestation.[21,22] A confusional state may appear within 24 hours of initiating treatment with L-asparaginase, and may persist for as long as a treatment course is given, or clear spontaneously within a few days even as the drug continues to be given. Alterations in the level of consciousness may be severe, however, resulting in stupor or in frank coma. Disorientation, hallucinations, and severe depression have been noted. These cerebral dysfunctions have occured during treatments with a wide variety of doses and schedules.[23] Diffuse slowing of the electroencephalogram has been noted, with improvement recorded after cessation of therapy.[24]

The cerebral dysfunction noted with L-asparaginase does not appear to be related to the physical properties of the enzyme itself. The drug does not cross the blood–brain barrier, and therefore the mode of action appears related to systemic metabolic abnormalities, involving amino acid depletions (L-asparagine and L-glutamine) and/or excesses (L-aspartic acid, L-glutamic acid).

The acute confusional state appears to be tolerable, for in one study of

110 children with advanced leukemia, only in 7 cases was the drug withheld.[123] However, since central nervous system leukemia, infections, and metabolic derangements (as heaptic coma) may be implicated in the etiology of the confusional state, careful investigations must be made before placing the blame with L-asparaginase.

Methotrexate

Cerebral dysfunction has been reported with chronic intrathecal administration of methotrexate as well as with systemic drug administration in meningeal leukemia.[25] Kay et al. described 7 children with acute leukemia in whom confusion, somnolence, and dementia developed after prolonged courses of oral and intrathecal treatment.[26] One patient died, and at postmortem no evidence of active leukemia or viral encephalitis was found. There were areas of infarction in the temporal and parietal lobes.

Many other neurologic toxicities have been reported with methotrexate therapy, but these are not in the purview of this chapter. Those interested are referred to a most comprehensive review.[19]

Procarbazine

Procarbazine is a methylhydrazine derivative that was originally synthesized as a potential monoamine oxidase inhibitor, but was found to have antineoplastic properties. In the occasional patient, lethargy, confusion, transient hallucinations, agitation, and manic psychosis have been reported.[27,28] Recovery has been the rule; drug discontinuation and serious psychologic reactions seem rare. Many other neurotoxicities occur with this agent and one should be especially aware of the synergistic interactions with barbituates, phenothiazines, and alcohol, acting through the monoamine oxidase inhibitor pathway, as well as through inhibition of many other enzymes.[29]

Symptomatic management of the acutely confused patient is both pharmacologic and psychosupportive. The patient should be nursed in a well-lit, quiet room, with a reassurance that the acute phase will pass. Since the orienting properties of the brain are disturbed, the patient may become panicky because of misinterpretation of sounds or sights that are usually normally understood. The patient feels endangered by such incidents. It is important for the medical staff to take such incidents seriously, to question the patient as to what they are perceiving as frightening, and to change the environment, if possible, to minimize the signals. Constant reassurance, clarification, and presence of staff go a long way.

When drugs seem involved as causative factors, they should be eliminated. But if the confusional state appears secondary to a disease-state alteration, or to a specific agent (as one of the aforementioned chemotherapeutic drugs), pharmacologic support may be found in the judicious use of the butyrophenones, phenothiazines, anxiolytics, and soporifics. Haloperidol, 2.0 mg 2–3 times a day, may be initiated, but the drug should be carefully titrated to the patient's needs and responses—the dose may be elevated, or decresaed, but daily monitoring is necessary.

Cancer and the Family

At the point where the physician communicates the diagnosis of neoplastic disease or of change in status, especially of recurrence or worsening, there are a number of crisis reactions which can occur in the family of the patient. Some of them are obvious while others may be well hidden under any number of seemingly unrelated symptoms. The attending physician is not expected to be an expert psychiatric diagnostician but should be alert to these disguised potential problems.

What are some of the forms that family adjustment difficulties can take? First of all, there are several generally negative reactions: shock, anxiety, confusion, denial, depression, and rejection of the patient. In addition, anger and resentment at the patient for being chronically and debilitatingly ill and interfering with routines or plans for the future is not at all unusual. Family members are often deeply ashamed of these emotions welling up inside them. Anger at the patient can show up later as self-hate or depression, especially if the patient dies.[30] It seems that a central unifying concept in all these is that of loss. The cancer patient has to deal with a variety of losses throughout his or her illness and the family must also find a way to cope with these losses, real or imagined, experienced or anticipated.[31]

Secondly, there are a number of specific reactions for which the physician should be alert. One might be classified as concentration difficulties: the student described as daydreaming, the employee whose productivity gradually decreases, etc. If there is a mention of such difficulty, the issue should be explored in terms of severity. Is that student, for example, occasionally sleepy in school or have there been a number of truancies or have there been reports of frequent and severe emotional outbursts in school? Various somatic complaints may also arise: the child may suffer loss of appetite or the spouse may complain of headaches. Often they will need encouragement to verbalize these complaints, because the severity of the patient's disease may tend to make them minimize their own problems. Similarly, the family member may employ a wide variety of drugs to help control their emotional pain and the physician should be alert to the possibilities for abuse. If their anxiety achieves overwhelming proportions, we may see the suicidal manifestations discussed in other parts of this chapter.

Problems can arise over financial matters. For example, a fairly wealthy patient may have decided to leave his wealth to his oldest son. At the time of his illness, this son may be living in a distant part of the country and the day-to-day care of the patient is carried out by his second son. We hear vague reports that the two sons had "a fight" when the oldest visited his father and we are tempted to pass it off as "sibling rivalry" or something else of minor importance. Two days later, however, we hear that the younger son has not been in to visit his father; on his next visit, there is the smell of alcohol on his breath. Time taken to talk with him helps him to unburden his feelings and conflicts. It would certainly be appropriate to set an appointment to see him again and to begin to investigate resources for supportive counseling. In this way, the physician is alert to signs that might otherwise be ignored, assisting in getting help for a troubled person.

This awareness of family process might also make visible a teenager's problems, for the adolescent appears to be especially vulnerable to deep psychologic disturbance when cancer strikes in a parent. Delinquent acting-out may become a serious problem as a teenager tries to tap his anxiety through actions for which "the consequences do at least pertain to realms of known cause and effect."[32] Long-term psychopathology may emerge after the parents' death.[33]

Finally, the physician often becomes the target for family tensions. Anger, resentment, and fear which is felt toward the illness is directed at the house officer, for example, and one study has shown that the doctor's reaction to this onslaught of blame was to feel angry, find fault with the family and spend less time with the patient.[34]

There are a number of factors which will influence the intensity with which these reactions will occur. The time period since the diagnosis can have two effects: first, the period immediately following the communication of the diagnosis is generally a time of high risk for crisis reactions.[35] Another period arises late in the prolonged chronic illness when coping mechanisms are taxed to the limit. Issues related to dying are those least shared by families.[36]

Generally, the younger the patient, the greater the degree of risk of family crisis, although this is related to many other factors as well. The role of the patient in relationship to others in the family, for example, is critical. The occurrence of childhood leukemia will have a serious and specific effect on the family,[37] while the illness of a parent will have other effects, which may vary inversely with the age of that parent's children.[38] The overall pattern of closeness in the family will influence the intensity of their reactions. It is not our experience that serious disease will "draw the family together"; rather, that the lines of communication that predated the onset will prevail and that those who cannot share their pain and fear will cope less well with it. The presence of ambivalent relationships between family members is predictive of difficulty in dealing with increased stress, especially among the members of the nuclear family, who have no others close by to dilute the stress. Where preexisting psychopathology has been evident, the liklihood of augmented severity is considerable. Thus, if there has been a history of chronic depression, neurosis, alcoholism, or other disturbance in a family member prior to the diagnosis of cancer one can expect a worsening of that condition at certain nodal points in the trajectory of the patient, especially if there is a period of recurrence, or in the period of late-stage disease.

As suggested in the example above, the financial resources of the family make them more or less vulnerable to problems. The ability to bear the cost of chronic illness will affect the family's ability to cope with the stress of it. Medicare provides good hospital coverage but leaves much responsibility on the family if the patient is at home. Private health insurance has no home care provisions at all in some cases. Social Security/Medicaid provides for the truly indigent, but the embarrassment and the delay add to the frustration.

Attention to family dynamics will also often reveal the presence or absence of other supports the family can use in times of crisis. The presence of a priest, minister, or rabbi can be of great assistance and can be a real ally to the physician when crisis intervention is called for. Home health agencies play a central role in patient care and can often provide "inside" information about family stress since they are with the patient perhaps several hours each day. Although they are often understaffed, especially in rural areas, they can constitute a vital link in the intervention team.

Individuals in a family nexus may need to feel that the medical system is concerned about them as people in need rather than as appendages to a sick patient. Reaching out to inquire how the family and its members are functioning, and what their needs may be, is not the behavior of most hospital units. Much disturbance in psychologic and social health is made visible, or even prevented, when a family-centered therapeutic team exists whose job is to evaluate family-member function during crisis points in a cancer patient's chronic course, and to plan interventions when stress was felt to be present. Controlled clinical trials in family crisis in cancer are not known to exist; nevertheless, the use of principles such as open communication, structural support, concerned and accurate empathy, and family-network support building is probably significantly therapeutic. The key is outreach and assessment. If the physician, or medical team, waits to hear of a family member in crisis, the chance for intervention will be lost. Exploring a family's coping styles needs to be an integral part of cancer care.

References

1. Robbins GF, MacDonald MD, Pack GT: Delay in the diagnosis and treatment of physicians with cancer. Cancer 6:624, 1953
2. Henderson JG: Denial and depression as factors in the delay of patients with cancer presenting themselves to the physician. Ann NY Acad Sci 125:856–864, 1966
3. Klein N: Sunshine. Based upon the audiotapes of Lynn Helton. New York, Avon, 1974, p 46
4. Fiore N: Fighting cancer: One patient's perspective. NEJM 300:284–289, 1978
5. Louhivouri KA, Hakama M: Risk of suicide among cancer patients. Am J Epidemiol 109:59–65, 1979
6. Leigh H: Psychotherapy as a suicidal terminal cancer patient. Int J Psychiat Med 5:173–181, 1974
7. Farberow NL, Shneidman ES, Leonard CV: Suicide among general medical and surgical hospital patients with malignant neoplasms. The New Physician 13:38–44, 1964
8. Johnston L: Artist's death: A last statement in a thesis on "Self-Termination." New York Times, June 17, 1979, p 1
9. Ervin CJ: Psychological adjustment to mastectomy. Med Asp Human Sex 7:42–65, 1973
10. Jameson KR, Wellisch DK, Pasnau RP: Psychological aspects of mastectomy. The woman's perspective. Ann J Psych 135:432–436, 1978
11. Morris T, Greer TS, Pettingale KW: Psychological and social adjustment to mastectomy: A two-year follow-up study. Cancer 40:2381–2387, 1977
12. Murphy GE: The physician's responsibility for suicide. Errors of omission. Ann Intern Med 82:305–309, 1975

13. Robins E, Gassner S, Kayes J, et al: The communication of suicidal intent: A study of 134 consecutive cases of successful (completed) suicide. Am J Psych 115:724–733, 1959

14. Delong W, Robins E: The communciation of suicidal intent prior to psychiatric hospitalization: A study of 87 patients. Am J Psych 117:695–705, 1961

15. DeRogatis R: Cancer patients and their physicians in the perception of psychological symptoms. Psychosomatics 17:197–206, 1976

16. Coping with Diagnosis, in Breast Cancer Digest. Office of Cancer Communications, April, 1979, p 62

17. Quint TC: The impact of mastectomy. Am J Nursing 63:88–92, 1963

18. Stedeford A: Understanding confusional states. Br J Hosp Med 20(6):694–698, 1978

19. Weiss HD, Walker MD, Wiernick PH: Neurotoxicity of commonly used antineoplastic agents. N Engl J Med 291:75–81, 1974

20. Oettgen HF, Stephenson PA, Schwartz MK, et al: Toxicity of E. coli L-asparaginase in man. Cancer 25:253–278, 1970

21. Moure TB, Whitecar JP, Bodey GP: Electroencephalogram changes secondary to asparaginase. Arch Neurol 23:365–368, 1970

22. Ohnuma T, Holland JG, Freeman A, et al: Biochemical and pharmacological studies with asparaginase in man. Cancer Res 30:2297–2305, 1970

23. Land VJ, Sutow WW, Fernbach DJ, et al: Toxicity of L-asparaginase in children with advanced leukemia. Cancer 30:339–347, 1972

24. Whitecar JP Jr, Bodey GP, Harris JT, et al: L-Asparaginase New Engl J Med 281:1028–1034, 1969

25. Bleyer WA, Drake TC, Chabner BA: Neurotoxicity and elevated cerebrospinal fluid methotrexate concentration in meningeal leukemia. N Engl J Med 289:770–773, 1973

26. Kay H, Knapton PJ, O'Sullivan JP, et al: Encephalopathy in acute leukemia associated with methotrexate therapy. Arch Dis Child 47:344–354, 1972

27. Greenwald HS: Cancer chemotherapy Part II. NY State J Med 66:2670–2681, 1966

28. Mann AM, Hutchinson JL: Manic reaction associated with porcarbazine hydrochloride therapy of Hodgkin's disease. Can Med Assoc J 97:1350–1353, 1967

29. Jardick NE: Drugs used in the treatment of psychiatric disorders, in Goodman LS, Gilman A (eds): The Pharmacological Basis of Therapeutics. 4th Ed. MacMillen, New York, 1970, p 151–203

30. Orcutt BA: Stress on family interaction when a member is dying, in

Pritchard ER et al. (eds): Social Work with the Dying Patient and the Family. New York, Columbia University Press, 1977, pp 23–37

31. Currier LM: Psychological impact of cancer. Rocky Mount Med J 63:43–48, 1966

32. Bonnard A: Truancy and pilfering associated with bereavement, in Lorand S, Schneer H (eds): Adolescents. New York, Paul Hoeber, 1961

33. Tallmer M: Childhood bereavement, in Schoenberg B et al: Bereavement. New York, Columbia University Press, 1975, pp 164–171

34. Schowalter JE: Death and the pediatric house officer. J Pediatrics 76:706–710, 1970

35. Lindemann E: Symptomatology and management of acute grief. Am J Psychiatry 101:141–148, 1944

36. Krant MJ, Johnson L: Family members' perception of communication in late stage cancer. Int J Psychiat Med 8:203–216, 1977–8

37. Bozman MF, et al: Psychological impact of cancer and its treatment. Cancer 8:1–19, 1955

38. Lifshitz M: Long range effects of father's loss. Br J Med Psychol 49:189–197, 1976

INDEX